Geopolitics in Health

GEOPOLITICS IN HEALTH

Confronting Obesity,
AIDS, and Tuberculosis
in the Emerging BRICS Economies

EDUARDO J. GÓMEZ

Johns Hopkins University Press
BALTIMORE

Johns Hopkins University Press
2715 North Charles Street
Baltimore, Maryland 21218-4363
www.press.jhu.edu

Library of Congress Cataloging-in-Publication Data

Names: Gómez, Eduardo J., 1973–, author.
Title: Geopolitics in health : confronting obesity, AIDS, and
    tuberculosis in the emerging BRICS economies /
    Eduardo J. Gómez.
Description: Baltimore : Johns Hopkins University Press, [2017] |
    Includes bibliographical references and index.
Identifiers: LCCN 2017008833| ISBN 9781421423616
    (pbk. : alk. paper) | ISBN 9781421423623 (electronic)
Subjects: | MESH: HIV Infections—epidemiology | Tuberculosis—
    epidemiology | Obesity—epidemiology | Epidemics—prevention &
    control | Health Policy | International Cooperation
Classification: LCC RA644.A25 | NLM WC 503.41 |
    DDC 614.5/99392—dc23
LC record available at https://lccn.loc.gov/2017008833

A catalog record for this book is available from the British Library.

Special discounts are available for bulk purchases of this book. For more information, please contact Special Sales at 410-516-6936 or specialsales@press.jhu.edu.

Johns Hopkins University Press uses environmentally friendly book materials, including recycled text paper that is composed of at least 30 percent post-consumer waste, whenever possible.

To the memory of my wonderful grandfather, Januario Gómez
Without his love and sacrifice, my opportunity and success would
never have been possible

Contents

Abbreviations

ABC   Agencia Brasiliera de Cooperaçãoê (Brazil)
ANC   African National Congress
ARV   antiretroviral
ASBRAN   Brazilian Association of Nutrition
ATICC   AIDS Training, Information, and Counseling Center
                (South Africa)
BJP   Bharatiya Janata Party (India)
BMI   body mass index
BRICS   Brazil, Russia, India, China, and South Africa
CAMS   Commission for Articulation with Social Movements (Brazil)
CARES   Comprehensive AIDS Response (China)
CCDC   Chinese Center for Disease Control and Prevention
CDC   Centers for Disease Control and Prevention (US)
CELAFISCS   Centro de Estudos do Laboratório de Aptidão Física de São
                Caetano do Sul (Brazil)
CONBRAN   Congresso Brasileiro de Nutrição
CONSEA   National Council on Food and Nutrition Security (Brazil)
DCNT   Plano de Ações Estratégicas para o Enfrentamento das
                Doenças Crônicas não transmissíveis (Brazil)
DFID   Department for International Development (UK)
DGSP   Diretoria Geral de Saúde Pública (Brazil)
DOH   Department of Health (South Africa)
DOTS   directly observed treatment, short course
FAO   Food and Agricultural Organization of the United Nations
FHP   Family Health Program (Brazil)

GONGO	Government-Organized Non-Governmental Organization (China)
GUIA	Guide for Useful Interventions for Activity in Brazil and Latin America
HAST	HIV/AIDS/STI/TB Initiative (South Africa)
HKASO	Hong Kong Association for the Study of Obesity
ICTS	International Centre for Technical Cooperation for HIV/AIDS Initiatives (Brazil)
IDEC	Instituto Brasileiro de Defesa do Consumidor
IDU	intravenous/injecting drug user
IIAA	Institute of Inter-American Affairs
IMF	International Monetary Fund
MACs	Municipal AIDS Commissions (Brazil)
MDR-TB	multi-drug resistant tuberculosis
MEA	Ministry of External Affairs (India)
MESP	Ministério de Educação e Saúde Pública (Brazil)
MHFW	Ministry of Health and Family Welfare (India)
MOH	ministry of health
MSM	men who have sex with men
NACO	National AIDS Control Organization (India)
NACOSA	National AIDS Convention of South Africa
NACP	National AIDS Control Plan (India)
NAP	national AIDS program
NASF	Núcleo de Apoio á Saúde da Família (Brazil)
NGO	nongovernmental organization
NHFPC	National Health and Family Planning Commission (China)
NPCDCS	National Program for Prevention and Control of Diabetes, Cardiovascular Disease, and Stroke (India)
NSP	National Strategic Plan (South Africa)
NTBP	National TB Program (South Africa)
PACs	Provincial AIDS Commissions (South Africa)
PAHO	Pan American Health Organization
PMTCT	prevention of mother-to-child transmission
PNAN	Política Nacional de Alimentação (Brazil)
PSE	Programa Saúde nas Escolas (Brazil)
RHF	Russia Healthcare Foundation

RMNCH	Reproductive, Maternal, Newborn and Child Health Coalition (India)
SACSs	State AIDS Prevention and Control Societies (India)
SANAC	South African National AIDS Council
SARS	severe acute respiratory syndrome
SCAWCO	State Council AIDS Working Committee Office (China)
STD/STI	sexually transmitted disease / sexually transmitted infection
SUS	Sistema Único de Saúde (Brazil)
TAC	Treatment Action Campaign (South Africa)
TB	tuberculosis
TSPSA	Tuberculosis Strategic Plan for South Africa
UN	United Nations
UNAIDS	United Nations Programme on HIV/AIDS
UNDP	United Nations Development Programme
USAID	United States Agency for International Development
VIGISUS	Health and Disease Surveillance System (Brazil)
WHO	World Health Organization
WTO	World Trade Organization
XDR-TB	extensively drug-resistant TB

Acknowledgments

This book was the product of not only my imagination, research, and writing but also the encouragement and help of many others. This project started just as I was leaving Rutgers University in 2013 to join the faculty in the Department of International Development at King's College London. I also thank my colleagues in the Department of International Development for providing me with excellent feedback during earlier presentations of this project. Throughout the final stages of this project, my research assistant, Josh Lomax at King's College London, provided invaluable editorial assistance. At other universities and institutions, colleagues Matthew McCaffrey, David McBride, Joe Harris, Benjamin Mason Meier, Lawrence Saez, Leslie Vinjamuri, Yanzhong Huang, and Stephan Haggard also provided wonderful comments and suggestions.

At Johns Hopkins University Press, I would like to thank my editor, Robin Coleman, for providing me with the opportunity to share my ideas and research, while being patient and encouraging throughout the writing process.

And finally, outside of academia, I wish to thank my dear friends at the Roger Gracie Brazilian Jiu-Jitsu academy in London for reaffirming the values of discipline and perseverance and staying cool under pressure, while providing daily respite from work. And finally, I am eternally grateful to my dearest father, Guillermo Leon Gómez, the best man that I know, for providing much encouragement and support throughout this project.

Geopolitics in Health

1

Introduction

The Geopolitics of Public Health in the BRICS Nations

In recent years, political leaders in Brazil, Russia, India, China, and South Africa, a group of nations known as the BRICS, have aspired to become world leaders in political and economic development. Their growing economies, cultural influence, and heightened participation in foreign affairs have earned the respect of the international community. This exclusive group of countries has worked together to reformulate international discussions and policies on issues ranging from fair and free trade to human rights, while defending the interests of less developed nations. The BRICS, empathizing with countries perceived as being controlled and manipulated by international creditors such as the International Monetary Fund (IMF) and the World Bank, have gone so far as to create their own regional development bank as a counterweight to these institutions (Pilling, 2014). And the tables have turned. In 2011, the IMF asked the BRICS for their assistance in helping save Greece, Portugal, and Spain, all on the brink of financial collapse (Soto and Murphy, 2011). Ironically, in 2003, it was Brazil that approached the IMF for help in rejuvenating its flagging economy (BBC, 2003). In short, the BRICS have aligned with one another based on their similar interests and success in reforming their foreign policies and achieving global prominence.

When it comes to health policy, however, the BRICS nations have not behaved as similarly, nor have their policy achievements been as impressive. As figure 1.1 illustrates, these governments have differed considerably in their commitment to healthcare spending, highlighting key differences in their approaches to improving the health and wellbeing of their citizens. Furthermore,

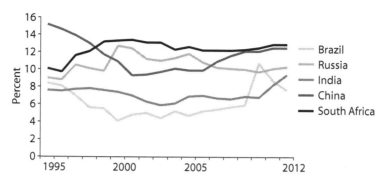

Figure 1.1. BRICS general government expenditure on health (as percentage of total government expenditure), 1995–2012. Source: WHO, 2015.

the BRICS have failed to prioritize the strengthening of the institutions and policies that undergird their healthcare systems, not only by ensuring that policies are effectively implemented, but also by ensuring that federal and state funding is allocated efficiently, that health officials are held accountable, and that everyone—especially women and minorities—is treated equally with respect to healthcare needs (Gómez, 2015b).

But were the BRICS as different when it came to responding to public health crises, such as epidemics? One could easily assume that, given the BRICS' increased prominence on the world stage and striving for greater political and economic influence, they would similarly take an interest in aggressively responding to diseases that threaten their economic performance and growth potential. One could further assume that such potentially devastating threats would increase political interest in responding through immediate and aggressive bureaucratic and policy reforms—especially when compared with responses to diseases perceived as less severe and catastrophic, such as diabetes, hypertension, and cancer, and broader health systems challenges. However, even when faced with disease epidemics, none of these nations immediately responded.

By the early 1990s, the HIV/AIDS epidemic was sweeping across the BRICS nations, generating fear, discrimination, and social instability and contributing to thousands of deaths in a short period of time. A foreign-born virus, HIV/AIDS had several modes of transmission, ranging from sexual relations and poorly managed blood transfusion processes to the sharing of needles in intravenous drug use. Tuberculosis (TB) resurfaced shortly thereafter because of the immune system deficiencies caused by HIV and because of increased poverty and urbanization. And as a consequence of accelerated economic growth, international trade, and changes in daily lifestyle—in essence, the very products of the BRICS' success as emerging economies—obesity emerged as a serious public health threat by the turn of the twenty-first century, contributing to a host of related diseases such as hypertension, diabetes, and cancer.

The BRICS differed in how they responded to these epidemics, highlighting important differences in their political commitment to meeting healthcare needs and safeguarding their societies. The BRICS' responses ranged from the limited introduction of prevention and treatment policies, mainly during the early 1990s, to a stronger policy response by the mid-1990s, which entailed a rise in administrative and policy spending on prevention and treatment programs. By the mid-2000s, the BRICS differed in the key outcome of interest in this book: developing a *centrist policy response*. This response, as I explain in greater detail shortly, entails continuously expanding the funding and administrative capacity of public health programs, consistently financing effective and innovative prevention and treatment programs, and introducing innovative policies to increase the national government's influence over implementation of policy at the subnational level. During the early 1990s, in all of the BRICS nations, the introduction of prevention and treatment programs was limited, drawing considerable international and domestic criticism and pressure. By the mid-1990s, Brazil, India, and China were the first and only BRICS nations to exhibit a stronger policy response, mainly by boosting their financial and administrative commitments to HIV/AIDS and obesity prevention and treatment programs. By the early 2000s, Brazil was the only BRICS nation to engage in a centrist policy response. In contrast, Russia and South Africa have never engaged in a stronger policy response, nor have they achieved a centrist policy response.

These findings lead us to question to what extent the BRICS are emerging as successful and equitable economies. By carefully unraveling how these governments have responded to different types of public health threats, we can see that the BRICS have not been entirely committed to introducing policy innovations that will help safeguard their population from disease, produce healthy and productive citizens, and contribute to sustainable levels of economic growth; if most of the BRICS are not adequately investing in public health, then to what extent are they fully committed to achieving these objectives (Clements, Coady, and Gupta, 2012)? Why haven't politicians taken public health seriously?

And will this lack of attention eventually undermine their growth prospects and influence? I address these questions in greater depth at the end of this book (chapter 7), arguing that in a context where several of the BRICS are experiencing economic recession and political and social instability, the failure to take healthcare more seriously may further undermine their ability to achieve their global economic and political aspirations.

Why were the BRICS nations so different in their response to disease epidemics? I argue that answering this question requires a comparative historical analysis of the BRICS' evolutionary policy responses to disease and their relationship with the international community. More specifically, I argue that the BRICS' geopolitical positioning mattered most when accounting for differences in the timing of government response to epidemics and their capacity to achieve a centrist policy response.

I define *geopolitical positioning* as explaining the interests and incentives of political leaders to respond to international criticism and pressure for an improved response to epidemics through a stronger policy response, the different domestic and foreign policy strategies that this response entails, and leaders' willingness to pursue international financial and technical assistance to achieve their policy objectives. More specifically, geopolitical positioning entails both positive and negative elements. On the one hand, *positive* geopolitical positioning emerges when political leaders respond positively to international criticism and pressure by immediately pursuing stronger domestic bureaucratic and policy reforms to increase their international reputation in health,[1] while at the same time proactively seeking the financial and technical assistance of the international community to achieve their objectives.[2] These efforts build on a long foreign policy tradition of enhancing the government's international reputation in development more broadly and in public health, while working in cooperative, reciprocal partnerships with international institutions in periods of health crisis. Positive geopolitical positioning also emerges when political leaders make public statements about their interest in increasing their government's reputation in health, while proactively marketing their policy success by inviting international officials to government meetings to display the government's commitment to reform. Finally, positive geopolitical positioning emerges when leaders provide foreign aid in health to further advance their international reputation—that is, they strive to help other developing nations respond to epidemics by sharing their successful policy ideas and experiences at international meetings, collectively working with other nations to ensure access to essential medicines, and providing financial and technical assistance. These efforts, in turn, further reinforce the government's international reputation as one that is capable of eradicating disease while helping other nations achieve the same. Such was the case for Brazil, India, and China, eventually prompting these governments to strengthen their response to HIV/AIDS and the more recent obesity epidemic.

Why were these nations concerned about building their international reputation in health, and which audience were they addressing? Brazil, India, and China were mainly targeting the West in their reputation-building endeavors, for several reasons. First, building a strong reputation in health facilitated the ability to increase international investor confidence and to establish trade and diplomatic relations with prosperous western nations (Bava, 2007; Y. Huang, 2013; Roberto de Almeida, 2013). Second, establishing a reputation of complying with the international policy norms and expectations established by influential western institutions, such as the United Nations (UN) and the World Health Organization (WHO), was perceived as a means for Brazil, India, and China to increase their legitimacy and influence within these institutions, while helping marshal UN support for their election to important UN bodies such as the UN Security Council and the World Trade Organization (WTO) (Bremmer, 2012; Jabeen, 2010). And third, in a context where these nations were seeking assistance to modernize their economies, they believed that by solidifying their reputation as states capable of controlling the economic consequences of disease, they could gain the trust and assistance of UN financial institutions such as the World Bank and the IMF (Finch, 2007; Roberto de Almeida, 2013).

On the other hand, *negative* geopolitical positioning emerges when political leaders ignore international criticism and pressure and have no interest in building their international reputation in health through a stronger policy response. In this context, political leaders position their nations as sovereign states, believing that they have the knowledge and capacity to respond on their own, at their own pace, and questioning the assistance of international institutions. This builds on a foreign policy tradition of global and regional leadership, striving to strengthen their bilateral influence rather than seeking cooperative, reciprocal partnerships with the international community. Consequently, negative geopolitical positioning also emerges when leaders decide not to pursue international financial and technical assistance when public health threats emerge, while rejecting alternative policy ideas that do not comport with the government's preexisting approaches to disease prevention and treatment. Although political leaders may provide foreign aid assistance in health to other nations, the purpose of these actions is to solidify their position as global leaders rather than attempting to be perceived as benevolent, caring nations that are also striving to improve their reputation in health. In this geopolitical context, leaders pursue an improved policy response to epidemics only when they pose clear threats to the national security, such as military readiness and economic stability. As I show in this book, Russia's and South Africa's responses to HIV/AIDS and TB fit this mold nicely, leading to a correspondingly delayed and ineffective policy response when compared with Brazil, India, and China.

It is important to note, however, that there are historical precedents shaping the emergence of positive and negative geopolitical positioning. With respect to positive geopolitical positioning, governments that are interested in international reputation building are often shaped by a foreign policy tradition of achieving this objective, repeatedly marketing their government's political stability, economic capacity, technical expertise, and cultural richness while being peaceful partners in international multilateral relationships in diplomacy, national security, economic cooperation, and global health policy. At no point have these nations historically perceived themselves as world leaders, superpowers, or the makers of international diplomacy, peace, and institutions. What's more, these nations often have a foreign policy tradition of receiving international financial and technical assistance for economic development and public health, realizing that they cannot achieve their policy goals without the help of the international community—this smacks of humility, an eagerness to learn from others. Taken together, and as table 1.1 here illustrates, it is the presence of three primary historical precedents that eventually contributes to the formation of positive geopolitical positioning: first, a historic foreign policy commitment to increasing a government's international reputation in economic and social development, as well as public health; second, a historic foreign policy commitment to engaging in peaceful international cooperation and multilateral partnerships in general and in public health; and, finally, government receptivity to international financial and technical assistance for development and health policy reform. In this book, Brazil, India, and China provide good examples of these historical precedents.

Negative geopolitical positioning is also often shaped by several historical precedents. The first of these is a historic government commitment to pursuing foreign policies in international leadership and world power in general and in

Table 1.1.   Geopolitical Positioning in the BRICS Nations

	Historical Precedents	Positive Positioning	Negative Positioning
Brazil, India, and China	• Historical foreign policy commitment to international reputation building in development and in public health • Historical foreign policy commitment to peaceful international cooperation and multilateral partnerships in general and in public health • Government receptivity to international financial and technical assistance	• Positive response to international criticism and pressure, and an interest in reputation building; pursuit of international financial and technical assistance for health policy reform	
Russia and South Africa	• Foreign policy legacies in international leadership and world power and in public health • Foreign policy legacies of government independence, sovereignty, and autonomy from external influence		• Government apathy toward international criticism and pressure, and lack of interest in international reputation building • Lack of receptivity to international financial and technical assistance for policy reform

public health. Here, a foreign policy of international leadership takes the form of governments seeking to establish world peace through the creation of treaties and institutions, establishing international economic trade agreements while providing international funding and technical assistance for a variety of economic and social welfare sectors, including public health; with respect to foreign policies of world power, this entails a government's historic commitment to developing foreign policy strategies for strengthening and sustaining its international influence, such as pursuing high levels of economic growth, investing in military capacity, engaging in foreign military campaigns, and providing military aid to other nations. The second historical precedent entails a foreign policy legacy of ensuring state independence, sovereignty, and autonomy from international interference, especially when such interference conflicts with preexisting domestic policy beliefs and preferences. When taken together, these historical precedents contribute to the formation of a government that is not influenced by a rise in international criticisms and pressures. Consequently, governments with these precedents have no interest in pursuing a stronger policy response in order to increase their international reputation in health. At the same time, as powerful, independent nations, they see no need to pursue international financial and technical assistance for their public health programs, as these nations consider themselves to have the experience, knowledge, and capacity needed to effectively respond to epidemics on their own. In this context, rather than receiving foreign aid assistance to enhance their policy response to health epidemics, governments will instead view themselves as donors of such financial and technical assistance—at times, even at the expense of neglecting to invest in their own policy response to the same disease. As we will see in this book, the countries of Russia and South Africa provide good examples of these processes.

Differences in geopolitical positioning provide necessary but insufficient causal conditions for ultimately achieving a centrist policy response. Also important is the type of *bureaucratic–civil societal partnerships* present. As the recent literature emphasizes, when these partnerships are strong, health bureaucrats can obtain the political support, financial resources, and information needed to ensure that policies are well funded and implemented (Garcia and Parker, 2011; Gómez, 2013b; Rich, 2010; Rich and Gómez, 2012). Scholars specifically claim that the bureaucracy needs civic organizations, such as nongovernmental organizations (NGOs), to strengthen its political legitimacy within government, thus allowing the formation of policy networks and coalitions. Bureaucrats, as a result, receive both political and financial support for their health programs (Carpenter, 2001). And yet, the bureaucracy also needs to work closely with NGOs to obtain information about ongoing healthcare needs and cultural and/or local institutional challenges to implementing federal (or international) policy guidelines (Garcia and Parker, 2011; Rich and Gómez, 2012). Under these conditions, the bureaucracy can both sustain and create effective policy responses to epidemics.

The BRICS countries vary considerably in the strength of the bureaucracy's partnership with NGOs. This, in turn, reflects differences in history, culture, institutions, and therefore political and civil societal expectations of how the bureaucracy relates to activists in the domain of public health. These unique backdrops have also shaped how NGOs view public health bureaucrats in response to disease outbreak; the bureaucracy's roles, responsibilities, and relationship with NGOs; and the issue of whether citizens should work with the government in response to public health threats.

In Brazil, there has been a strong historical partnership between the bureaucracy and civil society in the area of public health. This is mainly due to the bureaucracy's efforts since the early nineteenth century to work closely with social health movements, public health associations, and local communities to increase the bureaucracy's political legitimacy, support, and policy influence. This close working partnership facilitated the expansion of public health policies and federal intervention in helping local governments respond to epidemics. Federal bureaucrats also developed a high degree of cohesiveness and trust with these civil societal organizations, in the process aiding bureaucrats' ability to obtain important health information, learn about local needs, and design effective policy strategies. I argue that this strong bureaucratic–civil societal partnership persisted over time, eventually facilitating the emergence of a centrist policy response to HIV/AIDS and obesity.

None of the other BRICS nations have this long history of bureaucratic–civil societal partnerships. In India, China, Russia, and South Africa, for different historical, cultural, and political reasons, the public health bureaucracy was highly autonomous from civil societal influence, devising policies and imposing them on subnational governments. Consequently, local communities preferred to respond to diseases on their own, never seeking to challenge government policy and/or to volunteer information for better policy prescriptions. In South Africa, under apartheid, the government was divided in its partnership with activists, private physicians, and healthcare workers on racial grounds: white communities often benefited from public health bureaucrats' working with them in response to epidemics, while black communities often responded on their own. In India, China, Russia, and South Africa, then, unique historical contexts engendered weak bureaucratic partnerships with NGOs in response to the HIV/AIDS, obesity, and TB epidemics. These weak partnerships challenged their government's ability to sustain and deepen their policy response.

Bureaucratic–civil societal partnerships are not the only role that NGOs can play in response to epidemics. NGOs may also be effective at independently and aggressively pressuring the state for a policy response. As I explain in this book, however, this occurs only *after* national governments have already responded to epidemics and for their own geopolitical or domestic reasons—as seen in Brazil and South Africa, respectively. In contrast, in India, China, and Russia, NGOs are still comparatively weak and not nearly as effective in organizing and pressuring the government for policy responses to HIV/AIDS and other diseases (Gómez and Harris, 2015). Because of NGOs' limited role in instigating a policy response, I decided to focus in this book on the geopolitical incentives motivating governing elites to do so, as well as bureaucrats' subsequent efforts to seek out and establish partnerships with NGOs—but only after the bureaucrats were already committed to policy reform and were seeking allies to further consolidate their policy interests.

I argue that a *centrist policy response* to disease epidemics requires a combination of both positive geopolitical positioning and health bureaucrats' strong partnerships with civil society. However, geopolitical positioning emerges as the first and most important variable in our causal sequence of events, followed by the strength of bureaucratic–civil societal partnerships. This is because it is geopolitical positioning that first determines the incentives for governing elites to support the public health bureaucracy and its reform efforts. For instance, with regard to positive geopolitical positioning, political leaders will be motivated to proactively support bureaucratic reforms to achieve their international reputation-building interests. In the absence of these interests and political support, bureaucrats will not be incentivized to pursue stronger partnerships with NGOs, in the expectation that they will not be able to strategically use NGOs for the acquisition of financial resources. This is because, even if bureaucrats did succeed in establishing strong partnerships with NGOs, in the absence of political leaders' geopolitical incentives to support their cause, bureaucratic calls for reform would not be supported. Moreover, on their own, strong bureaucratic–civil societal partnerships will not enhance a nation's international reputation in health, especially when, due to a lack of political attention and support, they do not lead to the introduction of innovative prevention and treatment programs.

As table 1.2 illustrates, when the BRICS nations are compared, Brazil illustrates both causal conditions: positive geopolitical positioning and strong bureaucratic–civil societal partnerships. In contrast, while positive geopolitical positioning was present in India and China, they had no strong bureaucratic–civil societal partnerships. Meanwhile, in Russia and South Africa, neither of these causal conditions was present, thus leading to weaker policy responses.

My proposed geopolitical positioning framework is dynamic in nature: it assumes that different governments are not exposed to the same kinds of inter-

Table 1.2.   The Argument: Factors Affecting Responses to Epidemics in the BRICS Nations

	Positive Geopolitical Positioning	Negative Geopolitical Positioning	Strong Bureaucratic–Civil Societal Partnerships	Centrist Policy Response
Brazil	X		X	X
Russia		X		
India	X			
China	X			
South Africa		X		

national policy expectations and pressures at the same time and that, consequently, they vary in when they respond to health epidemics and their capacity to achieve a centrist policy response. My argument rests on the notion that international health agencies and donors respond to epidemics at different points in time, reflecting not only differences in the epidemiological nature of diseases and their social construction but also the varied influence of international institutions in policy-framing and agenda-setting processes (Shiffman, 2009). My proposed analytical framework therefore assumes that differences in the timing of these international expectations and pressures lead to differences in the timing of government response to epidemics, with some governments responding earlier than others. Reputation sensitive political leaders in some nations will support changes to prevention and treatment policies earlier in response to epidemics when compared to other nations, while bureaucrats in the former nations will do the same when it comes to establishing strong partnerships with NGOs to advance their policy interests. However, some governments may be delayed in their encounter with international policy expectations and pressures, reflecting differences in the timing of the epidemiological emergence of a disease in their country relative to others, with political leaders consequently supporting the creation of prevention and treatment programs at later times. Bureaucrats may similarly be delayed in their pursuit of a stronger partnership with NGOs for ongoing funding and support for policy innovation and implementation—though this depends, of course, on where political leaders position themselves geopolitically.

For instance, with respect to HIV/AIDS, Brazil's government encountered these international policy expectations and pressures by the late 1980s, several years before India and China, which encountered them in the early to mid-1990s; South Africa and Russia first encountered these pressures in the late 1990s and early 2000s, respectively. Consequently, Brazil's political leaders responded earlier to HIV/AIDS than these other nations and were willing to support a stronger policy response to it, and bureaucrats pursued a stronger partnership with NGOs for ongoing policy innovation and implementation, earlier than in these other nations.

These differences in the timing of international policy expectations, pressures, and government response to health epidemics vary for different types of health threats. For example, HIV/AIDS emerged and was recognized by the international community much earlier (by the mid-1980s) than obesity (early 2000s) and TB (late 1990s), and these differences account for the differences in the timing of government response to them both within and between nations.

This book's main dependent variable of interest, then, is *building a centrist policy response.* I define this centrist policy response as the creation and *ongoing* financial and administrative expansion of federal agencies, the development of effective prevention and treatment policies (in particular, and where applicable, universal access to essential medicines), and formal and informal strategies to increase the central government's policy influence in a context of healthcare decentralization; all three of these components are necessary for a successful centrist policy response. Formal strategies to increase the central government's policy influence are distinct from an *ongoing* increase in spending and administrative expansion for national programs because the former entails specific policy initiatives focused on conditional fiscal transfers to municipal governments in need of financial assistance, as well as informal strategies that entail the central government's contracting with NGOs to monitor and pressure local governments into compliance with federal policy guidelines. I highlight the word *ongoing* here because merely introducing public health policies in response to international criticism and pressure is not perceived as a successful centrist policy response. Nations may introduce policies but never follow through in continuing to finance and enforce them. To achieve a centrist policy response, health bureaucrats must prove capable of obtaining political and financial support for their programs on a continuing basis.

But why would a centrist policy response be necessary? Shouldn't healthcare decentralization provide a more effective approach to policy implementation? After all, theorists have long emphasized that politicians' electoral accountability, better access to information about citizens' needs, interstate competition, and civic participation in policymaking processes lead to more efficient subnational spending and policy implementation (Manor, 1999; Musgrave, 1959; Oates, 1999). Moreover, all of the BRICS nations—as well as most governments—have pursued a decentralized approach to healthcare financing and administration, thus suggesting a high level of confidence in this health systems approach.

Recent research nevertheless suggests that healthcare decentralization is not very effective in rendering public health services (Gauri and Khaleghian, 2002; Gómez, 2011a; Nathanson, 1996; Rich and Gómez, 2012; Saltman, 2008; UNAIDS, 1999; WHO, 1992). Indeed, it has been the repeated absence of political and bureaucratic accountability, ongoing corruption, and insufficient human resources that have challenged the ability of decentralization to adequately respond to disease epidemics—and other social welfare needs (Rich and Gómez, 2012; Smoke, Gómez, and Peterson, 2006). In fact, even the most vitriolic critics of a centralized government response to social welfare policy have argued that when it comes to public health, centralization is needed to ensure the timely provision of medical treatment (Pritchett and Wilcock, 2004).

This is not to say that decentralization has been a complete failure. Several scholars have pointed out that decentralization has both incentivized and encouraged increased healthcare expenditures and policy innovations at the subnational level in the BRICS and other developing nations (Capuno, 2011; Danishevski et al., 2006; Ho, 2010; Osterkatz, 2011). But this spending and policy experimentation is often limited to wealthier state governments, leading to a major source of regional inequality in service provision among the states—especially in the BRICS nations (Gómez, 2015b; Zhang and Liu, 2013). Moreover, and relatedly, healthcare decentralization in the BRICS has not led to a uniform increase in state-level expenditures for healthcare (Gómez, 2015b). Many state governments in the BRICS have in fact experienced ongoing deficits and debts and have not been able to afford increased spending for healthcare (Pahwa and Beland, 2013; Uchimura and Jütting, 2007). Consequently, among the BRICS, there is a consistently high level of inequality in subnational healthcare financing and policy innovation (Gómez, 2015b).

But why should we expect all of the BRICS nations to pursue a centrist policy response to epidemics? Given their vast differences in historical political institutions, culture, and economic performance, shouldn't we expect each of the BRICS to pursue its own unique kind of policy response? This may certainly be the case. Nevertheless, there is no disputing that since the late 1990s, a scholarly and international policy consensus and expectation has emerged asserting that in response to public health crisis, governments should strive for a more centrist policy response. Indeed, several scholars have argued that policy centralization facilitates implementation processes precisely because, in situations where local governments lack experience, technical expertise, and financial resources, experienced central government administrators with more resources and experience can be more effective at implementing policy. Central administrators are also less prone to corruption by local politicians and constituent interests (Gauri and Khaleghian, 2002; Prud'Homme, 1995; Rich and Gómez, 2012), while being more exposed to national media and political criticisms (Prud'Homme, 1995).

It was this very confidence in a centralized bureaucratic and policy approach to disease epidemics that led to the emergence of an international consensus within the UN in 2003 claiming that effective government responses to HIV/AIDS, for example, require a strong, well-coordinated, centralized policy response—more specifically, a "3-ones approach to AIDS policy." In this approach, nations have one agreed-upon HIV/AIDS national action framework that facilitates coordination for all parties involved, one national AIDS coordinating authority supporting a broad multisectoral mandate, and one agreed-upon country-level monitoring and evaluation system (UNAIDS, 2003).[3] In sum, this international scholarly and policy consensus can have a strong impact on domestic policy responses to epidemics, especially among emerging nations that are striving to engage in multilateral cooperation, obtain financial and technical assistance, establish international partnerships, and be perceived as cooperative, influential actors at the global level.

At the same time, we should also be mindful that the BRICS have a long history of providing a centralized government response to public health threats and that the decentralization of public health responsibilities is a recent policy phenomenon (Y. Huang, 2010b; Mushtaq, 2009). In this context, we should expect the BRICS to have a greater tendency to rely on a centralized response even when healthcare decentralization has been pursued (Rich and Gómez, 2012). And there has been a burgeoning realization within these nations that the central government needs to play a bigger role in ensuring that state and local governments have sufficient funding and administrative capacity and are responsive to civil societal healthcare needs (Chen and Jin, 2011; Yip et al., 2012).

Democracy, Historical Institutions, and Civil Society

But how does my argument about the importance of geopolitical positioning relate to the existing literature discussing the international and domestic political, institutional, and civil societal contexts incentivizing governments to respond to health epidemics? One school of thought emphasizes the importance of transitions to democracy and political regime type. Given the high level of domestic and international pressures associated with the rise of epidemics, incessant media attention, and technocrats advocating for an immediate government response, some claim that democratically elected forms of government will have incentives to immediately respond (Ruger, 2005b; Sen, 1999). This assumption is predicated on the belief that the presence of national elections and a high degree of political accountability, facilitated through a free press, creates incentives for politicians to immediately implement aggressive health prevention and treatment policies (Folayan, 2004; McGuire, 2010; Ruger, 2005b; Sen 1999; Whiteside, 1999). Especially within nations exhibiting high levels of disease prevalence, these electoral pressures are often too overwhelming to ignore (Putzel, 2004). Furthermore, some claim that the media's coverage of an epidemic's debilitating effect, such as HIV/AIDS, reinforces the need to respond, thus prompting aggressive bureaucratic and policy expansion (Bor, 2007; Sen, 1999). At the same time, a long history of politicians' interest in providing public health services can create social expectations and demands for a continued policy response, in turn generating further incentives to immediately do so (McGuire, 2010).

Nevertheless, others claim that the presence of an electoral democracy is not necessary for an effective policy response. In fact, nondemocratic governments are often more effective at quickly targeting epidemics and responding, either by quarantining individuals—the case of Cuba stands out (Gorry, 2008)—or by providing immunization treatment (Gauri and Khaleghian, 2002). In contrast, the presence of multiple veto actors within democracies, such as political parties, heightened media coverage and debate, and the infiltration of conservative moral views within these institutions has been known to stall democratic responses to epidemics (D. Altman, 1986; Shilts, 1987). Recent scholarship—as well as subsequent chapters in this book—also emphasizes that the presence of national elections does not prompt an immediate and effective policy response. In Brazil, for example, the work of Gauri and Lieberman (2006) and Lieberman (2009) shows that at no point did presidents campaign on the

HIV/AIDS epidemic, and that the first time a presidential candidate mentioned HIV/AIDS was several years after the government had already responded. Research by Putzel (2004) on Uganda's response to HIV/AIDS in the late 1980s similarly finds that HIV/AIDS was so prevalent and such an obvious problem that it was no longer perceived as a partisan issue.

Some scholars claim that the presence of historical institutional and policy legacies as an explanation for timely government responses to epidemics may provide a better alternative than political regime type (Skocpol and Amenta, 1986). Indeed, the work of McGuire (2010) suggests that even within previous authoritarian governments throughout the 1970s and 1980s, such as in Chile, Thailand, and Brazil, historic legacies of state-led public health programs serving the poor, women, and children led to aggressive policy responses to more contemporary diseases, such as malnutrition and eventually HIV/AIDS. Nathanson (1996) has also put forth the argument that a deep history and culture of bureaucratic technocratic capacity and political and health policy centralization in France facilitated and indeed encouraged the creation of autonomous, centralized public health agencies in response to HIV/AIDS. Alternatively, some claim that in Brazil, the historic presence and institutional legacy of a centralized bureaucratic approach to disease containment prompted and facilitated the government's subsequent ability to respond to HIV/AIDS (Gómez, 2015a). According to this view, public health officials wield a great deal of capacity, legitimacy, and autonomy, in turn convincing the government of the need to immediately respond to epidemics. This is often facilitated by the presence of a supportive president, who at times may have a personal interest in public health or is empathetic to the needs of the poor (McGuire, 2010).

The problem with this theoretical approach is that even if nations have an impressive historical institutional and policy legacy in providing public health services, this by no means guarantees *ongoing* bureaucratic and policy effectiveness. As the work of McGuire (2010) explains, even in countries in which historically progressive state-led public health programs existed, such as Argentina, Brazil, Taiwan, and Thailand, the subsequent failure of the president and the ministry of health (MOH) to consistently provide adequate funding, healthcare training, and salaries eventually led to poor policy implementation. And this occurred despite the presence of highly competent public health bureaucrats who pressured the national government to scale up its assistance to the states. Other scholars—as well as this book—maintain that in the case of Brazil, notwithstanding the presence of highly skilled and experienced public health bureaucrats working within a historically revered, centralized ministry of health, when the HIV/AIDS and obesity epidemics emerged, none of this history and experience helped public health bureaucrats in their ability to persuade the president and congress to provide ongoing financial and technical support (Nascimento, 2005; also see chapter 2 of this book). Thus, the notion that historical institutional and policy legacies matter in positively shaping how governments respond to epidemics is questionable.

If it is not democratic electoral incentives and historical institutional and policy legacies that eventually prompt a national government response, then perhaps it is civil society? A plethora of literature suggests that the presence of proactive NGOs is necessary for displaying civil society's discontent through proactive demonstrations, lobbying, and pressuring the government for the creation of prevention and treatment policies for HIV/AIDS and other diseases (D. Altman, 1986; Barnett and Whiteside, 2006; Boone and Batsell, 2001; Gould, 2009; Lucker, 2004; Parker, 2003; Rau, 2006; Whiteside, 1999). NGOs are also important for raising awareness, disseminating information, organizing meetings and focus groups, and providing prevention and treatment services in the absence of government intervention (Barnett and Whiteside, 2006; Boone and Batsell, 2001; Gould, 2009; Parker, 2003). With respect to HIV/AIDS, NGOs in Latin America and Africa were vital for providing services that were not provided by national and local health departments, such as condoms and sex education (Rau, 2006). In addition, others argue that AIDS NGOs have been instrumental in working with local health departments to not only create state-level heath agencies and programs but also successfully pressure the national government to create an effective HIV/AIDS program (Gauri and Lieberman, 2006; Lieberman, 2009; Parker 2003, 2009).

This "bottom-up" civil societal approach to explaining government response to epidemics also has several limitations. First, case study evidence in this book, as well as other scholarly research, suggests that regardless of how well organized and effective NGOs are, they are not the most important factor contributing to a government response to epidemics. For example, the work of Rau (2006) claims that while HIV/AIDS NGOs and their mobilization in Uganda and South Africa were encouraged by the national political leadership, ultimately the latter never respected and paid heed to NGOs' demands for constructing a national HIV/AIDS program (Gauri and Lieberman, 2006; Rau, 2006). Uganda's leadership often viewed NGOs as threats to the ruling elite's control over society, considering NGOs' growing popularity and collusion with international organizations (Rau, 2006). Others claim that in Brazil, while influential in helping construct municipal AIDS programs, NGOs did not succeed at pressuring the national government to provide adequate prevention and treatment services (Teixeira, 1997). And even after the national AIDS program was created in 1986, as chapter 2 explains, despite the creation of a national AIDS commission within the national AIDS program, which was explicitly designed to represent the interests of NGOs and incorporate their views into the policy-making process, few NGOs and people living with HIV/AIDS were present on the commission and were capable of influencing policy.

If democratic electoral incentives, historical institutions, policy legacies, and civil societal pressures do not motivate governments to respond to health epidemics, then which factors do? Findings in this book critique and build on the literature by suggesting that the impetus for a government response to health epidemics resides more at the international than the domestic level and concerns how nations have historically responded to the international community in times of health crisis. More specifically, it is a nation's *geopolitical positioning*, followed by the presence of strong bureaucratic–civil societal partnerships, that matters most when accounting for differences in the timing of government response to epidemics, as well as their capacity to engage in a centrist policy response.

It is important to emphasize, however, that my argument about the importance of geopolitical positioning focuses on public health issues, not other policy areas. Indeed, the BRICS vary considerably in their geopolitical alignment on other social welfare, economic, and security issues. In contrast to HIV/AIDS policy, for many years China, for example, was not interested in bolstering its international reputation in environmental policy, nor has the government sought to comply with international treaty protocols, such as reduced greenhouse gas emissions, while receiving international financial and technical guidance in crafting environmental legislation (Combes, 2012); the same can be said for some of Brazil's and India's policies on education (Dréze and Sen, 2013). That said, we should not expect that my argument about geopolitical positioning applies to *all* policy sectors; indeed, different policy sectors often possess their own unique histories and domestic and international political interests. Global public health may be unique in this regard, considering the longer history of international cooperation and state-led policies in public health—especially in disease eradication—when compared to education, the environment, and national security.

But is my theoretical argument about international reputation building in health grounded in empirical reality? This does appear to be the case, as much of the academic literature has discussed how nations strategically use domestic health policy reforms in order to enhance their international reputation in successfully addressing healthcare challenges (Chan, Chen, and Xu, 2010; McGuire, 2010; Smallman, 2007). For example, McGuire (2010) suggests that historically governments have strengthened domestic public health programs in order to save face with an international community when confronted with human rights violations, as well as government-led civil conflict and strife. In Latin America and East Asia, for example, military governments criticized by the international community for violating international protocols of human rights often invested heavily in public health programs focusing on women and children. In so doing, these nations believed that they could subdue international criticism and rejuvenate their international credibility (McGuire, 2010). Other nations have emphasized their investment in public health policies in order to bolster their government's international reputation for being committed to healthcare as a human right (Chan, Chen, and Xu, 2010; Y. Huang, 2006). As Yanzhong Huang (2006) has argued, in response to international criticisms of having a poor government response to the SARS epidemic in 2003, as well as a weak public health system in general, the Chinese government began to invest heavily in its public health system in the hopes of rejuvenating its international reputation for safeguarding citizens' healthcare needs and for having an effective public health system (Chan, Chen, and Xu, 2010).

However, when emerging nations positively position themselves in the world, *how* do they go about increasing their international reputation for having an effective public health system? First, I argue that reputation building is achieved when policymakers increase their political and financial support for a stronger policy response to epidemics; this is perceived by policymakers as the primary means through which they can increase their international reputation. Second, policymakers will seek to wine and dine with the best of them: that is, they will invite officials from international health agencies and scientists to their country in order to show these guests their successful policy strategies and to confirm that they are indeed curbing the spread of disease. These efforts can take place at meetings within ministries of health or international conferences hosted by the country. And, with respect to negative geopolitical positioning, political leaders will ignore international criticism, policy warnings, and suggestions for improvement, deciding instead to respond to epidemics at their own pace and, ultimately, in response to an epidemic's national security concerns. Moreover, political leaders will not try to meet proactively with international donors to obtain loans or technical assistance for policy reform. In an effort to bolster their position as global leaders, these leaders will instead provide foreign aid and technical assistance to combat diseases in other nations, even when they are neglecting their own domestic policies.

When compared to the existing literature discussing the international factors motivating governments to respond to epidemics, my argument about the importance of geopolitical positioning takes a rather different approach. My approach combines theories that for the most part have been treated as separate, isolated methods for explaining the international circumstances motivating governments to respond to health epidemics.

Indeed, works emphasizing the role of international criticism and pressure, and the literature discussing international reputation building in global health, have been treated as different approaches to explaining government responses to epidemics. With regard to international criticism and pressure, studies taking this approach tend to emphasize the coercive elements of international agency pressures, such as those of the WHO, UNAIDS, and the World Bank, on domestic health policy reform. Work by Lieberman (2009), for example, maintains that at the height of the HIV/AIDS epidemic, not only did UNAIDS impose its best practices on developing nations—such as the strengthening of national AIDS programs, prevention, and treatment policy (especially harm reduction)—but UNAIDS officials also met with health ministers at conferences, criticized, and coerced them—in essence through peer pressure—into adopting their policy prescriptions. Others claim that criticism and pressure from the WHO and the World Bank have been instrumental in motivating policymakers in Asia and Latin America to discover and address their bureaucratic and policy obstacles to reforming their public health system, as well as policies toward HIV/AIDS (Gómez, 2009; Y. Huang, 2006, 2010; Kaufman, 2010). The work of Okuonzi and Macrae (1995) emphasizes how the World Bank often used aid conditionally to essentially pressure developing nations into adopting its recommendations for health systems reform, such as privatization.

Other studies have instead focused on foreign policy in health as a means to increase government legitimacy and international policy influence. To achieve this, for example, governments often create bilateral aid programs to help other nations combat HIV/AIDS and other diseases (Feldbaum, Lee, and Michaud, 2010; Feldbaum and Michaud, 2010; Fidler, 2005, 2009; Labonte and Gagnon, 2010). Feldbaum and Michaud (2010) claim that the United States has for years provided medical training, infrastructural resources, and supplies to developing nations in order to restore the United States' image as an altruistic, peace-loving nation; and that, moreover, this has been important in the unpopular context of an Iraqi invasion (K. Lee, 2009). Similarly, others highlight China's and Cuba's efforts to provide medical assistance and medicine in order to "win the hearts and minds" of developing nations, mainly in Latin America and Africa, respectively, though these efforts were strategic moves to gain access to key resources, such as oil (Chan, Chen, and Xu, 2010; Feinsilver, 2008; Y. Huang, 2010).

My emphasis on geopolitical positioning combines these two strands of previously isolated literature. That is, positive geopolitical positioning combines the literature emphasizing the importance of international criticism and pressure for policy reform with the literature emphasizing the creation of health policy as a means to international reputation building in health. In so doing, my argument builds on the rich constructivist tradition in international relations by claiming that governments devise the idea and expectation that international reputation and ambition are important reasons for them to pursue policy reform (Ruggie, 1998).

Geopolitical positioning's merger of these two areas of research in turn reflects the unique nature of the emerging nations. For, unlike the advanced industrialized nations or less developed nations, because the BRICS are often perceived—and indeed perceive themselves (Hurrell, 2006)—as in the process of becoming potential world powers, they are more likely to be self-conscious of their developmental status and are often sensitive to world opinion. The advanced industrialized nations, such as the United States, the United Kingdom, France, and Germany, are not as sensitive to world opinion because of their high level of development and track record in leading the world in response to disease (Bliss, 2012). On the other hand, less developed nations may perceive their global development status as too low to have an impact on international economic and political affairs, believing that, regardless of international criticism and their interest in reform, they simply do not have the financial and infrastructural means needed to engage in a stronger policy response. The BRICS fall in between these two polar ends of the international development spectrum;

it is their unique status in the world that makes my argument about the importance of geopolitical positioning possible and potentially helpful.

Responding to Epidemics in the BRICS

Brazil, India, and China, as described above, were initially delayed in their responses to disease epidemics, and these nations differed in both the timing of
their response to epidemics and ultimately their capacity to pursue a centrist
policy response. During the first few years of the HIV/AIDS and obesity epidemics, in all three nations, several factors—the absence of credible epidemiological evidence suggesting that these diseases posed serious public health
threats, preexisting commitments to decentralization, and the presence of moral
and racial discriminatory views, especially toward the HIV/AIDS community—
delayed effective policy responses. Consequently, the international community,
mainly led by the WHO, began to criticize and pressure these governments to
implement more prevention and treatment programs.

In these three BRICS countries, international criticism and pressure had a
profound impact on achieving this objective. In Brazil, the government viewed
these criticisms and pressures as an opportunity to use policy reform as a means
to increase its international reputation as a government capable of successfully responding to HIV/AIDS and obesity; these reputation-building incentives
and response emerged earlier for HIV/AIDS than for obesity, however, because
of the international community's earlier response to HIV/AIDS. The government wanted to reveal that Brazil had the political commitment and resources
to quickly eradicate disease and to develop. It wanted to show western-based
institutions such as the UN and the WHO that they were wholeheartedly
committed to implementing international norms of access to healthcare as a
human right (Da Costa Marques, 2003; Gómez, 2015a). With this in mind,
and facilitated by the provision of a World Bank loan in 1993 (Teodorescu and
Teixeira, 2015), the government pursued a stronger, and eventually a centrist,
policy response to HIV/AIDS and obesity. Expanding the size of the national
AIDS and obesity programs; providing these programs with greater financial
and policymaking autonomy; enacting universal medical treatment policies; introducing conditional fiscal transfer programs and NGO partnerships for monitoring and holding local governments accountable to the central government—
all were centrist policy responses implemented to overcome the challenges of
poorly planned decentralization processes.

By the early to mid-1990s, India's and China's leaders also viewed the rise of international criticism and pressure as an opportunity to pass muster as nations capable of getting rid of disease. When these criticisms emerged, with the assistance of international donors and technical assistance, China's leadership immediately sought to restore the government's international reputation by providing new levels of financial and political support to the government's national AIDS program (Y. Huang, 2010). With respect to obesity, the government enacted a series of policy mandates emphasizing greater physical activity in schools and nutritional policy guidelines (Cheng, 2007). India followed a similar path. In response to international criticism, the government wanted to show the WHO and western governments that India could join them in containing the spread of HIV/AIDS and obesity. Facilitated by World Bank loans, parliament immediately began to ensure that the National AIDS Commission had ample financial and political support for prevention and universal antiretroviral (ARV) treatment programs (Lieberman, 2009). And, in response to obesity, India's Ministry of Health and Social Welfare confronted pressures from the WHO in 2005 by immediately engaging in a series of prevention initiatives (Reddy et al., 2005).

Although Brazil, India, and China reacted similarly to international criticism and pressure, they differed in the types of bureaucratic–civil societal partnerships needed to pursue a centrist policy response. In Brazil, seeking ongoing financial and political support from the congress to achieve this objective, MOH bureaucrats strategically sought and established strong partnerships with NGOs and social health movements that advocated centrist policy ideas with a long track record of success; this built on the MOH's historic tradition of working in close partnership with social health movements in response to disease (Hochman, 1988). By periodically meeting with NGOs and social health activists, creating national committees that guaranteed the groups' say in federal legislation, and periodically visiting with NGOs at the local level, Brazil's health bureaucrats succeeded in garnering the attention and support of the congress. Consequently, they were able to finance and consolidate their centrist policy response.

In contrast, India's and China's health bureaucrats never established this kind of partnership with NGOs. Neither nation had a long history of close bureaucratic–civil societal partnerships in response to disease; the absence of such a history was the result of a centralized, autonomous public health system with no interest in seeking civic participation in the policymaking process (Y. Huang, 2013; Mushtaq, 2009). In China and India, moreover, historically, social health movements preferred to work on their own, drawing from unique medical cultures and traditions (Andharia, 2009; Yang Da-hua, 2004), while in the case of China, cultural reverence for the state generated few incentives to question its policymaking authority (Pye, 1996). By the time the HIV/AIDS and obesity epidemics took hold in both nations, although NGOs and social health movements emerged in response, they did not proffer historically proven centrist policy ideas or have an interest in pressuring the government for policy reform, nor did health bureaucrats have any incentive to establish partnerships with NGOs in order to bolster bureaucratic legitimacy and capacity to obtain ongoing funding for policy innovation. Thus, while China's and India's ministries of health were eventually able to strengthen their policy response after the emergence of international criticism, their health bureaucrats did not have the ongoing support needed to introduce a centrist policy response. The similarity of these outcomes, one in a nascent democracy, India, and the other in a nondemocracy, China, further suggests that political regime type does not matter when it comes to establishing partnerships between the bureaucracy and NGOs; this may be due to the bureaucracy's decision to sustain its tradition of being highly autonomous in health policymaking in both nations, a lack of political commitment to incorporate NGOs' policy views in India, and the reluctance of political leaders in India and China to prioritize improvements in public health policy (Dréze and Sen, 2013).

In Russia and South Africa, the governments responded to epidemics in a different way. Although the two countries joined their emerging counterparts in exhibiting an initially weak government response to their respective healthcare challenges, in contrast to the situation in the other BRICS nations, Russian and South African presidents and senior health bureaucrats, historically, never cared about increasing their international reputation in health. Regardless of how much the WHO criticized and questioned their lackluster policy responses, these governments sought to respond on their own terms, at their own pace, at times introducing prevention and treatment policies that blatantly contradicted international policy advice (Wallander, 2005). In contrast to their emerging counterparts, Russian and South African political elites viewed and positioned themselves as world and regional leaders, too advanced for external assistance, and instead joining the advanced industrialized nations in leading the global fight against disease (Bakalova and Spanger, 2013). Russia's and South

Africa's political leaders were also not interested in constantly borrowing money from international creditors and establishing partnerships with them and with other international agencies in order to adopt new policy ideas. In essence, I argue that these policy views stemmed in both nations from a foreign policy tradition of being highly involved in international diplomacy, constantly conjuring up peace treaties, participating in and helping end world wars, and striving to shape rather than follow international discourse and geopolitical trends.

In this context, Russia and South Africa responded to disease epidemics only when they posed a clear threat to national security, and, even then, this threat was insufficient for eliciting a strong policy response. In Russia, the government essentially ignored HIV/AIDS until it was clear that it threatened the military's ability to recruit and retain soldiers (Sjostedt, 2008). Nevertheless, while federal funding began to increase, it was consistently deemed insufficient, eventually began to decline, and failed to facilitate the pursuit of any effective prevention and treatment programs (Schwirtz, 2011). Although a TB epidemic emerged due in part to HIV, because TB did not threaten military readiness or the economy, the government never pursued a stronger policy response. South Africa responded in a similar manner. Notwithstanding the end of apartheid rule and a transition to democracy, the national government began to respond to HIV/AIDS only when it threatened not just to damage military capabilities but also to foment economic and social unrest (Baleta, 1998). After these problems emerged, the government began to take HIV/AIDS more seriously, improving funding and policy reforms, though continuing to fall short of providing adequate funding and effective prevention and treatment programs, as well as much-needed investments in human resources and healthcare infrastructure (SAPA, 1998b). Although TB resurfaced due to HIV, as in Russia, its failure to threaten national security in South Africa meant, again, that it did not elicit a strong government response.

If the threat of HIV/AIDS to national security in Russia and South Africa began to increase politicians' interest in responding to the epidemic, why didn't their health ministries engage in a stronger—possibly even a centrist—policy response? As in India and China, part of the problem also stemmed from the absence of a strong partnership between the national health bureaucracy and NGOs in Russia and South Africa. Historically, in both nations, in addition to the government's disinterest in incorporating healthcare activists' and concerned citizens' views into the policymaking process, social heath movements and community-based organizations preferred to work on their own, believing that they had greater knowledge and public health expertise than the government, while in South Africa, apartheid's racial segregation and discrimination toward black communities further compelled the latter to work on their own (Conroy, 2006; Hosking, 2001; Kalipeni, 2000). Consequently, in both nations social health movements were uninterested in proposing that the central government interfere in their health affairs, while health officials were essentially apathetic in partnering with them in response to disease. In Russia, when state communism emerged during the early twentieth century, the state also suppressed various social movements, viewing them as suspect, influenced by pro-democratic western forces. By the 1990s, when the HIV/AIDS and TB epidemics emerged, societal fears of state suppression endured, in turn leading to the absence of progressive, well-organized NGOs that responded to these diseases. In South Africa, due to historic racial divisions and government suppression of activists criticizing the government, even after the transition back to democracy under African National Congress (ANC) rule, no national-level unifying social health movement, or group of well-organized, funded NGOs, emerged in the area of public health (Schneider, 2002). Because of their respective challenges, then, neither nation's HIV/AIDS and TB bureaucrats viewed NGOs and social health movements as potential allies in their quest to strengthen the government's policy response (Gauri and Lieberman, 2006). Consequently, and similar to what we saw in India and China, a well-organized group of NGOs that Russian and South African public health bureaucrats could strategically use to engender a stronger or even centrist policy response never emerged.

Methodology

When conducting my research for this book, I employed a qualitative comparative case study design. The methodological purpose of the study was to examine the effectiveness of my proposed analytical framework across several different types of political, social, and cultural contexts. This approach is emblematic of what Lijphart (1971) and Przeworski and Teune (1970) referred to as a "most different systems" research design. Here, case studies exhibiting differences in broader contextual variables are selected to see whether a theoretical framework applies and whether it explains reforms in diverse settings, thus illustrating the argument's potential generalizability. For my research, I selected the BRICS because of their different political, cultural, and institutional structures. My argument about the importance of geopolitical positioning and strong bureaucratic–

civil societal partnerships was applied to these cases to see whether this analytical approach could help to explain variation in the timing of government response to health epidemics and capacity to pursue a centrist policy response.

The goal of this study was to establish a theoretical framework that explains when and how the BRICS responded to epidemics. My approach therefore resembles what other comparative scholars have referred to as a middle-range generalizable claim (Ziblatt, 2006), in which the scope of the analytical concepts—in this case, geopolitical positioning and strong bureaucratic–civil societal partnerships—and their causal mechanisms pertains to only a select group of cases (Mahoney and Gertz, 2004; Ziblatt, 2006). This middle-range approach allows for a more focused theoretical framework while providing claims that can be subsequently falsified through the introduction of other, similar types of case studies.

Selection of Countries and Epidemics

Why study the BRICS' response to HIV/AIDS, TB, and obesity? At first glance, it may appear that these are very different types of public health threats, given their modes of epidemiological transmission, the emergence of illness and death, and the different types of prevention and treatment needed in response. Levels of international financial and political attention are also significantly different for each of these diseases, with HIV/AIDS receiving by far the most international funding and attention (Sridhar and Gómez, 2010).

In this book, I view the HIV/AIDS, TB, and obesity epidemics from a different perspective, seeing them as more similar than different. In so doing, I focus not on the epidemiology of and international responses to these diseases,[4] but on how domestic politicians and bureaucrats *initially perceive* and respond to these threats. In this process, politicians and bureaucrats initially consider several factors. The first is the extent to which a new disease poses a threat to the entire nation versus a particular community. As seen in chapters 2 to 6, evidence of these political/bureaucratic elite perceptions is provided through the reporting of such views in scholarly publications, policy reports, and, in some instances, quoted statements from politicians expressing their views on a disease's threat to society. The second factor is elite views about which level of government should be responsible for initially responding, the central or state governments—an issue that is relevant in a context of federalism and decentralization, which is present in all of the BRICS nations, where the states are responsible for financing and administering public health policies, though they vary in level of responsibility. And the third factor is the moral views and beliefs associated with particular diseases. When holding conservative beliefs, for example, some politicians and bureaucrats may perceive epidemics such as HIV/AIDS, obesity, and TB as being associated with immoral acts, such as sexual promiscuity (HIV/AIDS), gluttony (obesity), and laziness, an unwillingness to work, and thus poverty (TB) (D. Altman, 1986; Courtwright and Turner, 2010; Puhl and Heuer, 2010). With such views, conservative elites may be unwilling to immediately respond and help communities afflicted by these ailments; the opposite situation may also occur, especially within the bureaucracy, thus leading to conflicting views, debates, and a policy stalemate between politicians and bureaucrats. These conflicting views and debates may also be attributed to other factors, such as the epidemiological character of disease, as well as ease of treatment (Shiffman and Smith, 2007).

When simultaneously considering these three factors, the emergence of a public health threat can instigate a great deal of contestation and a lack of consensus between politicians and bureaucrats over how and when the government should respond. This contestation, in turn, provides an opportunity for the emergence of a critical juncture that shifts elite perceptions in different ways, such as the rise of international criticism and pressure—which, as I posit in this book, instigates the rise of positive and negative geopolitical positioning. Other kinds of epidemics, such as avian flu or bioterrorism events, are more commonly and immediately perceived by political and bureaucratic elites as serious national-level threats with no moral implications. Consequently, these "flash epidemics" are rarely contested among governing elites and often elicit an immediate government response (Ostergard, 2007). It is therefore the politically contested nature of the HIV/AIDS, TB, and obesity epidemics that makes these diseases more similar than different with respect to domestic politicians' and bureaucrats' initial perceptions—which is why they were selected for comparative analysis.

But why focus on some epidemics in some countries but not others—that is, HIV/AIDS and obesity in Brazil, India, and China, versus HIV/AIDS and TB in Russia and South Africa? First, obesity was examined in Brazil, India, and China only because of its earlier emergence among adults and children in these countries, during the 1990s, compared with its later emergence in Russia and South Africa at the turn of the twenty-first century (Branka, Nikogosian, and Lobstein, 2007; Nordling, 2016). Obesity's delayed emergence was the result, in Russia, of a decline in the consumption of energy-dense diets in periods of economic recession during the 1990s, and, in South Africa, of the delayed emergence of urbanization and access to previously denied imported foods for black communities under apartheid (Branka, Nikogosian, and Lobstein, 2007; Nordling, 2016; Youfa Wang, Monteiro, and Popkin, 2002). Thus, in contrast to Brazil, India, and China, the governments of South Africa and Russia did not pay much attention to rising obesity cases until the last five years, and clear national policy strategies and goals focused on obesity prevention have yet to emerge (Branka, Nikogosian, and Lobstein, 2007; Motsoeneng, 2014; Nordling, 2016). For this reason, I did not compare obesity in Russia and South Africa with that in the other BRICS nations. Also, given the earlier policy responses in Brazil, India, and China, I focused on obesity in these nations because of the larger amount of published academic literature and media attention on the epidemic in these nations.

Tuberculosis was examined only in Russia and South Africa because of the higher prevalence rates, especially in its association with HIV/AIDS, compared with Brazil, India, and China (Dimitrova et al., 2006; Loveday and Zweigenthal, 2011). Due to earlier and successful prevention and treatment programs in Brazil, India, and China, TB cases have decreased and stabilized in these nations (Gómez, 2013b; R. S. Gupta, 2015; Long, Qu, and Lucas, 2016). As I show in later chapters, however, the Russian and South African governments still have not strengthened their policy response to TB, with the specter of deadlier forms of drug-resistant TB increasing and posing a global pandemic threat. It is not, moreover, the shameful nature of the disease, that is, TB's association with poverty and inequality, that has generated a lack of government attention in Russia and South Africa; instead, political leaders have not prioritized a stronger policy response mainly because of their apathy toward international criticism and pressure, a product of the negative geopolitical positioning of the leaders' respective countries, and the resulting lack of geopolitical incentives to achieve this policy outcome. In Brazil, in contrast, despite the historical stigma associated with TB, the government has positively responded to its resurgence and viewed this response as a way to bolster its international reputation in health (Gómez, 2013a).[5] Despite the more effective response to TB in Brazil, China, and India, prevalence rates are still high in these nations, and recent political crises and economic recessions may challenge these governments' ability to sustain their national TB programs.

Finally, I compared the HIV/AIDS epidemic across all of the BRICS nations. It was important to select at least one disease that all five nations confronted, though with varying degrees of success. This revealed key differences in geopolitical positioning and bureaucratic–civil societal partnerships.

The HIV/AIDS, obesity, and TB epidemics were also selected for study because of the heightened international attention they have received and thus the potential for some nations to build their international reputation in health. As discussed in chapters 2 to 6, the importance of these epidemics to the international community, specifically to UN institutions such as the WHO and UNAIDS, was exemplified through criticism of governments and pressure to strengthen their response. Nevertheless, and as mentioned above, these international pressures emerged earlier for HIV/AIDS, by the early 1990s, than for TB and obesity, in the early 2000s. Some would argue that the importance of obesity to the WHO, its policy prescriptions and pressures on member states, emerged earlier (W. James, 2008), through several regional WHO meetings— held mainly in the Asia Pacific—and policy reports. These reports included *Obesity: Preventing and Managing the Global Epidemic* (WHO, 1998) and the ensuing report of the same name in the WHO Technical Report Series (WHO, 2000). Nevertheless, others recognize *Global Strategy on Diet, Physical Activity, and Health* (WHO, 2004b) as marking a critical juncture in the WHO's pressuring of and policy expectations for its member states (Cannon, 2004; Gómez, 2013a).

These epidemics were also selected in order to better understand the international and domestic politics of how governments respond to different types of public health threats. Most of the scholarly work on the politics of government response to disease epidemics has focused on HIV/AIDS.[6] Yet this provides us with but a narrow glimpse of the international and domestic factors shaping government responses to epidemics, as well as the different public and private sector interests involved. Comparing the HIV/AIDS, TB, and obesity epidemics provides a more robust understanding of the politics of government responses to epidemics in the BRICS nations.

Finally, readers may be questioning whether the author engaged in a process of selection bias by purposefully selecting only those epidemics that would have led to the outcome of interest. Was an analysis of TB in Brazil, for example, omitted because it would not have provided an example of positive geopolitical positioning and strong bureaucratic–civil societal partnerships? This certainly was not the case. For, as Gómez (2013b) explains, notwithstanding a delayed government response to TB, soon after the emergence of international pressures from the WHO and the Global Stop TB Campaign by the late 1990s, political leaders positively responded by recentralizing the National TB Program in 1998 while increasing funding for drug distribution and directly observed treatment, short course (DOTS). Facilitated by the acquisition of a grant from the Global Fund to Fight AIDS, Tuberculosis, and Malaria, moreover, national TB officials also started to work closely with NGOs on TB (Santos Filho and Gomes, 2007). In China, the government also positively responded to TB and other infectious diseases after the emergence of international pressures stemming from the SARS epidemic (Y. Huang, 2013). However, as we saw with HIV/AIDS and obesity, to my knowledge the government still has not pursued a stronger partnership with TB NGOs.

Sources of Data

For this study I relied on several different types of qualitative and quantitative data sources. The qualitative evidence derives from archival newspaper clippings and articles obtained from research institutions and more recently published articles, books, and policy reports. I also relied on newspaper clippings obtained from various news engines, such as *Access World News*, *World News Connection*, and Google. These searches located articles published between the late 1980s and the end of 2016; several different types of keyword search terms were used in quotation marks to find articles. Because the *Access World News* and *World News Connection* databases provide articles translated from different languages, by topic and date, they were helpful when conducting research on nations for which I do not know the language, such as Mandarin Chinese and Russian. A total of 26 interviews were conducted in Brazil, India, and South Africa at different times during the years 2007, 2008, 2012, 2013, 2015, and 2016. Those selected for interviews were either recommended by colleagues working on the issue or located via government and NGO websites. Interviewees were selected based on their extensive policy experience and knowledge of the topic; these individuals included former presidents, senior health officials, international agency officials, NGO representatives, and members of academia. Interviewees were not chosen for their specific point of view, as this would have biased the interview data. Interview themes ranged from the importance of international criticism, pressure, and reputation building, to policy design and implementation and the history and strength of bureaucratic-civil societal partnerships in health policy. All of the individuals interviewed gave consent to acknowledge their formal titles and positions. Data from these interviews were stored as MS Word documents, while some were also stored as voice-recorded files, with the interviewee's consent.

The study relied on several different types of quantitative information, such as archival and contemporary epidemiological data on various diseases obtained from public health institutions, mainly through official government websites and/or online reports. Budgetary data on federal government expenditures were obtained from online databases and published reports. While there were ample amounts of data from Brazil, I experienced difficulties collecting data for the other emerging nations, especially China and Russia.

Road Map

In the next chapter, I turn to an in-depth examination of Brazil's response to HIV/AIDS and obesity, followed by India's and China's responses to HIV/AIDS and obesity (chapters 3 and 4). Russia's response to HIV/AIDS and TB is then examined (chapter 5), followed by South Africa's response to the same epidemics (chapter 6). In chapter 7, I close with some broader theoretical and empirical lessons about the BRICS' responses to epidemics while reevaluating their emerging-nation status in the area of public health.

NOTES

1. This is not to say that governments concerned about increasing their international reputation in health are equally concerned about doing so in other social policy areas, such as education and the environment. My focus is instead on those nations focusing on domestic health policy as a means of enhancing their reputation.

2. Receptivity to international financial assistance is not the only factor comprising positive geopolitical positioning. If this were the case, essentially all nations receiving foreign aid in health would fall under this category. To be classified as a nation engaged in positive geopolitical positioning, governing elites must do more than receive foreign aid: they must also seek out and work closely with international agencies to learn and adopt their policies; they must proactively voice their interest in and commitment to building their international reputation in health; and they must engage in activities that further market their policy success, such as organizing conferences, while eventually providing foreign aid assistance to other nations.

3. Centralization is not the only approach to effectively responding to disease. This is especially the case when nations do not have the historical institutional experience, political culture, or expertise to engage in a centrist response. According to Nathanson (1996), for example, when compared with France, the United States does not have a long tradition of state-led health policy research and implementation. Instead, essentially all health policies were decentralized during the early twentieth century, engendering a federal government that had no tradition or interest in pursuing a centralized response to HIV/AIDS

and other diseases (Gómez, 2013). In other instances, decentralization has proven just fine in terms of implementing health policy (Tendler, 1997). As seen in Uganda and Botswana (Patterson, 2006), when they are well-experienced, committed, and accountable, local governments can effectively respond to HIV/AIDS. Though decentralization may work in these smaller nations, it faces far greater challenges within large geographical federations that possess a myriad of distant municipalities, which for the most part are bereft of sufficient resources and where intergovernmental coordination is an ongoing challenge.

4. The epidemiological and international financial factors associated with these epidemics certainly have an influence on elite perceptions at a later time, but this is not why I selected these epidemics. Rather, I chose them for their initially contested nature, which has more to do with the initial perceptions of countervailing elites.

5. We must keep in mind that HIV/AIDS was also initially viewed as a shameful disease in all of the BRICS' nations. And yet, Brazil's, India's, and China's leaders eventually positively responded, due to an increase in international criticism and pressure, while Russia's and South Africa's did not. Thus, it is not the domestic stigma of disease but rather political leaders' concern about international pressures and reputation building that matters most.

6. This focus largely stems from the greater attention that HIV/AIDS has received in recent years compared with other diseases, mainly due to the stigma and political and social conflict surrounding HIV/AIDS, the rapid increase in number of cases and deaths throughout the 1990s, and the higher levels of international funding for this disease relative to other diseases.

2

Brazil's Response to HIV/AIDS and Obesity

In the midst of its transition to democracy and introduction of free market reforms, at the turn of the twenty-first century, Brazil confronted the HIV/AIDS and obesity epidemics. The government's failure to respond immediately through effective prevention and treatment programs drew criticism and pressure from influential international institutions such as the UN and the WHO. Seeking to improve the government's international reputation in health, Brazil's political leaders immediately began to provide more political and financial support to the MOH for its prevention and treatment programs. To expedite this process, the government also requested the help of international donors such as the World Bank, through both financial and technical assistance. These efforts revealed the government's positive geopolitical positioning, which was built upon the historical precedent of the striving of Brazil's governments since the early twentieth century to enhance the nation's international reputation in development and public health while pursuing international donor assistance and collaboration to eradicate disease. Eventually, Brazil would begin to provide foreign aid assistance to other nations grappling with HIV/AIDS, with the intent of furthering its international reputation in health.

The government's ability to achieve a centrist policy response to HIV/AIDS and obesity was facilitated by the presence of strong bureaucratic–civil societal partnerships, which predated the arrival of these epidemics. Equipped with a reliable and informative working relationship with NGOs, bureaucrats strategically used this partnership to bolster the MOH's legitimacy and influence within government, thus securing bureaucrats' ability to obtain the ongoing funding and political support needed to implement their centrist policy response.

Responding to HIV/AIDS

The HIV/AIDS epidemic first emerged in Brazil in 1982 in the city of São Paulo and subsequently spread to Rio de Janeiro and other major cities. The disease first emerged within the gay community, then intravenous drug users (IDUs) and heterosexual couples. By the late 1980s, HIV/AIDS had begun to affect the lives of famous individuals, including intellectuals, artists, and politicians (*Veja*, 1985). In a context of heightened discrimination toward the gay community (Mott, 2003), the virus's emergence among famous individuals drew a considerable amount of media and political attention (Parker, 2003). Despite this greater media attention and the accompanying alarm and fear, the epidemic continued to spread throughout the nation, puzzling medical scientists and alarming politicians.

In July 2009, CNN's Sanjay Gupta reported that Brazil was the "envy of the world." He was referring neither to the economy nor to Brazil's vibrant culture and beautiful beaches. He was referring to the government's impressive policy response to HIV/AIDS that led to a massive decline in infection and death rates. What many may not know is that several years before Gupta's public commentary, Brazil's government had joined its BRICS counterparts in being substantially delayed and lackluster in its policy response (Da Costa Marques, 2003; Galvão, 2000). Several years would go by before the president publicly acknowledged the epidemic (Da Costa Marques, 2003; Galvão, 2000). In addition, in pruning government spending, stabilizing markets, and encouraging decentralization throughout the 1980s, the government allocated little of the federal budget for AIDS prevention and treatment programs. And the national AIDS program (NAP) that was eventually created, in 1986, was poorly organized and managed (Da Costa Marques, 2003). Many were of the view that the NAP was a hollow shell, with little funding and little political support and poorly managed from within (Teixeira, 1997; *Visão*, 1985). It was as if the government created an institution to give the impression that it was fully committed to eradicating HIV/AIDS, when in reality it was not. Even though the NAP began to provide information on prevention, the quality and effectiveness of the advice was deemed insufficient and questionable (Parker, 2003). Worse still, the minister of health at the time, Carlos Santana, publicly claimed that his ministry had more important healthcare matters to attend to, and senior health officials questioned whether HIV/AIDS actually posed a public health problem (Parker, 2003; Teodorescu and Teixeira, 2015).

Despite the government's commitment to healthcare decentralization as enshrined in the 1988 constitution, during the 1980s the state governments found themselves in need of financial and technical assistance to respond to HIV/AIDS. By 1985, several state health departments, beginning with São Paulo, had developed prevention and treatment programs (Parker, 2003; Teodorescu and Teixeira, 2015). The NAP, however, did not provide sufficient financial, human resource, and infrastructural assistance (e.g., beds and x-ray machines) to São Paulo and other state governments, notwithstanding repeated pressure from governors (*O Globo*, 1987). By 1986, the situation had become so dire that the individual in charge of São Paulo's state AIDS program, Paulo Teixeira, had to appeal to the Pan American Health Organization (PAHO) and the WHO for assistance—but to no avail, as these institutions did not at the time have policies for providing direct support for state government prevention and treatment programs (Teixeira, 1997).

To further complicate matters, during this period the NAP failed to develop a strong partnership with NGOs. Even after the program's creation in 1986, its first director, Lair Guerra Macedo Rodrigues, was far from enthusiastic about meeting with and providing assistance to people living with HIV/AIDS. In the AIDS community, the director's cold-hearted, seemingly apathetic character earned her the title of "the bitch" (E. Filho, 2006). She had little confidence in a participatory approach to AIDS policymaking. Instead, she preferred that experienced MOH bureaucrats take the lead in devising and implementing policies.

This tenuous partnership with NGOs emerged even after the creation of a formal committee within the NAP that was dedicated to incorporating NGOs' views on AIDS policy. In 1987, the national program created the National AIDS Commission. The commission's primary objective was to incorporate the views of NGOs, government officials, and the private sector to devise more effective HIV/AIDS prevention and treatment programs. It soon became apparent that few if any NGO representatives were present on the commission, and those that were present were mainly invited for their particular opinions rather than their substantive participation in designing policy (Da Costa Marques, 2003). The most important commission members in this regard were government officials, WHO and PAHO officials, academics, and select human rights activists (Nascimento, 2005).

Despite these challenges, NGOs were mobilizing. Building on a long history of social health activism and human rights, dovetailing with the fight for redemocratization during the early 1980s (Berkman et al., 2005; Parker, 2003), several AIDS NGOs began to emerge. The first, in São Paulo, was created by the gay community in 1985: the Grupo de Apoio á Prevenção á AIDS (Support Group for the Prevention of AIDS). This was followed by Associação Brasileira Interdisciplinar de AIDS (Interdisciplinary Association for AIDS) in Rio in 1986. By the end of 1985, there were an estimated 11 AIDS NGOs working throughout the nation (Parker, 2003). All of these NGOs were demanding that the government provide sufficient political and financial attention to public awareness campaigns—especially for groups at high risk, such as the gay and drug communities. At the same time, *sanitarista* activists, the business community, and even the Roman Catholic Church began to support several prevention efforts (Parker, 2003). As Rich (2010) claims, this period was marked by aggressive NGO pressure on the NAP to provide policy leadership, funding, and assistance to communities struggling with the HIV/AIDS epidemic.

Despite these efforts, throughout the 1980s and into the early twenty-first century, the NGO community did not have a significant impact on the design and implementation of AIDS policies (Nascimento, 2005; Gómez, 2015a). Although the NAP was gradually implementing several prevention programs, mainly information on safe sex and testing, and limited amounts of AZT medications were being funded and distributed through the MOH, the national program did little to empower NGOs, provide more funding to the states, and ensure the rapid containment of the epidemic. HIV/AIDS cases continued to burgeon in the early 1990s, leading the World Bank to claim that by 2010, Brazil would see approximately 1,200,000 cases (Brazil, Ministry of Health, 2005).

International Criticism and Pressure

The World Bank's predictions in the 1990s reflected the international community's concern about the quick spread of HIV/AIDS in Brazil and other developing nations. A critical juncture emerged at the international level when the UN, several other international organizations, and the scientific community began to evaluate, criticize, and provide policy recommendations (Lieberman, 2009). In this context, Brazil was singled out by international organizations such as the UN and the World Bank for its failure to respond adequately to the epidemic. The World Bank made it a point to criticize Brazil for failing to develop a strong health systems response—that is, failing to ensure that hospitals had adequate staff and infrastructure to treat people living with HIV/AIDS (*O Estado de São Paulo*, 1993). Highly acclaimed scientists from the United

States, such as Dr. Anthony Fauci of the National Institutes of Health, criticized the Brazilian government and advocated for a stronger policy response (*O Estado de São Paulo*, 1987). Fauci would soon join other scientists at international conferences that highlighted Brazil's challenges and policy limitations. At a major international AIDS conference in Puerto Rico in 1987, for example, Brazil was singled out as having the worst response to the epidemic in the entire Latin America region (*O Estado de São Paulo*, 1987).

The Brazilian government did not take this international criticism and pressure lightly. The office of the presidency was by far the most concerned with this situation (Cardoso, 2007; Gómez, 2015a). Striving to obtain closer economic and political relations with the United States and other western nations such as the United Kingdom and France, President Fernando H. Cardoso strove to improve his reputation with them. This was important in securing their trust and confidence in engaging in more trade with Brazil, investing in several of its newly privatized industries, consolidating relationships with Wall Street bankers, and ensuring greater regional security. With respect to the United States, this process was facilitated—and indeed, encouraged—by Cardoso's strong personal relationship with President Bill Clinton, Cardoso's experience teaching at the University of California, Berkeley, and his extensive experience working with the United States in developing diplomatic and business partnerships as senator and finance minister. Taking up the presidency at a time of deep economic recession, Cardoso also sought to gain the trust and confidence of important international lenders such as the World Bank and the IMF, which could provide the funding needed not only to stabilize the economy but also to help fund AIDS and other public health programs (Roberto de Almeida, 2013).

By 1994, Cardoso viewed his investment in strengthening the NAP as an effective strategy for bolstering his government's international reputation in health. He wanted to demonstrate that Brazil was fully committed to eradicating HIV/AIDS and meeting the nation's healthcare needs (Chequer, 2008; D'Avila, 2008). Cardoso viewed an improvement in AIDS policy as a means to achieve this objective (Chequer, 2008; D'Avila, 2008; Roberto de Almeida, 2013). But he also believed that Brazil needed to support the international community's normative consensus of establishing a more aggressive AIDS policy response, while emphasizing prevention and access to medicine and treatment as a human right. Cardoso was also mindful that Brazil had a long tradition, dating back to the early twentieth century, of working closely with international health organizations and philanthropic foundations to eradicate disease and share knowledge and resources, while working with other governments to construct multilateral health institutions such as the WHO (Gómez, 2015a).

In addition to introducing innovative prevention and treatment policies (as explained shortly), Cardoso organized and participated in several international events to raise Brazil's global profile. For instance, in the mid-1990s Cardoso began to attend international meetings and conferences to discuss Brazil's strategy against AIDS (Da Costa Marques, 2003; Galvão, 2000). He also invited delegates from the WHO and the World Bank to visit Brazil and assess its government's policies (Da Costa Marques, 2003; Galvão, 2000; Gómez, 2015a). The goal behind these endeavors was to prove to the West that Brazil's government was unwaveringly committed to strengthening its policy response to AIDS (Da Costa Marques, 2003; Gómez, 2015a). Indeed, Galvão (2000) claimed that this was a time when the government was trying to establish itself as a world pioneer in the fight against AIDS.

These international reputation-building interests would have a profound affect on domestic AIDS institutional and policy reforms. After these reforms were pursued, the government used their success as a justification for providing multilateral and bilateral assistance to other nations responding to HIV/AIDS—a strategy that was used to further improve the government's international reputation.

Was international reputation building the government's main concern during the Cardoso administration? Let's look at some alternative explanations. Perhaps it was the government's realization by the mid-1990s that a full-fledged AIDS epidemic had emerged that prompted Cardoso and the congress to initiate reforms. But this cannot be the case, given that the office of the presidency and the MOH had already known for several years that AIDS was a serious public health threat (Parker, 2009). So, perhaps Cardoso's interest in election to the presidency in 1994 and reelection in 1998 explains his motivation. This argument also does not hold. Cardoso at no point campaigned on the AIDS issue during the 1994 and 1998 presidential elections (Gauri and Lieberman, 2006). The first time any presidential candidate campaigned on AIDS was when Cardoso's minister of health, José Serra, ran for presidential office against Luiz Inacio Lula da Silva in 2001 (Gómez, 2015a). Perhaps, then, Cardoso was trying to increase the popularity and legitimacy of his office by strengthening his response to AIDS. This also cannot be true, because it is well documented that

Cardoso was already popular and revered for his success at taming hyperinflation through his introduction of the Plano Real (Real Plan) stabilization program as finance minister from 1992 to 1994 (Resende-Santos, 1997). Finally, perhaps it was the spread of HIV/AIDS among famous individuals in society that prompted government interest and response? This cannot be the case, however, because, although the government was aware of the situation as early as 1988, even the death of Henfil, a famous cartoon artist in Brazil, due to AIDS, as well as other notable members of society, did not motivate the government to strengthen its policy response (Parker, 2003).

Cardoso's international reputation-building interests therefore seem to be the most plausible explanation for his desire to encourage reform. Nevertheless, finding the means with which to pursue these interests proved difficult. With the introduction of the Real stabilization program in 1994 and efforts to reduce public spending, increasing the funding for AIDS programs proved to be difficult. In this context, Cardoso decided to engage in a partnership with the World Bank to achieve the necessary funding.

In 1994, Cardoso pursued a loan from the World Bank to fund the administrative and policy activities of the NAP (Galvão, 2000; Teodorescu and Teixeira, 2015). Bank officials agreed to provide Brazil with a loan of US$120 million; the loan could be extended for an additional five years, based on adherence to bank policy mandates and performance. This funding was mainly used to pay for hiring staff and technical consultants, HIV prevention activities, and NGO initiatives (Galvão, 2000; Parker, 2003). Funding for more medical treatment, such as for drugs manufacturing and disbursement, was expressly forbidden (Mattos, Terto, and Parker, 2003). Bank funding was therefore centralized, focusing on strengthening the government's administrative capacity and prevention initiatives—dovetailing with Cardoso's interest in the government's solidifying its renewed commitment to policy reform.

Positive Geopolitical Positioning

Where did Brazil's interest in international reputation building, working with international organizations, and receptivity to World Bank funding—in other words, its positive geopolitical positioning—come from? Was this response a product of the times: the urgency and need to respond to HIV/AIDS? Or did this reflect a preexisting historical precedent, a deep foreign policy legacy of political elites who positioned themselves as leaders in an emerging nation sensitive to international criticism and receptive to international collaboration and foreign aid assistance in achieving their government's health policy objectives?

There were certainly deep historical precedents in all of these areas. Since the 1920s, Brazil's presidents had been keen to create policies and engage in diplomatic activities that would improve the nation's international reputation (Garcia, 2012). Brazil's government wanted to show the world that it was not only a sovereign state but also one that had unlimited economic potential and international influence, a nation that could contain the spread of disease and could prosper (Garcia, 2012; Hochman, 2009). Shortly after independence from Portugal in 1822, and continuing through the First Democratic Republic (1889–1930), presidents and diplomatic officials became sensitive to other nations' views of Brazil, especially in a context that historian Roberto de Almeida (2012, 21) once described as "um sistema internacional fortemente discriminatório em relação a 'potências menores'" (an international system that strongly discriminates against "lesser powers"). In essence, it was a time when the world looked down on Brazil. This agitated political leaders (Roberto de Almeida, 2012), as they never wanted Brazil to be perceived as a second-rate nation (Cervo, 2011).

During the 1930s, President Getúlio Vargas (1930–45) strove to transform Brazil into a revered partner in international peace and development (Figueira, 2011). Vargas was incessantly worried about Brazil's international image and position in the world. He often lamented about previous governments' apathy toward building Brazil's international reputation: "A posição do Brasil na vida internacional nunca foi de tanto prestígo e segurança" (Brazil's position [in international politics] has never been about prestige and security) (quoted in Garcia, 2012, 256).

Vargas was a state builder and believed that Brazil had the potential to become an advanced industrialized nation, looked up to by many. He often attended and hosted international conferences, on issues ranging from economic trade to international peace and security. At these conferences, Vargas lectured about Brazil's fine achievements and its future plans, aspirations, and significance to the world (Figueira, 2011; Garcia, 2012). By the mid-1950s, Brazil's government was so confident in its international position that Vargas's diplomats allegedly boasted at international conferences about the United States' and Mexico's respect for Brazil's cooperative assistance in international trade and security (Garcia, 2012).

To further enhance the nation's international reputation, Vargas engaged in several diplomatic activities, while devising policies that would draw attention to Brazil. When the Second World War began, in 1939, Vargas decided to help US President Franklin D. Roosevelt by being the first (and only) Latin American nation to send troops in support of the allies' fight against the Nazis (Figueira, 2011). Vargas saw this as an opportunity to bolster Brazil's prestige as a nation that could be relied on to help defeat evil in the world and to safeguard human rights, individual freedom, and dignity (Garcia, 2012). Indeed, historians note that it was the international reputation-building effects of engaging in the Second World War that motivated Vargas to stay involved in international diplomacy (Cervo, 2011; Figueira, 2011).

But Vargas was also keen on creating public health policies that would garner the international community's respect. For instance, he pursued the creation of centralized bureaucratic institutions to eradicate diseases such as TB, syphilis, and yellow fever, while investing in public infrastructure and agricultural exports, mainly coffee—endeavors that earned Brazil international acclaim (Gómez, 2015a; Roberto de Almeida, 2012). Vargas also sponsored his most accomplished medical doctors to attend world conferences to display Brazil's success in combating disease (Carrara, 1997; Peard, 1999).

For example, Vargas sponsored the Sifilógrafo movement, a team of highly regarded medical doctors who worked on syphilis, to participate in international conferences. These endeavors allowed Vargas to reveal how the government was succeeding in limiting the spread of syphilis in major cities and ports (Carrara, 1997, 1999). Proud of his medical establishment, Vargas went so far as to send one of his prized medical doctors to San Francisco in 1945 to help establish the WHO (Clift, 2013). This was done to build up the government's international reputation as a state that was advanced in medical scientific discovery and public health policy and was in a strong position to help other nations respond to disease. Vargas was tired of the world's perceiving Brazil as an inferior, inconsequential nation, believing instead that it was a nation that Americans and Europeans could respect and be glad to work with. Future presidents shared Vargas's views and followed a similar geopolitical approach (Garcia, 2012).

The government's commitment to improving its international reputation in health persisted over the years, motivating subsequent governments to create programs for achieving the same objective. During the 1950s, President Juscelino Kubitschek de Oliveira, for example, was disappointed about Brazil's international reputation as being an underfunded, inept "huge hospital," a "sick country" with a weak healthcare system (Hochman, 2008). This motivated Kubitschek to declare "o Brasil não é só doença" (there is more to Brazil than disease) (quoted in Hochman, 2008). To overcome this international perception, Kubitschek followed Vargas's tradition of creating several federal institutions and campaigns to eradicate disease, including yellow fever, malaria, and smallpox (Hochman, 2008). Subsequent military governments, from 1964 to 1985, viewed investing in public health policy as a means to improve their reputation and legitimacy as a state capable of eradicating disease while meeting social needs (Hochman, 2009). This also helped to overcome the military's reputation as a government that did not respect human rights and civil liberties (Palmer and Hochman, 2010).

After independence from Portugal in 1822, Brazil had also been committed to international cooperation and partnerships (Cervo, 2011). During the First Republic, presidents emphasized international cooperation in the areas of trade, intellectual property, and technology (Roberto de Almeida, 2012). And despite a war with Paraguay (1864–70) and hostilities toward Argentina, by the early twentieth century Brazil sought to ameliorate its tensions with these nations (Figueira, 2011). But Vargas was also gifted at establishing diplomatic ties. He worked hard to protect his close economic relationship with the United States, viewing President Roosevelt as an ally and friend. Over the years, Brazil would engage in several endeavors to provide technical assistance and social welfare services to lesser-developed nations. Between 1960 and 1990, for example, Brazilian scientists cooperated in approximately 1,300 developmental projects throughout Latin America and Asia (Cervo, 2011). International cooperation for ensuring social welfare needs such as health care, narcotics regulation, and the punishment of those responsible for trafficking women and girls in the sex trade throughout the Americas was also of importance (Garcia, 2012).

Brazil's government was also committed to establishing collaborative partnerships with the international community in response to disease. In addition to sending teams of medical doctors to international conferences to develop a stronger response to syphilis and TB (Carrara, 1997), the government worked closely with the international philanthropic sector. During the 1920s and 1930s, the MOH, at that time the Diretoria Geral de Saúde Pública (DGSP), partnered with the David Rockefeller and Irene Diamond foundations and the Red Cross to eradicate hookworm, yellow fever, and malaria (Stepan, 1976). With respect to yellow fever, the DGSP worked with the Rockefeller Foundation's

International Health Board during the 1920s to create a national yellow fever program and establish local health units and programs (Stapleton, 2005). The DGSP also worked with the Rockefeller Foundation to eradicate malaria. In addition to co-financing several projects, it worked with foundation officials to adopt several eradication strategies successfully pursued in the United States. The Rockefeller Foundation and the DGSP also established several autonomous public health institutions focused on malaria control in the northeast of Brazil, such as the Northeast Malaria Service, created in 1938 (Griffing et al., 2015). In the late 1950s, the government decided to work closely with the WHO and its World Health Assembly to adopt its suggested measures for eradicating malaria (Hochman, 2008; Silva and Paiva, 2015), eventually leading to the creation of the MOH's Malaria Control and Eradication Working Group in 1958. Silva and Paiva (2015) write that this working group was created to work with and to accommodate the needs of the WHO while strengthening Brazil's relationship with the United States.

Finally, when it came to smallpox—historically, a highly prevalent disease throughout the nation—despite a lull in the government's attention to the disease between the 1920s and 1950s,[1] as soon as the WHO and PAHO began to establish an international consensus on the need to completely eradicate smallpox in 1959, presidents João Goulart (1961–64) and Humberto de Alencar Castello Branco (1964–67) began to collaborate with the WHO to increase Brazil's policy response. In 1962, for example, President Goulart instructed the MOH to create the National Campaign Against Smallpox, which facilitated the MOH's work with the WHO, the United States, and private foundations such as the Rockefeller Foundation (Silva and Paiva, 2015). Brazil's collaboration with the international community therefore emerged in response to a rise in international attention to a previously neglected disease—as would happen with its response to AIDS and, as we will see, obesity.

Engaging in international technical cooperation also became a key aspect of Brazilian foreign policy. To that end, beginning in 1969, the government established several federal agencies dedicated to providing technical assistance to other developing nations, with a focus on training, research, and the production and conservation of foods. Brazil would also strategically use this technical assistance as a means to enhance its image as a benevolent state, one that could help other nations develop and prosper—a foreign policy tradition that would reemerge with AIDS (Silva and Paiva, 2015).

But Brazil was also committed to working with other nations to help establish postwar peace and international institutions. In 1918, Brazil had been one of the founding members of the League of Nations in Paris (Garcia, 2012). Brazil eventually withdrew from the league, however, after realizing in 1926 that other member states were too domineering and disrespectful toward smaller participating nations—a move that smacked of Brazil's unwavering principles of defending state sovereignty, mutual respect, global equality, and multilateral cooperation (Garcia, 2012; Roberto de Almeida, 2012). Following the Second World War, President Vargas cooperated with President Roosevelt and European leaders to establish an agreement for international peace (Garcia, 2012). To that end, in 1944 Brazil collaborated with the United States, Norway, England, and China to help form the UN and, two years later, the WHO (Garcia, 2012). After Vargas's presidency, the government remained committed to avoiding any hostilities toward other nations, seeking to remain neutral during the Cold War (Cervo, 2011). This view was held even under the phalanx of military dictatorships that governed Brazil from 1964 to 1985. By 1979, under the leadership of President Ernesto Geisel (1974–79), the government made it a point not to take sides between socialist and capitalist nations, while increasing the number of presidential and diplomatic visits to maintain international cooperative peace (Figueira, 2011). It was under Geisel that the government sought to reduce its political and economic dependence on the United States and to establish diplomatic ties with other nations (Cervo, 2011; Figueira, 2011).

Indeed, Brazil's presidents and diplomatic elites never viewed themselves as world leaders and powers, eager to shape international discourse and policy (Cervo, 2011). Instead, Brazil always considered the United States to be the regional and global hegemon, and it worked alongside the United States as a supportive ally (Garcia, 2012). Pacifism, nonintervention, partnership, mutual respect, equality, and peace were always the guiding principles shaping Brazil's foreign policy endeavors (Cervo, 2011; Garcia, 2012). During formation of the UN in 1944, for example, Brazil's delegates made it clear that the UN's laws should prohibit states from acting in a unilateral manner to safeguard state sovereignty (Cervo, 2011; Garcia, 2012). Brazil believed that no nation had the right and responsibility to govern the world on its own (Roberto de Almeida, 2012).

For several decades, then, Brazil's government was committed to multilateralism in international negotiations (Cervo, 2011; Figueira, 2011; Garcia, 2012;

Roberto de Almeida, 2012). Beginning with the Vargas administration, the government believed that nothing could be achieved in the world without peaceful multilateral cooperation, without mutual understanding and trust. Cervo (2011) maintains that Brazil's commitment to multilateralism stemmed from its social diversity: politicians had to learn to adjust to a burgeoning hodgepodge of cultural, social, and economic interests and needs. By the 1950s, Vargas's successor, President Jânio Quadros (1955–59), and his diplomats strongly believed that Brazil's opinion and voice mattered in the world, that it needed to be involved in every major policy decision at the UN, and that other nations should work with Brazil to resolve international conflict (Cervo, 2011; Garcia, 2012).

Adding further credence to Brazil's belief in international cooperation was its interest in receiving financial and technical assistance from other nations. By the mid-twentieth century, Brazil had established a reputation for borrowing from other nations and capital markets and for repaying loans on time (Roberto de Almeida, 2012). Humble yet eager to develop Brazil's economy, Vargas at one point claimed that there was simply no way that Brazil would be able to develop without the support of the United States and European leaders (Garcia, 2012). Vargas once commented: "Sem a colaboração de um país industrializado, e dispondo de technologia avançada, o Brasil não poderá levar avante, com a rapidez necessária, a reconstrução econômica" (Without the collaboration of an industrialized country, featuring advanced technology, Brazil cannot carry on, quick enough, for economic reconstruction) (quoted in Garcia, 2012, 79). By 1947, Brazil had become the first nation in Latin America to borrow money from the World Bank—an estimated US$79 million to build the government's electrical sector (Figueira, 2011; Roberto de Almeida, 2012).

When it came to public health, Brazil's political leaders would once again turn to the international community for financial assistance. Facing austere budget cuts in public health due to increased government spending for economic development (Hochman, 2009), by the early to mid-twentieth century—in response to public health threats such as smallpox, yellow fever, and malaria—the government approached the WHO, PAHO, Rockefeller Foundation, and United States for assistance in funding prevention and eradication programs (Silva and Paiva, 2015). For instance, Brazil's Special Public Health Service of the Amazons, created in 1942 to provide sanitation services throughout the northeastern states and the Amazon, was partially funded by the US Institute of Inter-American Affairs (IIAA), with the coordinating assistance of Rockefeller

Foundation staff. By 1944, approximately 80% of this funding came from the IIAA (Griffing et al., 2015). The government also turned to PAHO, the WHO, and the United States for funding the government response to smallpox. Hochman (2008) reports that by the late 1960s, approximately one-third of Brazil's smallpox eradication budget came from the United States. During this period, the MOH also acquired approximately 230 vehicles from PAHO and the WHO, as well as clean needles for providing vaccinations.

The Brazilian government's receptivity toward international financial assistance in the area of public health persisted through most of the twentieth century. It was a foreign policy tradition that had a long-term precedent, as mentioned earlier. The government's receptivity to international assistance reflected its humility and willingness to learn and work with the international community in response to disease. Although these efforts would subside with the emergence of more conservative and isolationist governments during the 1980s (Parker, 2003), it would emerge again later, positively influencing the government's geopolitical positioning and receptivity to international assistance in response to HIV/AIDS and obesity.

In sum, there were deep historical precedents to Brazil's positive geopolitical positioning. Brazil was always a nation that was conscious of its government's image in the world, eager to build its international reputation as a modern state capable of developing and eradicating disease, while working closely with other nations to learn and to acquire resources. Brazil never sought to lead the world in politics and power; rather, it sought to work closely with the international community, repeatedly humbling itself and acknowledging that the government needed assistance from other nations to achieve its goals. When the HIV/AIDS epidemic emerged, the government's response followed a long tradition of using state building, health policy, and, ultimately, the provision of financial and technical assistance to other nations as a means to bolster its international reputation while working closely with international donors and philanthropists to achieve its domestic policy objectives. Equipped with international financial support and strong presidential backing, Brazil would now engage in a series of impressive centrist policy reforms.

Pursuing a Centrist Policy Response

By the mid-1990s, reinvigorated by its positive geopolitical positioning and aspirations, the government moved to bolster the NAP, in essence creating a highly centralized, autonomous, and influential agency. The first step along this path was to delegate a high level of policymaking autonomy to the program. President Cardoso and his health minister, José Serra, believed that the NAP had the technical expertise and experience needed to enact effective prevention programs and to work with the states in implementing them. In this context, Cardoso and Serra felt comfortable giving NAP directors the authority not only to devise policy but also to seek direct funding from the congress. For unlike any of its agency counterparts within the MOH, the NAP was allowed to bypass the traditional reams of paperwork entailed in obtaining federal funding from the national treasury through the congressional committees (Cardoso, 2007; Galvão, 2000; Teixeira, 1997). This greatly facilitated the NAP's ability to fund several prevention activities.

To enable the NAP's imposition of policies onto the states, it also created the Comissões Municipais de AIDS (Municipal AIDS Commissions, MACs). The MACs essentially acted as bureaucratic arms of the NAP, receiving orders and working with municipal health bureaucrats to carry them out (Teixeira, 1997). This initiative underscored the NAP's belief that the states had to follow its policy directives, even in a context of increased healthcare decentralization under the Sistema Único de Saúde (SUS) (Da Costa Marques, 2003; Gómez, 2011a). In essence, the MACs were delegated the responsibility of closely monitoring municipal health department's adherence to NAP policy guidelines, providing technical assistance in the implementation of prevention programs, and reporting any discrepancies back to the NAP (Teixeira, 1997).

By the mid-1990s, the NAP had also introduced several prevention programs targeting the groups at highest risk, such as the gay community and women. In 2002, Brazil became one of the first nations to create media awareness campaigns for the young gay community (Levi and Vitoria, 2002). In 2007, it did the same for women, creating the Plano Integrado de Enfrentamento da Feminização da Epidemia de Aids e otras DST (Integrated Plan Confronting the Feminization of AIDS and Other STDs). Through this program for women, NGOs provided free HIV testing, female condoms, and sex education materials (Brazil, National AIDS Program, 2007; Gómez, 2015a). Furthermore, in 2009 the NAP instituted a host of sex education initiatives, not only through the media, such as in television infomercials and on billboards, but also through the educational curriculum in schools (Arnquist, Ellner, and Weintraub, 2011). In 1994, the NAP began to distribute condoms, with the goal of providing approximately three billion to all state governments (Lieberman, 2009). And in

2000, in an effort to curb the growth of infections in IDUs, the congress passed legislation allowing the federal provision of clean needles to state health departments through the NAP (Paiva, Pupo, and Barboza, 2006).

The NAP also emphasized its centrist governing structure through the provision of ARV medications. In 1996, Brazil became the first nation in the world to mandate the universal distribution of ARVs (Paiva, Pupo, and Barboza, 2006). Through presidential decree act no. 9313, by federal law the NAP was given the authority to distribute medications to all state health departments (Mattos, Terto, and Parker, 2003; Paiva, Pupo, and Barboza, 2006). A state or municipal government's failure to adhere to this law permitted citizens to take the government to court—an option that some citizens used both for the delayed distribution of medications and for issues concerning HIV testing (Berkman et al., 2005).

The NAP soon realized, however, that to ensure that its prevention and treatment programs worked effectively, it also had to overcome the challenges of decentralization and create incentives for municipal governments to adhere to its policy mandates. In the late 1990s, state and municipal health departments were given a considerable amount of administrative, policy, and financial discretion in providing healthcare services through SUS (Arretche and Marques, 2002). In 2002, moreover, the NAP began to decentralize more financial and administrative responsibility to municipal health departments (Rich and Gómez, 2012). However, in some instances this led to poor management of hospital administration and health services provision (La Forgia and Couttolenc, 2008). To ensure that these challenges did not hamper HIV/AIDS prevention and treatment programs, in 2003 the NAP created an intergovernmental fiscal program that increased its ability to persuade mayors and local health administrators into compliance with NAP policies.

It is through this initiative, the ministerial ordinance no. 2313 Fundo-a-Fundo Incentivos program, that the NAP would provide financial grants to municipal health departments in need of assistance, as long as they complied with national NAP policy recommendations (Barboza, 2006; Brazil, Ministry of Health, 2010). To qualify for a grant, municipal health departments had to meet the following conditions: (1) a high HIV and AIDS epidemiological burden—approximately 50,000 cases; (2) the municipality's participation in the first two World Bank loans, provided in 1994 and 1999; and (3) evidence that a municipal health department was already trying to obtain financial and administrative help (Barboza, 2006; Gómez, 2011a). Other stipulations required municipal governments to improve their human resources and infrastructure for health, improve existing prevention and treatment programs and their work with NGOs, and ensure the purchase and supply of ARV medications (Barboza, 2006; Pires, 2006).

To ensure that grant recipients adhered to these conditions, the NAP often sent bureaucrats to municipal health departments to monitor how the money was being spent. This led to an increase in federal accountability and motivated mayors to adhere to policy guidelines (Gómez, 2015a). At the same time, the NAP dispersed federal manuals and technical norms to the municipalities to ensure that they were continuously up to speed on the policies and procedures they should be pursuing (Barboza, 2006). This endeavor signaled the NAP's commitment to strengthening oversight and accountability in Fundo-a-Fundo funding and municipal government compliance with the NAP's policy priorities.

Over the years, federal funding for the Fundo-a-Fundo program increased. As figure 2.1 illustrates, transfers from the MOH to the municipalities increased from almost R$58 million (reais) in 2003 to just over R$178 million in 2013. Most of this funding went to those municipalities in greatest need of assistance. For example, the city of São Paulo, Brazil's largest metropolitan area, received the lion's share of funding, an estimated 33.4% of total Fundo-a-Fundo funding from 2002 to 2011 (Gómez, 2015a). Moreover, by 2010, approximately 26 states and 489 municipalities received Fundo-a-Fundo funding (Gómez, 2011a).

In addition to creating intergovernmental fiscal policies, the NAP also began to increase its "informal" policy influence. That is, AIDS bureaucrats began to contract with NGOs to closely monitor municipal health departments' usage of Fundo-a-Fundo funding, as well as monitoring their general policy performance. By periodically obtaining information from NGOs and visiting them on a regular basis, AIDS bureaucrats were able to increase municipal governments' accountability to the MOH and thus incentivize greater compliance with national policy guidelines (Gómez, 2015a; Rich and Gómez, 2012). By the turn of the twenty-first century, with many NGOs being unemployed and in search of funding, these bureaucrats took advantage of the opportunity to contract out to NGOs to work as the eyes, ears, and arms of the NAP at the municipal level (Gómez, 2015a; Rich, 2010; Rich and Gómez, 2012).

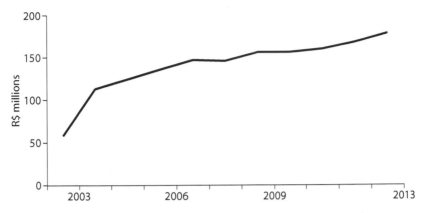

Figure 2.1. Fundo-a-Fundo Incentivo transfers to municipalities in Brazil (R$ millions), 2003–13. Sources: Abong, Portal dos Fundos Públicos, National AIDS Program, 2012, www.abong.org.br; Brazil, Ministry of Health, 2010; Diário Oficial de União, 2013.

Thus, by the early 2000s, the government had succeeded in building a strong centrist policy response. As explained in the previous chapter, such a response requires three components: the creation and ongoing financial and administrative expansion of federal agencies, the development of effective prevention and treatment programs (particularly, universal access to medicines), and formal and informal strategies to increase the central government's policy influence in a context of healthcare decentralization. In Brazil, the congress continued to authorize an increase in spending and administrative expansion of the NAP and created effective prevention and universal ARV treatment policies, while the national program formally and informally increased its subnational policy influence by providing conditional fiscal transfers and working with NGOs to monitor municipal government compliance with national program mandates.

Building on the success of the government's centrist policy response, by the early 2000s the Lula administration began to pursue foreign policies that would help to further improve Brazil's international reputation, while at the same time expanding the government's health policy beliefs and experiences at the global level. One such policy was the government's decision to take a leading role in working with other nations to establish declarations of nations' rights to essential medicines and to engage in negotiations with pharmaceutical companies for increased access to more affordable ARV medicines (Watt, Gómez, and McKee, 2014). The Lula administration believed that not only did these efforts help to bolster the government's international reputation as an empathetic emerging power (Heijstek, 2015), but Brazil also had an ethical obligation to assist other nations—by applying its principled beliefs in universal access to medicine as a human right to the international community and by applying the lessons learned from its domestic policy experiences (Heijstek, 2015; Watt, Gómez, and McKee, 2014).

For example, in 2001 in Doha, Qatar, President Lula's health minister, Paulo Teixeira, took the lead in working with India and other emerging nations to establish an international declaration allowing developing nations to reinterpret flexibilities in the WTO's TRIPS Article 31 rulings regarding conditions for the issue of compulsory licenses: these would now include "public health crisis" such as HIV/AIDS as one such justifiable condition. This would essentially allow developing nations to obtain generic medication such as ARVs at a lower price (Correa, 2002). In 2004, Brazil also worked with other nations at the International AIDS Conference in Bangkok, Thailand, to create the International Technical Cooperation Network, an agreement that facilitated the sharing of financial and technical resources between nations to encourage the production of generic medications. And in 2005, building on the 2001 Doha declaration, Brazil worked with several Latin American governments through the Union of South American Nations to collectively pressure pharmaceutical companies, including Merck, Abbot, and Roche, into agreeing to lower their prices for ARV medications throughout the region (Passarelli and Pimenta, 2012). All the while, Brazil led by example through its engagement in several rounds of intensive negotiations with these companies, which eventually led to a reduction in the prices of ARVs: Abbot's lopinavir/ritonavir by 56.2%, Roche's nelfinavir by 73.8%, and Merck's efavirenz by 73%. The government even went as far as to issue a compulsory license in 2007 for Merck's efavirenz (Salama and Benoliel, 2010). Moreover, according to WikiLeaks information disclosed by Edward Snowden in 2010, in 2003 Lula sought to increase his bargaining power with pharmaceutical companies by issuing an executive order amending Article 71 of the 1996 Patent Law for Medications. This amendment allowed for the production of generics without the consent of pharmaceutical companies as previously stipulated under TRIPS rulings (Dickinson, 2010). Because of all these efforts, by the end of Lula's term in office, several international health agencies and NGOs, including Médecins sans Frontières, praised Brazil for its success in taking an aggressive stance against the pharmaceutical sector while helping other nations gain access to more affordable medications (Gómez, 2015a).

The Lula administration realized that providing bilateral aid to other nations could help to promote the government's international reputation (Russo, Cabral, and Ferrinho, 2013). Building on its success in producing and universally distributing ARV medicines through SUS, in 2002 the NAP began to donate medications and provide technical assistance in the areas of prevention and treatment to Bolivia and Paraguay. It did so through the MOH's International Collaboration Program for the Control and Prevention of HIV in Developing Nations, with provision extending to other nations through the program's renewal in 2005 (Passarelli and Pimenta, 2012). And in 2003, in Africa—a region that some claim was intentionally pursued by the president to help build Brazil's international profile in donor assistance (Carrillo et al., 2011)—Lula worked with Brazil's Ministry of Foreign Affairs, MOH, and Agência Brasileira de Cooperação (ABC; Brazilian Cooperation Agency, the government's primary agency for managing overseas development assistance) to help Mozambique. Initiated at the request of the Mozambique government, the goal was to help construct a pharmaceutical plant for the production of ARV medications in the city of Mobato, along with a "mini-FIOCRUZ" infectious diseases research institute. In addition to sending AIDS technicians to Mobato, Lula also invited Mozambican health officials to Brasília to receive technical training (Gómez, 2009).

Lula also agreed to help construct pharmaceutical plants in Nigeria (in 2005) and Angola (in 2007). And in 2005, the International Center for Technical Cooperation for HIV/AIDS Initiatives (ICTS) was created, housed within the NAP and co-financed by the NAP, UNAIDS (the Joint United Nations Programme on HIV/AIDS), and the Department for International Development (DfID) in London. Staff from the ICTS continued to travel to Mozambique, Nigeria, and Angola to provide training in monitoring and evaluation, drug procurement, supply chain management, and HIV awareness and education through the program Harmonization of Policies for Sexual Education, HIV/AIDS Prevention, and Drugs in the School Environment. This program also provided assistance to several Latin American countries, including Argentina, Chile, Peru, and Uruguay (Gómez, 2009). By providing this kind of bilateral assistance to Latin American and African nations, Lula succeeded in increasing Brazil's international reputation as an influential aid donor, one that could help other nations respond to AIDS, while at the same time bolstering its ability to shape international policy discussions and motivate other nations to provide similar types of bilateral assistance (Carrillo et al., 2011; K. Lee and Gómez, 2011). These bilateral efforts won considerable praise from the international community (K. Lee and Gómez, 2011), eventually compelling Brazil's minister of foreign affairs at the time, Celso Amorim, to comment that "technical cooperation is an essential tool of foreign policy" (quoted in Carrillo et al., 2015).

Noticing the success of this policy strategy, Lula's government continued to invest in bilateral and even multilateral assistance in health. From 2005 to 2009, the federal budget for these activities tripled (Alves, 2013). By 2011, the NAP, through the ICTS, had established 19 technical collaboration projects with Latin American, Caribbean, and African nation's (Passarelli and Pimenta, 2012), while the MOH had established 53 bilateral arrangements across several health sectors with 22 African countries (Carrillo et al., 2011). During this period, the MOH also began to donate a considerable amount of funding to multilateral institutions such as the WHO, PAHO, Global Alliance for Vaccine Initiative (later renamed Gavi, the Vaccine Alliance), and Global Fund to Fight AIDS, Tuberculosis, and Malaria (Passarelli and Pimenta, 2012). It was a time when the Lula administration was striving to solidify Brazil's position in the world as a caring, benevolent state, one incessantly working with other nations to eradicate disease and poverty.

The Dilma Rousseff administration (2011–16) did not share Lula's foreign policy interests. Instead, due to an ongoing economic recession and increased civil societal demands for improved social services, Rousseff paid less attention to foreign policy and was focused more on domestic issues (Burges, 2014; Di Ciommo and Amorim, 2015). Consequently, the federal budget for ABC and other MOH bilateral and multilateral programs decreased considerably (Burges, 2014; Di Ciommo and Amorim, 2015; Gómez and Perez, 2016). In the past two years, because of this situation, the NAP has had to start denying the provision of bilateral assistance to several African nations (Burges, 2014). As I discuss in chapter 7, Brazil's recent economic recession, when combined with Rousseff's obsessive focus on fostering her government's domestic legitimacy in a context of potential presidential impeachment, hampered the MOH's ability to continue helping other developing nations combat disease while further solidifying the government's international reputation.

The Advantages of Strong Bureaucratic-Civil Societal Partnerships

How was Brazil able to succeed in building a strong centrist policy response, one that brought both domestic policy advantages and international prestige? The response was made possible by the formation of a strong bureaucratic–civil societal partnership, which enabled bureaucrats to obtain ongoing financial and political support from the congress. The emergence of this partnership was made possible, in turn, through the historical presence of well-organized social health movements responding to disease while working with public health officials to contain their spread.

For example, in the early twentieth century, in response to syphilis and TB, the Sifilógrafo and Liga Contra a Tuberculose social health movements emerged in the cities of Rio de Janeiro and São Paulo. Organized by medical doctors, healthcare activists, professors, and public health bureaucrats, these movements strove to work closely with the national government through the Diretoria Geral de Saúde Pública, in operation from 1889 to the end of the First Republic in 1930, and the Ministério da Educação e Saúde Pública (MESP) during the Estado do Novo under President Vargas from 1930 to 1945. The Sifilógrafo and Liga Contra a Tuberculose emerged to raise awareness about these diseases and propose policy solutions. These movements were particularly adamant about creating universal prevention and treatment policies managed and implemented by the central government (Carrara, 1997; Gómez, 2015a). The Sifilógrafo, for example, became world famous for advocating sex education in schools and working with federal health bureaucrats and private businesses to inform the public about safe sex practices (Carrara, 1997; Fernandes, 1931). Both movements also required that the DGSP universally distribute free medications (Araujo, 1939; Gómez, 2015a), while advocating for nondiscriminatory views toward those groups particularly afflicted by these diseases, such as the black community (Carrara, 1997). It was a time when doctors, activists, and educators were working proactively with the public health bureaucracy to establish a strong central government response to health epidemics (Gómez, 2015a).

During this period, public health bureaucrats also worked closely with these social health movements. In 1906, the director of the DGSP, Oswaldo Cruz, worked with the Sifilógrafo and Liga Contra a Tuberculose to pressure the president of the republic to create specialized federal programs to eradicate TB and syphilis (Nascimento, 2005). Cruz quickly realized that he could not work on his own and that he needed these organizations to strengthen his position and influence within government (Gómez, 2015a). Given the growing popularity and influence of the Sifilógrafo and Liga, both domestically and abroad through their participation in conferences (Carrara, 1997; Nascimento, 2005), Cruz believed that partnering with these social health movements would give him the credibility needed to pursue reforms. Such views within government persisted over time, motivating future DGSP and MESP bureaucrats to work closely with these and other social health movements to create a strong, centralized government response to disease (Gómez, 2015a).

When the HIV/AIDS epidemic emerged in the 1980s, Brazil's rich tradition of proactive social health movements advocating for a universal, effective, and equitable policy response persisted. This period benefited from the presence of the *sanitarista* social health movement, which arose during the 1960s as a prodemocratization movement advocating for the creation of a universal healthcare system (Weyland, 1996). Consisting of local politicians, activists, medical doctors, and university professors, the *sanitaristas* mobilized to address HIV/AIDS by increasing public awareness and working with at-risk groups such as the gay community to mobilize a strong policy response. As previously mentioned, AIDS NGOs emerged during this time in Rio and São Paulo to help people living with HIV/AIDS, provide medical care and psychological counseling, and lobby the government for assistance (Barreira, 2012; Brito, 2012; Galvão, 2000).

As they had done since the early twentieth century, these social health movements worked closely with public health bureaucrats. In addition to continuously lobbying the MOH under the military and the new democratic government, beginning in the late 1980s, *sanitarista* and AIDS NGO leaders realized that to become successful they needed to forge strong partnerships with AIDS bureaucrats to build a solid network of supporters within government (Gómez, 2015a). These activists approached AIDS bureaucrats mainly by taking advantage of preexisting participatory institutions within the NAP, such as the National AIDS Commission, while meeting with bureaucrats in government-sponsored workshops and meetings at the local level (Rich, 2010; Rich and Gómez, 2012).

Nevertheless, bureaucratic efforts to work closely with these NGOs did not occur until after the Cardoso administration had positively responded to international criticisms and pressures through policies focused on improving the government's international reputation (recall earlier that, prior to Cardoso's response, the MOH was not working closely with NGOs, notwithstanding collective protests and pressures for policy reform). The Cardoso administration's reputation-building interests and the heightened level of support that he gave to the NAP therefore provided an opportunity and incentive for bureaucrats to finally engage in a stronger partnership with NGOs.

Indeed, by the late 1990s, the bureaucrats benefited from forging a strong partnership with the *sanitarista* and AIDS NGO community. NGOs became the eyes and ears of bureaucrats at the local level, which helped not only in learning about local needs and in improving policy (Rich, 2010) but also in finding out what it took to build a strong bond and sense of trust with local communities. Much of this learning was made easier by bureaucrats periodically meeting with activists through local participatory institutions such as the Commission for Articulation with Social Movements (CAMS), present in several cities and organized by national AIDS bureaucrats, NGOs, and community members (Rich and Gómez, 2012). The CAMS, as well as facilitating informal meetings between AIDS bureaucrats and NGOs, helped to establish a sense of trust between the state and NGOs. They were therefore critical for ensuring that prevention and treatment programs worked effectively (Rich, 2010; Rich and Gómez, 2012), especially in contexts where cultural traditions and religious beliefs offered alternative, traditional medical approaches to treating AIDS (Garcia and Parker, 2011).

Establishing a strong partnership with NGOs helped to bolster national AIDS bureaucrats' legitimacy and influence within government, enabling them to obtain ongoing presidential and congressional support for their centrist policy reforms (Barreira, 2012; Brito, 2012; Campos, 2012; Dhalia, 2012). This legitimacy was enhanced because several senators and congressmen were familiar with the *sanitarista* and NGO movement (several politicians at the time were medical doctors and were previously involved in the *sanitaristas*), its dedication to achieving universal healthcare, its historical success in working with the government and international community in response to disease (Carrara, 1997), and its commitment to partnering with the public bureaucracy in response to epidemics. These were traits deemed impressive and helpful in the fight against HIV/AIDS (Barreira, 2012; Brito, 2012; Campos, 2012; C. Filho, 2012; Grangeiro, 2012; Shaffer, 2012). Over time, this congressional support enabled AIDS bureaucrats to secure funding, not only for hiring more staff and part-time consultants, but also for several innovative AIDS programs such as the Fundo-a-Fundo program to hire NGOs, to conduct prevention campaigns, and for the universal distribution of ARV medications (Barbosa, 2008; Barreira, 2012; Brito, 2012; Campos, 2012; Dhalia, 2012). Finally, international donors at the time, including the World Bank, were advocating for stronger partnerships between national AIDS programs and NGOs. Thus bureaucrats could consistently obtain World Bank funding and technical support, while increasing their credibility within the congress Gómez (2015a).

Responding to Obesity

Around the time that the national government was consolidating its centrist policy response to HIV/AIDS, yet another epidemic was emerging in a somewhat clandestine but expeditious manner, reflecting Brazil's gradual economic prosperity, openness to international trade, and food culture: an epidemic of obesity. How did the government respond to this?

If one had argued two or three decades earlier that Brazil would confront an obesity epidemic, the idea would have been viewed as absurd and vehemently challenged by the scientific community. During the 1980s, worsening poverty levels and malnutrition riddled the nation, a byproduct of years of government neglect in developing the economy and introducing effective social welfare programs for the poor—including healthcare. In the late 1990s, however, the socioeconomic environment quickly changed. The introduction of a successful macroeconomic stabilization program, the Plano Real, along with the privatization of state-owned enterprises and increased international trade, ushered in a period of rapid economic growth and opportunity. Brazilians would for the first time have access to new kinds of imported foods, new technological innovations such as computers and cellphones, and new employment opportunities, which came with longer working hours and increased stress levels. The broader economic and social context changed and set the stage for a steady rise in adult and, especially, childhood obesity (fig. 2.2).

By the late 1990s, the sudden influx of imported cheap and high-caloric foods, the increased availability and marketing of such products (Monteiro, Conde, and Popkin, 2007; Sichieri, 2002), and the ability of the poor to readily obtain these foods through conditional cash-transfer programs that provided food vouchers (such as the Bolsa Família program)—all were closely associated with an increase in overweight and obesity (Freitas, Sousa, and Jones, 2014; Veloso and Santana, 2002). Furthermore, increased access to technological devices,

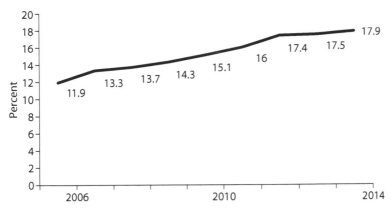

Figure 2.2. Obesity cases in Brazil (as percentage of population), 2006–14.
Source: Brazil, Ministry of Health, 2016.

greater employment opportunities, work-related stress, and constraints on individual time led to less physical activity and increasingly sedentary lifestyles (Veloso and Santana, 2002). This was further reinforced by Brazil's food culture, which traditionally emphasized the consumption of starchy vegetables (rice, potatoes, and beans), carbohydrates (breads and cereals), and sugar (Monteiro and Cannon, 2012).

According to government statistics, the percentage of overweight individuals increased from 43% in 2006 to 53% in 2014, with an increase in obesity cases from 11.9% to 17.9% over the same period (Vigitel, 2014). In 1975, approximately 19% of men and 29% of women were overweight; by 2011, these figures had increased to 54% and 48% (Senthilingam, 2014). The number of obese individuals increased in urban and rural areas, with a marked increase in rates among the rural poor (Gómez, 2015c). The number of poor that are malnourished is still high, but within the past decade, because of the rapid growth of overweight and obesity, the government has considered obesity to be a priority focus. In 2010, the minister of health, José Gomes Temporão, claimed that "the problem of Brazil is no longer malnutrition but childhood obesity and the increase in weight" (quoted in Yapp, 2010).

As with HIV/AIDS, the government did not immediately respond to obesity. Although the government had a long tradition of establishing sound nutritional policies and increasing public awareness of good health, wellness, and physical fitness, it took several years for the MOH to recognize and respond to the obesity epidemic (Gómez, 2015c). This was mainly because, during Brazil's

economic recovery, politicians were more preoccupied with addressing malnutrition and poverty (Wanjek, 2005). The rise in obesity was acknowledged
for the first time by some health bureaucrats and the scientific community at
the 1996 Congresso Nacional de Nutrição (National Congress of Nutrition),
but it was not until 1999 that the congress took action. That year, the congress
passed the Política Nacional de Alimentação (PNAN; National Policy of Nutrition). With this policy, the MOH began to address obesity through a variety
of prevention initiatives, such as increasing public awareness through media
campaigns and funding the provision of healthier foods in schools. And, in addition to conducting surveys and collecting data on the geographic spread of
obesity, PNAN began to train healthcare professionals in obesity prevention
and treatment for its related ailments such as hypertension and diabetes
(Monteiro, Conde, and Popkin, 2002). In 2000, PNAN also mandated that approximately 70% of all foods provided by schools be fresh and minimally
processed. To achieve this, the MOH began to provide grants to schools that
agreed to work with local farmers in providing nutritious foods (Coitinho, Monteiro, and Popkin, 2002; Monteiro, Conde, and Popkin, 2002). Finally, in 2000
the congress passed legislation requiring that all processed foods carry labels
listing their nutritional content (Coitinho, Monteiro, and Popkin, 2002).

While these preventive efforts were certainly important, the government was
still not fully committed to supporting the MOH's work on obesity and increasing the funding for prevention programs. In addition, few state and municipal
governments were receiving the financial and administrative support needed to
address the epidemic (Gómez, 2013a). In a context of increased healthcare decentralization and municipal governments' greater fiscal constraints, as well as
a corresponding decline in municipal governments' ability to adequately fund
and manage healthcare services (La Forgia and Couttolenc, 2008), more federal
support was needed to help ensure that schools—and especially families—
could learn about the causes and consequences of obesity.

International Criticism and Pressure

These domestic challenges drew a considerable amount of international attention. But compared with the response to HIV/AIDS, the timing of international
pressure and criticism was considerably delayed for the obesity epidemic, emerging mainly in the early 2000s. This delayed response reflected the international
community's unwillingness at first to recognize obesity as an international health
threat. Some claim that this delay was attributable to the international commu-

nity's obsession with tackling more mysterious and salient communicable diseases such as HIV/AIDS, as well as the absence of well-organized NGOs and social health movements successfully lobbying the UN to address obesity (Gómez, 2011b).

At this time, several academic researchers and consultants at international health organizations highlighted Brazil's unwillingness to respond promptly to obesity and introduce legislation (Monteiro, Conde, and Popkin, 2002; Norum, 2005; Swinburn et al., 2004). Scholarly articles emerged emphasizing the Brazilian population's ongoing weight problem (Norum, 2005; Sichieri, 2002), the thriving sugar and fast-food industry ("floating Nestlé" snack-bar boats sailing up and down the Amazon drew heated attention; see Mangu-Ward, 2010), the rising prevalence of ailments associated with obesity, such as type 2 diabetes (Rigby, 2006), and a weak political commitment to policy reform (Gómez, 2013a).

As was seen with HIV/AIDS, the government eventually began to take these criticisms more seriously. In an emerging nation seeking to pass muster as having an effective public health system and a healthy and prosperous work environment, government officials sought to improve Brazil's international reputation as a state committed to reducing obesity. And, again as we saw with HIV/AIDS, the government also focused on improving its reputation among the western industrialized nations such as the United States (for the economic and political reasons described earlier in the chapter) and the western-based international institutions, such as the WHO, that were critiquing Brazil's response to obesity.

These reputation-building interests became most apparent as soon as senior health officials began to worry that Brazil was perceived as similar to other nations struggling with the obesity epidemic. Indeed, by 2010, Brazil's MOH "feared that Brazil would soon join the U.S. in having a reputation as an obese nation" (Gómez, 2013a, 84). In an interview published by the London *Telegraph*, Otaliba Libanio Neto, director of the MOH's Department of Health Analysis, stated that if Brazil's obesity cases continued to surge, the nation's situation would approximate that in the United States by 2012 (Yapp, 2010). Neto's comments underscored the government's concern about being seen as resembling the United States in its struggle to combat obesity, and they revealed a desire to overcome international criticism for not effectively responding to obesity. For, as mentioned earlier, the government at the time did not have a reputation for successfully controlling the epidemic (Monteiro, Conde, and Popkin, 2002; Norum, 2005; Swinburn et al., 2004).

Other health officials began to express similar views. In 2010, Health Minister José Temporão commented that "if we stay at this pace, in 10 years we will have two-third[s] of the population overweight (or obese), as has happened in the United States" (quoted in Reuters, 2010). In 2012, Temporão's successor, Alexandre Padilha, stated: "Now is the time to act to ensure we don't reach the levels of countries like the U.S., where more than 20% of the population is obese" (quoted in *BBC News*, 2012). And, "There is a tendency toward increased weight and obesity in the country. It's time to reverse the trend to avoid becoming a country like the United States" (quoted in Ghosh, 2012). NGO activists and scholars confirmed Padilha's position, claiming that the MOH's concern with improving Brazil's international reputation as a healthy and prosperous nation, free of the obesity challenges seen in the United States and other industrialized nations, was a key factor motivating its response to the epidemic (Coutinho, 2016; Jones, 2016). At the same time, the media were also referring to Brazil's ongoing obesity problem, emphasizing how embarrassing it looked for a nation preparing to host the 2016 Olympic Games (Yapp, 2010).

Brazil's governing elites were also committed to working with international health agencies to address obesity. This became evident through the MOH's proactive involvement in creating the WHO's report *Global Strategy on Diet, Physical Activity, and Health*. In fact, during the 2004 meetings of the Group of 77 (G77), Brazil's delegates chaired the working group on nutrition and diet and collaborated with other nations to build a consensus on the policy strategies governments should follow to address obesity and other noncommunicable diseases (Norum, 2005). In 2006, Brazil sent four delegates to the United Nations Standing Committee on Nutrition, meeting in Geneva. Brazil's delegates worked closely with government officials and civil societal organizations to provide more effective nutritional guidelines for addressing the double burden of malnutrition—overconsumption and underconsumption of calories—with a large component dedicated to improved childhood nutrition, nutrition as a human right, and food security. At the meetings, Brazil co-chaired, along with representatives of South Africa and Canada, the civil societal working group on these nutritional issues (United Nations, 2006). A year later Brazil returned to the same UN working group, convening a joint session on national guidelines for improving children's diet and providing nutritious school meals as a human right. Consistent with the government's historical track record in engaging in peaceful multilateral cooperation and partnerships, these efforts once again revealed Brazil's ongoing commitment to working collaboratively with other nations rather than striving to take the lead in creating and imposing its government's policy views (United Nations, 2007).

Brazil's MOH bureaucrats also used their relationship with the WHO through the *Global Strategy* to reveal to the world the government's strong commitment to reducing obesity and other noncommunicable diseases. During this period, for example, an anonymous health official working with the WHO on the *Global Strategy* stated: "We brought the various experiences of [Brazilian] states and municipalities to show WHO representatives what we were doing in Brazil" (Brazil, Ministry of Health, 2006, 51).

Brazil's health bureaucrats and the research community were also committed to establishing bilateral and regional partnerships to share policy ideas and experiences and to learn from each other in the area of obesity prevention. For example, since 2006 the US Centers for Disease Control and Prevention (CDC), with an office located in Brazil's MOH, has provided technical assistance in developing a noncommunicable disease risk factor surveillance system and in policy design, planning, and the evaluation of physical activity. The CDC has also provided funding for these efforts, which are managed through Brazil's MOH Health and Disease Surveillance System (VIGISUS) (CDC, 2015). Since 2005, the MOH has also worked closely with the United States and with other Latin American nations to create an initiative called Project GUIA (Guide for Useful Interventions for Activity in Brazil and Latin America). The purpose of this initiative is to establish a network of academic and government institutions in the United States, Brazil, and other Latin American nations. Its intent is to share research and lessons from policy intervention strategies at the community level in the area of health and promotion of physical activity, with a focus first on Brazil, then on other countries in the region, including Colombia and Uruguay. This project was funded by the CDC as a Special Interest Project and consists of several partnership institutions: the Prevention Research Center in St. Louis (Missouri), Universidade Federal do São Paulo, Brazil's MOH, Universidade Federal de Pelotas, Pontificia Universidade Católica do Parana, CELAFISCS (Centro de Estudos do Laboratório de Aptidão Física de São Caetano do Sul), the CDC, and PAHO (Parra et al., 2013).

As we saw with the government response to HIV/AIDS, then, senior health bureaucrats' interest in bolstering the government's international reputation in health while working in close partnership with other nations demonstrates the government's positive geopolitical positioning. This incentivized the government to embark on a new round of obesity prevention initiatives, policies that were centrally controlled and primarily funded by the MOH.

But were these geopolitical interests the main reason that the government would begin to pursue a stronger policy response? Perhaps, instead, politicians such as the president were working with the congress to pass obesity legislation in order to win elections and increase their popularity in society. In fact, during this period, public opinion surveys revealed that rising obesity levels were a public concern, an issue that politicians could have capitalized on (Arbex et al., 2014). They chose not to, however; Lula's presidential campaign did not refer to Brazil's obesity problem during the 2002 and 2006 presidential elections. In fact, these campaigns were focused on the opposite health situation—poverty and malnourishment—perceived by some as an important strategy for winning these elections (Zucco and Power, 2013). Dilma Rousseff followed suit in her electoral tactics, strategically using Lula's social welfare programs to lock in popular support for her election to office in 2010 (*Economist*, 2010).

Alternatively, perhaps the MOH and the congress were responding to a spike in the number of overweight and obesity cases during the first few years of the twenty-first century. Again, this cannot be the case, as the government had been receiving in-depth reports about the rising overweight and obesity problem since the mid-1970s and 1980s (Soares and Ritto, 2010). This is further reflected in the fact that by 1996, the congress had already organized the National Congress on Nutrition, a national health conference consisting of legislative representatives, health officials, and civil societal activists that discussed—among other factors such as malnutrition, poverty, and food security—the ongoing rise in the overweight and obese population and associated ailments such as type 2 diabetes and heart disease (Souza et al., 2011). Moreover, PNAN was created in 1999 to increase interagency coordination and response to obesity and improved nutrition, reflecting the government's knowledge and concern about the problem by that time (Monteiro, Conde, and Popkin, 2002). Clearly, the government had known about the impending obesity epidemic for quite a while.

Finally, perhaps NGOs and activists mobilized to increase awareness and pressure the congress and the MOH for a policy response. But this, too, cannot be the case. Prior to the government's escalated policy response, little attention was being paid to civic activists, who through institutions such as the

Conselho Nacional de Segurança Alimentar e Nutricional (CONSEA; National Council on Food and Nutrition Security) were lobbying and trying to pressure the government into strengthening its policy response (Aranha et al., 2009; Maluf, 2011). As I discuss in more detail shortly, activists went as far as to organize national nutrition conferences to raise government awareness about the need to respond to obesity and related diseases (ICDA, 2006; Maluf, 2011). But these appeals fell on deaf ears during the first few years of the Lula administration (Recine, 2016), when the federal budget for most public health programs decreased due to reduced government spending, fiscal stabilization efforts, and a priority focus on other health and social welfare issues such as poverty alleviation and food security (Aranha et al., 2009; Maluf, 2011). Moreover, politicians' inattentiveness to civil societal demands primarily stemmed from their belief, as mentioned earlier, that obesity did not pose a national health threat and that poverty, malnutrition, and other infectious diseases required more attention. Furthermore, from the 1990s through the first few years of the Lula administration, while remaining committed to pressuring the government for policy reform, activists' ability to influence policy was challenged by their inability to effectively organize and create well-funded, influential NGOs focused on obesity. These organizations have only recently emerged, as explained below. However, and as we saw with HIV/AIDS, NGO's policy influence would be felt later, when MOH bureaucrats strategically partnered with activists to facilitate an expansion of their obesity prevention programs—but only *after* the MOH had already responded to the epidemic because of bureaucrats' primary focus on international reputation-building interests.

Pursuing a Centrist Policy Response

Motivated by the MOH's efforts to enhance the government's international reputation in obesity policy, the president and the congress eventually provided more political and financial support for the ministry's obesity prevention programs. In 2007, for example, through presidential decree no. 6.286, the MOH created the Programa Saúde nas Escolas (PSE; School Health Program). The PSE was managed by the MOH and the Ministry of Education and pursued several objectives: to increase the evaluation of children's health in schools; to promote better nutrition and health in schools; to provide better training to healthcare workers, focused on nutrition and health in schools; to monitor and evaluate school health programs; and to provide more information and awareness for children through several media and classroom initiatives (Brazil, Ministry of Education, 2012). Through the PSE, federal and local healthcare workers are committed to visiting schools to monitor children's overweight and obesity status and provide teachers and families with nutritional information, while ensuring adequate infrastructural and human resource support—such as a sufficient supply of healthcare workers (Brazil, Ministry of Health, 2012b).

In 2009, the MOH further enhanced its prevention policy efforts and influence over subnational policy by creating the Programa Dinheiro Direto na Escola (Direct Funding for Schools Program). Through this initiative, the MOH provided funds to schools from the Fundo Nacional de Desenvolvimento da Educação (National Development Fund for Education) to implement nutrition and obesity awareness programs. Schools participating in the program were required to ensure that approximately 30% of the funds were used to purchase agricultural products from farmers (Reis, Vasconcelos, and Faias de N. Barros, 2011). This program was similar to the PNAN initiative in that funding was conditional on adherence to MOH stipulations on purchasing farm products, emphasizing the MOH's ongoing effort to influence the design and implementation of local policy.

Further efforts were made to expand the MOH's work in obesity prevention in 2010, when the Plano de Ações Estratégicas para o Enfrentamento das Doenças Crônicas não transmissíveis (DCNT) was created. The DCNT established national policy guidelines and procedures for the next 10 years; it also entailed an increase in federal funding for obesity awareness and prevention activities in schools. Through this program, additional funding was supplied to train municipal SUS healthcare workers to provide prevention services (Brazil, Ministry of Health, 2012a). Through the DCNT, the MOH made it clear that the national government was escalating its policy influence and response to obesity.

This was made further explicit through the MOH's creation of the Academia da Saúde in the following year, 2011. The academia provided additional funding for 4,000 municipalities to construct recreational parks for exercise and fitness and free education programs, while hiring local healthcare workers to help supervise these parks and their programs (Parra et al., 2013). Similarly, in 2012, through the PNAN and PSE initiatives, the MOH provided additional funds for schools to purchase physical education structures such as gymnasiums and outdoor recreational sites, as well as equipment such as slides and climbing ladders (Pontodepauta, 2012). Once again, this funding was conditional: any school agreeing to accept the funds was required not only to adhere to PNAN and PSE policy guidelines but also to participate in the Semana de Mobilização na Escola (Week of School Mobilization) (Pontodepauta, 2012; Gómez, 2015c). In fact, the MOH's Family Health Program teams, consisting of teams of doctors, nurses, and healthcare workers that provided primary care services, were tasked with the responsibility of monitoring school compliance with this conditionality. This helped to increase both schools' accountability to the MOH and the ministry's policy influence (Gómez, 2015c).

In May 2014, the MOH, in partnership with the Núcleo de Pesquisas Epidemiológicas em Nutrição da Universidade de São Paulo (Core Epidemiological and Nutritional Research Unit of the University of São Paulo), together with the financial support of PAHO, established efforts to provide more information about enhanced nutrition and improved eating habits. In that year, to help stem the rise in obesity cases and to decrease malnutrition, the MOH created the *Guia Alimentar para a População Brasileira* (Feeding Guide for the Brazilian Population). The guide provides nutritional guidance and recommendations to families and the research community on the types of foods to eat and how to cook more nutritiously (Schmidt, 2014). During the announcement of this initiative, Minister of Health Arthur Chioro stated that the guide "was being implemented within the [WHO] global strategy to promote health and confront excess weight" (Schmidt, 2014, 1). And in 2015, the MOH, through the PNAN program, created the federal campaign Da Saúde se Cuida todos os Dias (Healthcare Is Every Day), which is focused on helping people make smart, healthy, daily decisions about nutrition and exercise (Brazil, Ministry of Health, 2016). In November 2015, through the Pacto Nacional para Alimentação Saudável (National Pact for Healthy Food), President Dilma Rousseff and the MOH spearheaded a new federal program that encourages families to produce and consume organic foods, while ensuring the increased availability of these foods in markets. And in 2016, in partnership with several NGOs and the private sector, the MOH created another public awareness campaign: Campanha Brasil Saudável e Sustentável (Brazil Healthy and Sustainable Campaign). This campaign provides information and sponsors activities encouraging healthy eating and individual self-reflection on eating habits, while alerting individuals about their particular health risks (Portal Brasil, 2016).

The introduction of these obesity prevention programs was made possible through MOH bureaucrats' ability to secure consistent financial support from the congress. The Departamento de Atenção Básica (Department of Basic Health), which manages the Programa Saúde Nas Escolas and Academia da Saúde programs, obtained an increase in its budget from R$7.5 billion in 2006 to R$24.3 billion in 2015. More specifically, the allocation for the department's educational funding from this budget saw an increase from R$388.2 million in 2013 to R$437.1 million in 2015 (Brazil, Ministry of Planning, Budget, and Spending, 2016). At the same time, bureaucrats working within the Ministry of Education, through the Fundo Nacional de Desenvolvimento da Educação, were able to secure an increase in funding for the Programa Direto na Escola, from R$2.38 billion in 2013 to R$2.9 billion in 2015 (FNDE, 2016). Congressional funding for the MOH's general nutrition and feeding programs also increased, from R$3.45 million in 2006 to R$4.3 million in 2015 (Brazil, General Accounting Office, 2016).

In addition, during this period the MOH started to strengthen preexisting federal institutions to enhance its ability to implement obesity prevention programs at the local level. In the mid-2000s, the ministry began to repurpose the MOH Family Health Program (FHP) to include among its repertoire of primary care services efforts to provide nutritional and physical fitness guidelines at the community level (Gómez, 2015c). The FHP was created in 1994 as a national- and state-funded SUS initiative that organized teams of doctors, nurses, and healthcare professionals for visiting households in hard-to-reach areas to provide primary care services, vaccinations, and public health information. Building on the FHP's success in locating these hard-to-reach communities, the MOH assigned the teams the additional task of providing information about better nutrition, healthy lifestyles, weight reduction, avoiding weight gain, and obesity-related ailments such as type 2 diabetes, hypertension, heart disease, and cancer (Gómez, 2015c). The FHP teams also began to visit schools and work with teachers to provide training and assistance in developing prevention awareness campaigns. They supplied information on better nutrition for children, healthier lifestyles, and media campaigns to increase students' awareness of good nutrition, through movie clips and other visual aids (Gómez, 2015c). The FHP's new focus on obesity prevention has been critical in helping prevent a further rise in childhood obesity.

Nevertheless, by 2008 the MOH realized that the FHP needed additional help in the area of obesity awareness and prevention. To help ensure that the FHP achieved its objectives, the ministry created the Núcleo de Apoio á Saúde da Família (NASF; Nucleus of Support for Family Health). Through this program the MOH provided teams of nutritionists, psychologists, physical therapists, and educators to help FHP teams provide additional nutritional and physical fitness information (Jaime, Feldenheimer, et al., 2011; Jaime, Silva, et al., 2013). The NASF teams not only support FHP personnel by providing additional, follow-up information for families but also are expected to provide further information in specialized areas such as psychological therapy (e.g., for depression and anxiety) and physical fitness. By 2011, the MOH provided approximately 1,371 NASF teams in 894 municipalities (Jaime, Feldenheimer, et al., 2011). This additional support has been vital for ensuring that the FHP and MOH locate target areas for obesity prevention services (Gómez, 2015c).

And finally, in order to help ensure that national obesity prevention programs were being effectively implemented at the municipal level, the MOH also began to work with NGOs to monitor municipal government performance and hold health officials accountable. MOH bureaucrats' partnership with NGOs also provided advantages for monitoring the implementation of policy guidelines and grant conditionalities imposed by the ministry (Bortoletto, 2016; Recine, 2016). As with the HIV/AIDS epidemic, while MOH bureaucrats were supportive, in principle, of healthcare decentralization through SUS, when working on obesity policy they were concerned that state and municipal health departments lacked the political commitment and resources needed to implement their policies. In an effort to overcome this challenge, bureaucrats began to work closely with NGOs to monitor state and municipal governments and hold them accountable for adherence to the grant conditionalities associated with several of the obesity prevention programs—such as the Programa Saúde nas Escolas and the Programa Dinheiro Direto nas Escolas (Bortoletto, 2016; Recine, 2016).

This monitoring and reporting process mainly occurred through the MOH's collaboration with NGOs present within state and municipal CONSEAs (Bandeira, 2016; Bortoletto, 2016; Karageorgiadis, 2016; Lessa de Oliveira, 2016; Recine, 2016). At periodic CONSEA meetings, activists questioned local health officials about their adherence to federal MOH guidelines and conditionalities. Activists then provided MOH bureaucrats with the information obtained from these meetings at the state and municipal level. Through this information-feedback process, because of the MOH's strong partnership with NGO activist leaders within CONSEA, health bureaucrats were able to increase the accountability of state and municipal health departments and therefore ensure that the grant money targeted for schools and other obesity prevention initiatives was being used effectively (Bandeira, 2016). Through this process, then, and similar to what we saw with HIV/AIDS, the MOH was able to sustain its centralized presence and influence within a decentralized context, a key ingredient of the government's successful centrist policy response.

Thus, soon after the arrival of international criticism and pressure, the MOH was able to achieve a strong centrist policy response. That is, the MOH received ongoing congressional funding and administrative expansion, continued to introduce effective and innovative prevention programs, and increased its formal and informal influence over municipal health departments by establishing conditional grant assistance for prevention programs while contracting NGOs to achieve the same objective.

In contrast to what we saw with the HIV/AIDS epidemic, because of the newness of the government's centrist policy response to obesity and its focus on implementing policy, it never attempted to build on its response by providing foreign aid in obesity prevention so as to enhance its international reputation in health (Recine, 2016). The only foreign policy that the government pursued in the area of obesity prevention was its successful attempt in 2003 to help build a consensus within Mercosul,[2] through the Committee on Food (Sub-Working Group 3; SWG3), for the adoption of RTM (Mercosul Trade Regulations) 04/10: "Declaration of Nutritional Properties." This declaration required Mercosul governments to implement regulations for the proper labeling of food and beverages for nutritional content and serving sizes. Brazil's leadership and commitment in this endeavor were inspired by the congress's passage of the same legislation in 2003 (Coutinho, 2016b). Brazil continued to work with other Mercosul nations on the need to prevent and control obesity, with periodic discussions in another Mercosul Working Group, WG FNS, which comes under the Strategy of Nutrition for Health and Food and National Security within Mercosul's Sub-Working Group 11 on Health (SWG11). The WG FNS meets twice every six months to share ideas and policy experiences and to encourage nations to invest more in obesity prevention (Coutinho, 2016b).

There were some limited attempts, however, to improve Brazil's international reputation in the area of children's nutrition through international cooperative funding efforts to improve nutrition in schools. In 2013, Brazil's National Fund for the Development of Education, Ministry of Education, and the ABC worked with the Food and Agricultural Organization (FAO) to create Strengthening School Feeding Programs in African Countries. In an effort to share policy ideas and experiences, knowledge, and resources for school feeding programs and family farming, with an initial budget of US$2 million, Brazil agreed to support children's nutrition and local farming businesses by providing funding and technical assistance and supplying schools with nutritious foods from local farmers (FAO, 2013). Consistent with what we saw in the government's bilateral assistance for HIV/AIDS, through all of these endeavors the government worked to share policy experiences and technical knowledge for sustainable development.

Although obesity prevention was not the explicit focus of this bilateral initiative, senior health officials recognized the associated geopolitical benefits. One such official was the president of Brazil's National Fund for the Development of Education, José Carlos Wanderley Dias de Freitas. He referred to Brazil's international reputation in school feeding programs to suggest that the fund would continue to improve this reputation through its bilateral assistance to Africa, while adding credibility to foreign policy efforts: "The most important aspect of this cooperation is to know that Brazil is recognized as a global benchmark in the field of school meals. Our work in terms of food security and family farmers [has] turned us into an example" (quoted in FAO, 2013, 1). Brazil and the United Kingdom were recognized at the International Congress on Obesity in 2010 as taking the lead in implementing effective obesity prevention programs. Receiving specific recognition were Brazil's regulation of food marketing, provision of nutritious foods in schools, promotion of healthy lifestyles through investments in parks, and monitoring of obesity trends (Gómez, 2015c). Perhaps, as we saw with HIV/AIDS, it is only a matter of time before the government strives to enhance its reputation through greater bilateral assistance to Africa in the area of obesity prevention.

The Emergence of Strong Bureaucratic–Civil Societal Partnerships

While Brazil's positive geopolitical positioning served as a necessary catalyst for the government's eventual centrist policy response, activists striving to increase government attention to obesity also played an important role. In Brazil, efforts by activists to mobilize in response to the obesity epidemic emerged from preexisting, well-organized social health movements dedicated to combating poverty, hunger, and malnutrition. The civil societal movement had a long history, was distinct from the *sanitaristas*, and was dedicated to the belief that access to quality food and sound nutrition is a human right (Aranha et al., 2009). The movement and its beliefs emerged as early as the 1930s and were reinforced by the government's views at the time that developing a hygienic, healthy, and productive society was necessary for economic growth and prosperity. Initial efforts to mobilize on these issues were led by housewives, farmers, nutritionists, and human rights activists; this mobilization fostered public demonstrations and led to the first Brazilian Conference of Nutrition, in 1958 (ICDA, 2010). The movement sustained itself throughout the 1960s, even under the duress of a despotic military government seeking to suppress civic activism (1964–85) (Takagi and Graziano da Silva, 2011).

The social movement's focus on access to nutritious food (deemed a food security issue), overall good nutrition, and health solidified over the years, leading to the organization of conferences and institutions that deepened society's commitment to proactive mobilization and government engagement. In 1982, for example, the first Brazilian Congress of Nutrition (Congresso Brasileiro de Nutrição; CONBRAN) was established in the city of Rio de Janeiro. CONBRAN was formed by the social movements, bringing together nutritionists, activists, and government officials to address poverty, hunger, and malnutrition—all seen as human rights issues. In 1988, the first Brazilian Food and National Security Forum was established in São Paulo (ICDA, 2010). And in 1993, the first CONSEA emerged as a federal- and state-level consultative body organized by activists, with the support of government officials, to provide advice on the creation of food and nutrition policies. CONSEA was initially composed of 10 state ministers and 21 civil societal activists and was chaired by an elected member of civil society; this governance structure helped to ensure civil society's influence in the design of legislation. CONSEA was the first civil societal organization to be established as a formal consultative body to the office of the president, which further enhanced CONSEA's fame and its ability to influence policy. CONSEA was temporarily dissolved under the Cardoso administration (due mainly to fiscal retrenchment through reduced government spending to stabilize the economy and reduce inflation), but it reemerged under the Lula administration in 2003 and, once again, was controlled mainly by civil societal representatives (Leão and Maluf, 2012).

Therefore, by the time the obesity epidemic emerged in Brazil, activists had already established a strong commitment to mobilizing and addressing nutritional issues, viewing access to quality food, good nutrition, and health as human rights. Although these activists did not realize it at the time, they were becoming well equipped to mobilize, pressure, and work with public health officials to create policies focused on the prevention of obesity and its related diseases.

For instance, by the 1990s, NGOs such as ACT+ (building off the ACT for Tobacco NGO) emerged to help increase government awareness and consensus around the issues of food regulation, improved nutrition, and obesity prevention (ACT+, 2014). Other NGOs emerged from preexisting organizations focused on poverty reduction, nutrition, and healthy living, such as the Associação Brasileira de Nutrição (ASBRAN; Brazilian Association of Nutrition), which was formed in 1949. NGOs also emerged from preexisting movements that addressed diseases closely related to obesity, such as the Sociedade Brasileira de Diabetes (Brazilian Diabetes Society), formed in Rio de Janeiro in the 1940s (Damaceno, 2013). However, throughout the 1990s, due to the government's lack of attentiveness to obesity (for the reasons outlined above), activists were unsuccessful in pressuring the government to introduce obesity legislation (Bandeira, 2016; Lessa de Oliveira, 2016; Recine, 2016).

Nevertheless, these organizations persisted in their efforts, and in the mid-2000s several new NGOs emerged to work with them and with a more receptive government. The Instituto Alana and the Instituto Brasileiro de Defesa do Consumidor (IDEC), for example, arose to increase public awareness, conduct research, and lobby the government for several prevention policies, such as regulating the advertising of fast foods to children. Other NGOs included ACTBr, which focuses on obesity and other noncommunicable diseases; ABESO, focusing on obesity research and treatment; Pastoral da Criança and CREN, both focusing on improving children's nutrition; and ABRASCO, with a focus on conducting research on obesity policies (Karageorgiadis, 2016).

By the time the Lula administration emerged in 2002, a long-held partnership between MOH bureaucrats and activists was focusing on the importance of good nutrition and poverty alleviation. But it was only during Lula's second term in office (2006–10) that MOH bureaucrats began to meet with these NGOs, at a time when the government was already strengthening its policy response to obesity. MOH bureaucrats whom I interviewed emphasized that they started to work closely with NGOs only after 2010, when Minister of Health José Temporão increased his interest in and focus on obesity (Bandeira, 2016; Lessa de Oliveira, 2016; Recine, 2016). Before then, even though activists were mobilizing and seeking to pressure the government to enact legislation, the partnership was not as strong, given that obesity was not yet a policy priority for the government. Again, as with HIV/AIDS, it was only *after* the government sought to bolster its international reputation in health—a byproduct of its positive geopolitical positioning—that we saw MOH bureaucrats seeking to work closely with the NGO community.

After 2010, MOH bureaucrats' primary strategy for forging a closer partnership with NGOs was achieved through regular meetings at national commissions on nutrition, national- and state-level CONSEA meetings, and periodic meetings with activist groups and the private sector (Karageorgiadis, 2016; Lessa de Oliveira, 2016; Recine, 2016; Takagi and Graziano da Silva, 2011). MOH bureaucrats, especially within the Departmento de Atenção Básica (Department of Basic Attention), periodically met with NGOs at meetings of these national commissions, which were cosponsored by the MOH and NGOs. The commissions organized several meetings throughout the year, and MOH bureaucrats were committed to meeting with NGOs at these events, thus showing their ongoing support and forging a stronger partnership (Bortoletto, 2016; Karageorgiadis, 2016; Lessa de Oliveira, 2016; Recine, 2016). In addition, CONSEA was instrumental in helping the MOH develop a close relationship with NGOs, as well as in influencing the policymaking process (Bandeira, 2016; Bortoletto, 2016; Karageorgiadis, 2016; Lessa de Oliveira, 2016; Recine, 2016).

During this period, MOH bureaucrats also worked closely with NGOs to obtain the information needed to formulate effective obesity prevention policies (Bandeira, 2016; Bortoletto, 2016; Jaime, Silva, et al., 2013; Karageorgiadis, 2016; Lessa de Oliveira, 2016; Recine, 2016). Information provided by NGOs at the national nutritional commission meetings, CONSEA meetings, and periodic meetings held through the National Health Council,[3] helped the health bureaucrats better understand the types of policies needed to increase social awareness of obesity and the government's prevention programs (Bandeira, 2016; Bortoletto, 2016; Karageorgiadis, 2016; Lessa de Oliveira, 2016; Recine, 2016; Takagi and Graziano da Silva, 2011). By meeting with NGOs, bureaucrats began to learn more about the realities that families faced in their daily nutritional and environmental challenges—details that helped to provide ideas for more effective obesity prevention efforts (Bandeira, 2016; Bortoletto, 2016; Karageorgiadis, 2016; Recine, 2016).

MOH bureaucrats also obtained important information through the FHP teams working at the municipal level. FHP teams could provide information and policy suggestions from the school administrators and families with which they worked, especially in the area of school nutrition and exercise.

The MOH's strong partnership with NGOs also helped to increase health bureaucrats' legitimacy within government, facilitating their ability to secure ongoing political and financial support. The MOH bureaucrats I interviewed emphasized this: that by working closely with NGOs, they were able to increase their legitimacy within government (Bandeira, 2016; Coutinho, 2016a; Lessa de Oliveira, 2016). NGO activists interviewed on this particular issue confirmed these views (Bortoletto, 2016; Karageorgiadis, 2016; Recine, 2016). Bureaucratic legitimacy increased because the president and the congress believed that these bureaucrats had the type of credible and reliable information needed to make informed and effective policy decisions. By emphasizing their repeated and ongoing dialogue with NGOs, moreover, health bureaucrats were able to show politicians that they were in tune with NGOs and could formulate policies that were effective and socially acceptable (Bandeira, 2016; Bartoletto, 2016; Coutinho, 2016a; Lessa de Oliveira, 2016; Recine, 2016). Through this repeated information gathering and dialogue, MOH bureaucrats were also showing congressional members that they had a justifiable need for their support. In addition, the office of the president and the congress recognized the widespread popularity of and civic support for these bureaucrats, which motivated the government to provide its support. In a context of democratic representation and preexisting government commitments to participatory governance in health, this social recognition and support mattered. As a consequence of their increased legitimacy and influence within government, MOH bureaucrats had an easier time obtaining the ongoing funding and political support necessary to create and implement their obesity prevention programs (Bandeira, 2016; Bartoletto, 2016; Recine, 2016).

Conclusion

Despite its delayed response to the HIV/AIDS and obesity epidemics and the international pressure that ensued, Brazil's positive geopolitical positioning and strong bureaucratic–civil societal partnerships facilitated the eventual introduction of a centrist policy response. Striving to develop and integrate into the global economy, political leaders worked to improve Brazil's international reputation in health through a stronger policy response, while pursuing international policy guidance and funding to help with this process. To improve the government's international reputation in health, the MOH later provided foreign aid to other nations seeking to eradicate HIV/AIDS, while working with the international community to increase access to essential medicines. This positive geopolitical positioning built upon the government's foreign policy tradition of committing to promoting its international reputation as an effective, developed state and a combatant against disease, while engaging in peaceful multilateral partnerships with other nations and pursuing international financial and technical assistance for disease eradication. In the context of challenges accompanying healthcare decentralization processes, health bureaucrats eventually introduced a centrist policy response to HIV/AIDS and obesity to augment the MOH's policy influence. This helped to ensure the successful implementation of prevention and treatment programs at the local level. Achievement of this centrist policy response is attributable to the strong partnership between MOH bureaucrats and NGOs, a partnership forged and strengthened since the early twentieth century.

NOTES

1. This lull was mainly due to the belief that smallpox had already been eradicated through aggressive federal programs (Hochman, 2009).

2. Mercosul, the South American Common Market, is a regional free trade agreement and institution, with representatives from Argentina, Brazil, Paraguay, Uruguay, and Venezuela.

3. Organized at the national, state, and municipal levels, the National Health Council consists of government officials, NGOs, activists, and academics, thus ensuring a participatory approach to the making of health policy.

3

India's Response to HIV/AIDS and Obesity

By the 1980s, India's emerging democratic and economic system, like Brazil's, was confronting the HIV/AIDS and obesity epidemics. With both epidemics highly contested among the country's politicians and bureaucrats, for a variety of reasons—often nothing to do with public health—India's government did not immediately respond. However, with the arrival of international criticism and pressure, by the early 1990s the situation began to change: politicians pursued a stronger policy response to HIV/AIDS and obesity in order to promote the government's international reputation for being capable of eradicating disease and of developing. Shortly thereafter, with the intent of furthering its international reputation, the government provided foreign aid assistance to other nations for HIV/AIDS prevention and the production of medications. These reputation-building interests, as well as a receptivity to international financial and technical assistance, reflected the government's positive geopolitical positioning. As we saw in Brazil, this positioning had a long historical precedent, spanning back to the early twentieth century when political leaders sought to enhance India's international image, importance, and position in the world. However, even though the government's positive geopolitical positioning served as an important catalyst for reform, the absence of strong bureaucratic–civil societal partnerships prohibited the emergence of a centrist policy response.

Responding to HIV/AIDS

The HIV/AIDS epidemic emerged later in India than in Brazil. The first reported case of AIDS in India arose in 1986, when an NGO in the city of Chennai (previously known as Madras), in the southern state of Tamil Nadu, reported

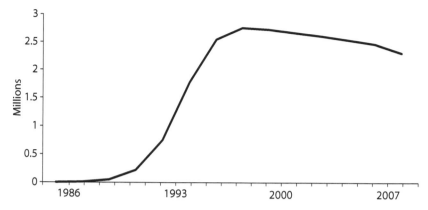

Figure 3.1. HIV/AIDS cases in India (millions). Source: India, Ministry of Health and Family Welfare, 2010.

a female sex worker with the virus. The virus subsequently spread throughout the southern states, hitting major urban centers such as Mumbai (formerly Bombay) in the state of Maharashtra (which by 1996 reported approximately 50% of all AIDS cases in India), Andhra Pradesh, Karnataka, and the northern states of Manipur and Nagaland (Lieberman, 2009; Solomon and Ganesh, 2002). AIDS was initially concentrated among sex workers, IDUs, and gay men, but by the early 2000s it had traveled to the rural population and blood transfusion recipients. Since the early 2000s, moreover, HIV/AIDS has been mainly concentrated among heterosexual couples, sex workers, and men who have sex with men (Solomon and Ganesh, 2002). Figure 3.1 shows the numbers of HIV/AIDS cases through 2007.

As occurred in Brazil, India's government did not immediately respond to the HIV/AIDS epidemic. The prime minister, parliament, and officials in the Ministry of Health and Family Welfare (MHFW) were essentially apathetic about the issue, even after these leaders became aware that HIV/AIDS was spreading like wildfire in other nations (Kadiyala and Barnett, 2004). In 1994, at the Twelfth Annual Convention of the American Association of Physicians in India, the government's health minister, B. Shankarahand, commented that "AIDS is not a problem in India," reflecting the government's denial of the new disease (quoted in Jayapal, 1996, 1). No elected politician publicly mentioned AIDS until 2001, when Prime Minister Atal Bihari Vajpayee proclaimed his commitment to what the government finally considered a "national crisis" (Lieberman, 2009). The government's initial inaction was mainly the result of conservative cultural beliefs—open discourse on sex was taboo—and of stigma that tainted the views of the parliament, the prime minister, and MHFW officials (Kadiyala and Barnett, 2004; Lieberman, 2009; Mawar et al., 2005; Schaffer and Mitra, 2004). People living with HIV/AIDS were seen as immoral outcasts, the "naughty them," subject to punishment for their embarrassing sins (Lieberman, 2009; Schaffer and Mitra, 2004), deemed unworthy of government support.

While the government did respond by creating the National Committee on AIDS in 1987, the National AIDS Control Organization (NACO) in 1992, and the first of three National AIDS Control Plans (NACPs) in 1992, these initiatives lacked the strong support of the prime minister and parliament and were poorly staffed and underfunded (Kadiyala and Barnett, 2004; Lieberman, 2009). Lieberman (2009, 183) describes NACO during this period as a mere "bureaucratic shell," hollow and inept. Others referred to NACO as a "semi-autonomous" agency (Mitra, Haté, and Schaffer, 2007), falling under the auspices of the MHFW, designed to devise national policy and monitor the epidemic and the blood supply, while providing epidemiological information (Solomon and Ganesh, 2002). With respect to the first NACP, a former NACO official later admitted that "NACP 1 was basically an administrative response, because the country was not ready to face up to the challenge" (quoted in Tran et al., 2013, 4). During this period, NGOs were invited to help construct the NACP and NACO (Lo et al., 2005). Yet, in practice, NACO bureaucrats neglected to work closely with NGOs (Gómez and Harris, 2015; Motihar and Mahendra, 2003). And although NACO helped to increase awareness and implemented prevention programs throughout the 1990s, it failed to provide sufficient financial and technical support to the states, especially for medical training (Kadiyala and Barnett, 2004).

The national government's first impulse—much as in Brazil—was to rely on the states as the initial policy responders. By 1999, when the second NACP was created, which emphasized targeting at-risk groups (Lo et al., 2005), NACO officials decided to decentralize the implementation of policy by creating State AIDS Prevention and Control Societies (SACSs). Others, however, claimed that this policy underscored New Delhi's apathy toward constructing an effective national AIDS program (Lieberman, 2009). The SACSs were the arms and ears of federal NACO bureaucrats, financially dependent on the latter yet responsible for subnational policy implementation (Lo et al., 2005). Despite their importance, the SACSs consistently received inadequate financial and technical assistance from the center; consequently, they exhibited low levels of managerial and technical capacity (Chandrasekaran et al., 2006; Lo et al., 2005).

International Criticism, Pressure, and Reputation Building

By the early 1990s, international criticism and pressure for a more effective government response to HIV/AIDS had begun to emerge, reaching an apogee by the early to mid-2000s. In 1992, the director of the WHO's Global Program on AIDS, Michael Merson, warned that if India did not ramp up its response to HIV/AIDS, prevalence rates could reach those of Africa (Lieberman, 2009). Gradual, periodic pressure throughout the 1990s turned into what Lieberman (2009) and others describe as a critical juncture in international pressure for a more aggressive response to AIDS in India. In 1996, the head of UNAIDS commented at the Eleventh International AIDS Conference in Vancouver that India had the largest number of people infected with HIV and AIDS in the world (L. Altman, 1996). In 2003, Peter Piot, former director of UNAIDS, was quoted as stating that "India has a king-sized problem. AIDS is spreading rapidly in the country," while the BBC commented that "so far the government has been slow to tackle the problem" (*BBC News*, 2003, 1, 2). In 2003, Richard Feachem, then executive director of the Global Fund to Fight AIDS, Tuberculosis, and Malaria (Global Fund), added further criticism by stating that India had the world's largest number of HIV-infected people, surpassing South Africa's, and that India was "on an African Trajectory" (quoted in Boseley, 2003, 1). Feachem commented in the following year that "nothing serious enough was being done in India to prevent the spread of HIV" (quoted in Devraj, 2005, 1).

By the early 2000s, according to Lieberman (2009, 179), India had become "a country increasingly concerned with its place in the international political economy . . . [and] . . . faced pressure to control the growth of this pandemic." International criticism of India's lackluster response to HIV/AIDS succeeded in garnering the attention of senior political and bureaucratic officials, upsetting them and making them defensive. In 2002, for example, parliamentarians and MHFW bureaucrats vehemently criticized a report published by the CIA titled *The New Wave of HIV/AIDS: Nigeria, Ethiopia, Russia, India, and China*, which claimed that India would likely "have 20 to 25 million [infected] by 2010," leading to "the largest number of people with HIV/AIDS in the world" (CIA, 2002, 4, 13). Government officials argued that this CIA report was kindling unnecessary fears, "spreading panic" and "scares" (Perry 2005, 1), and gave "completely inaccurate data" (Kadiyala and Barnett, 2004, 1889). NACO officials became even more incensed when Bill Gates quoted these CIA figures when discussing India's situation and how he could help with his proposed Avahan project in 2002 (Perry 2005, 2). This prompted MHFW officials to unrealistically claim that they had successfully reduced the number of HIV infections by 95% within one year (Perry 2005, 1).

As I explained in chapter 1, there are several reasons that emerging economies have a desire to improve their international reputation in health. By overcoming international criticism through stronger policy reforms, these nations increase their international credibility and respect—an achievement and status that are essential to becoming constructive, influential partners in the global fight against disease.

These reputation-building incentives were certainly present in India. The government wanted to convince the international community—specifically, western industrialized nations and international institutions such as the World Bank, IMF, PAHO, and WHO—that it was capable of developing a sound economy and improving the nation's healthcare situation, particularly HIV/AIDS (Skolnick, 2013). Convincing the West was perceived as vital for enhancing the nation's international reputation as a successful emerging economy, one that was politically and economically stable, healthy, and prosperous enough to invest in and to work with as a coequal partner (De Milliano, 2007). Saving face with the West and building a strong reputation were also perceived as facilitating India's ability to gain more influence and support within important international institutions such as the UN National Security Council and the IMF (Jabeen, 2010).

Rajiv Misra, India's minister of health (1991–94), was particularly interested in building a stronger policy response to HIV/AIDS, efforts that he believed could improve the government's international reputation as a state committed to eradicating the disease (Misra, 2013). In an interview with the author, Misra indicated that despite his inability to obtain parliamentary support for his AIDS program for NACO during the early 1990s (prior to the aforementioned international pressures), parliament eventually authorized NACO to approach the World Bank for a loan in 2001. Richard Skolnick (2013), the senior economist responsible for providing the first World Bank loan package for India, totaling US$203 million, indicated that the government wanted to use its heightened response to AIDS—which was facilitated by the loan (Jha, 2013)—to bolster India's reputation as a nation that could not only generate a success-ful policy response to AIDS but also effectively invest in its public health sys-tem. Up to that point, India had a reputation of poorly funding its public health system (Skolnick, 2013). The government wanted to efface this negative im-age; aggressively responding to HIV/AIDS provided an opportunity to do so (Misra, 2013).

Other strategies were pursued to strengthen India's international reputation in HIV/AIDS. For example, at the Fifteenth International AIDS Conference, held in July 2004 in Bangkok, Sonia Gandhi, chairwoman of the Congress (I) Party, in the presence of former South African president Nelson Mandela, closed the conference with a speech emphasizing India's commitment to eradi-cating HIV/AIDS, claiming that "I would like to take this opportunity to categorically assert the determination and ability of the Government and the people of India to meet this daunting challenge, just as effectively as they did in the campaign to eradicate smallpox some decades ago. We have risen to meet social, political and technological challenges in the past and I am confident that we will do so again in the present context" (Gandhi, 2004, 1).

This was the first time that India had made an international commitment to combating HIV/AIDS. Gandhi was poised to attest to India's strong AIDS leadership (Mitra, 2004). The government also sought to demonstrate India's developmental potential as a nation having the medical and pharmaceutical ca-pacity needed to eradicate the epidemic. The time had come to reveal the con-fidence of a new India—a nation with the will and ability to curb the spread of disease and to develop and prosper.

Given this desire to raise India's profile as an emerging nation, international criticism of the country's AIDS strategy was a major source of consternation for India's political leaders (Skolnick, 2013). Despite their initial defensive pos-ture, officials began to speak more openly, not only about AIDS and their ca-pacity to engender a stronger policy response, but also about their commitment to start working together in a bipartisan manner. As Lieberman (2009) claims, by 2001, international pressure correlated highly with the efforts of the governing BJP (Bharatiya Janata Party) and opposition Congress (I) to display true politi-cal leadership on AIDS.

In an attempt to further build its international reputation, during this period the government also sponsored international conferences to draw atten-tion to NACO's AIDS policies. In July 2000, for example, NACO bureaucrats sponsored an international conference in Nagpur, Maharashtra, organized by medical practitioners and researchers: the International Conference on the Validity of HIV/AIDS Programs (*Rethinking AIDS*, 2000). In addition to presenting research on the causes of AIDS, this conference provided a venue to share NACO's and the Indian research community's research and policy accomplishments. More than a hundred participants from India and other nations attended the conference, providing a vast audience for India's AIDS bureaucrats to display their accomplishments (*Rethinking AIDS*, 2000). In November 2003, moreover, the MHFW and NACO sponsored a conference organized by the South Asian Association for Regional Cooperation (SAARC) on the issue of developing a common regional strategy to combat AIDS and TB (SAARC, 2009). Through this meeting, NACO bureaucrats could not only highlight their achievements but also reveal their strong commitment to multilateral partnership and cooperation in containing AIDS and TB (SAARC, 2009). And finally, in 2005, in an effort to confirm for the international community that HIV/AIDS cases were on the decline (following much skepticism from international experts), NACO invited WHO officials to New Delhi to show them epidemiological evidence suggesting that HIV and AIDS prevalence was waning, while highlighting the government's success in introducing new prevention and treatment policies (One World, 2005).

But were international criticism and reputation building the only factors motivating the government to pay more attention to the HIV/AIDS epidemic? One could easily argue that India's vibrant democracy and burgeoning electoral pressures motivated the government to do so. The problem with this argument, however, is that at no point did the national BJP or Congress (I) Party use the AIDS situation as an electoral strategy. Indeed, as Lieberman (2009) points out, the ruling BJP did not start to publicly address the HIV/AIDS issue until 2001, well after its election to parliament. Or, one could argue that the incidence of AIDS was so high by the early 2000s that the government had no choice but to strengthen its policy response. The problem with this argument is that the government knew about the gravity of the situation at a much earlier time (Jha, 2013; Lieberman, 2009; Sankaran, 2006). Indeed, Sankaran (2006, 1) writes that "the government recognized the seriousness of the problem quite early after the reporting of the first case of HIV/AIDS in 1986."

Finally, one could envision the possibility that HIV/AIDS prompted a more aggressive response during this period because it had touched the lives of influential individuals in India, such as the upper- and middle-income classes and famous actors, activists, and movie stars. Yet again, this does not apply in the case of India. AIDS first emerged among poor IDUs, sex workers, and eventually truck drivers and the gay community (Solomon and Ganesh, 2002). The disease began to emerge among high-risk groups only in the late 1990s, among a small, select population that was not well organized or vocal about its problems (Baria et al., 1997). To my knowledge, there were no instances of famous individuals infected with the virus who attracted media attention, and use of this to pressure the government for policy reform.

History and the Emergence of Positive Geopolitical Positioning

International reputation building seems to have been the more important catalyst for policy reform in India, but where did this interest come from? And why was the government so interested in working with the international community and financial lenders to strengthen its policy response to HIV/AIDS? It seems to have been historical precedent that shaped the government's interest in positioning India as an emerging nation, eager to build its international reputation in health, while peacefully cooperating with the international community and seeking financial assistance to achieve its policy objectives. Indeed, as we saw in Brazil, there was a deep historical precedent to India's positive geopolitical positioning.

Indian diplomatic thought and foreign policies essentially derived from historical religious and philosophical beliefs. Since the sacred Hindu writings of the *Bhagavad Gita*, the principles of truth and respectful discourse with other nations have been present in India (Dasgupta, 2005). Another enduring tradition is the state's concern with international opinion. Even before independence from British rule in 1950, India's politicians were sensitive to other nations' opinions of their nation, while always seeking international support for their endeavors (S. Cohen, 2002; Dasgupta, 2005; Kember, 1975). Some attribute these views to India's unique cultural and social structure—specifically, the caste system, with political and social elites at the top of the hierarchical chain—as explaining "why elitist leaders have been sensitive to the finest perceived slight to themselves, or their countries, by foreigners" (S. Cohen 2002, 22).

Many would claim that modern-day diplomatic thought has its origins in a particular individual: Jawaharlal Nehru. Nehru was India's first foreign minister under the British Raj, then post-independent India's first prime minister (1947–64). Like President Getúlio Vargas in Brazil (1930–45, 1951–54), Nehru was infatuated with foreign affairs. He was incessantly concerned with India's position in the world, how others perceived the nation, and how he could bolster India's reputation as a modern state, independent of other nations' influence—especially the colonizing West (S. Cohen, 2002). In response to India's "weak or at least highly variable reputation," Stephen Cohen (2002, 24) claims, Nehru "urged his fellow Indians (and the rest of the world) to recognize India's importance in the Middle East, Southeast Asia, and the Far East." Nehru was tired of hearing other statesmen claim that India was insignificant, a "British problem," not a serious world player—never on other nations' radar screens (Kember, 1975). Much of Nehru's anger stemmed from his realization that the advanced industrialized nations—as well as the British Dominions, such as Canada, New Zealand, and South Africa—essentially ignored India, even at important international venues such as the League of Nations. This motivated Nehru to refer to India's participation in the league as, simply put, "a farce" (Kember, 1975).

Nehru was so concerned about India's international reputation that he made establishing a favorable "world opinion" toward India an important aspect of his foreign policy objectives (Dasgupta, 2005). Coupled with this was his commitment to establishing peaceful and cooperative diplomatic negotiations as well as nonalignment with world powers (S. Cohen, 2002; Dasgupta, 2005). Through his various diplomatic missions and participation in international organizations such as the UN, which he firmly supported, Nehru sought to educate the world about India's future potential and geopolitical importance. He would not tolerate any more criticism about India's ability to develop into a modern and effective state.

These interests and endeavors did not stop with Nehru. Historians claim that his daughter, Prime Minister Indira Gandhi (1966–77, 1980–84), agreed with his foreign policy views; the same was said for his grandson, Prime Minister Rajiv Gandhi (1984–89) (S. Cohen, 2002). As members of Nehru's Congress (I) political party, Indira and Rajiv remained firmly committed to Nehru's foreign policy objectives and, as such, shared his concern for world opinion. They constantly sought to bolster India's reputation and global influence. Nehru's views and objectives would go on to shape the nation's foreign policy for decades to come (Tripathi, 2011).

Despite the government's interest in projecting India as a successful modern state, Nehru and subsequent government officials had no interest in becoming a global power, intervening in other nations, or shaping global policy and discourse. In fact, quite the opposite was true: Nehru had a deep disdain for selfish and imposing global powers and instead emphasized equality and fair treatment between nations (Alden and Vieira, 2005; Tripathi, 2011). Prior to and under Nehru's rule, the focus was always on India's defense against external threats (Cohen, 2002; Tripathi, 2011). Like Vargas in Brazil, Nehru never believed that one particular nation or small group of nations should dominate world opinion and geopolitics. This view motivated Nehru and subsequent administrations to pursue a policy of "nonalignment," in which India would refrain from taking sides with global powers such as the United States, England, and Russia (Alden and Vieira, 2005; S. Cohen, 2002; Ito, n.d.). This belief shaped India's diplomatic activities throughout the Cold War, convincing politicians to remain neutral, warmly nestled between the United States and Russia.

India had a long history of engaging in international cooperation and partnerships. Even before Nehru, peaceful international cooperation with other nations was a cornerstone of India's foreign policy objectives. Shortly after independence, Nehru worked closely with his Cabinet for External Affairs to engage in new cooperative partnerships with international organizations and other nations—in fact, these were explicit policy goals that he inscribed into India's constitution (S. Cohen, 2002). For example, Nehru was very supportive of the creation of the UN, and while not playing a formal role in its creation, India did support it and provided policy suggestions. All of these efforts underscored the fact that emerging India was, like Brazil, unwaveringly committed to international multilateral cooperation.

India's commitment to this kind of foreign policy was especially noticeable in the area of global health. In 1948, India became the first nation to cooperate with other nations in the creation of the South-East Asia Regional office of the WHO, and it has worked closely with the WHO since then to eradicate diseases in that region (WHO, 2009a). India worked closely with the WHO to help eradicate smallpox by strengthening India's National Smallpox Eradication Program (Srigyan, 2008). India also worked with the WHO and with other nations to develop a vaccine for smallpox (Welcome Trust Center, 2009). By 1954, India was sending delegates to the WHO's World Health Assembly to warn nations about an impending crisis of chronic diseases (such as heart disease, diabetes, and cancer) in developing nations, thus signaling the nation's proactive, visionary stance in global health (S. Rao, 2004).

India also joined other nations in signing the Alma Ata declaration (in 1978) on the need to make universal, equitable healthcare a human right (Elliot Armijo, 2007). In recent years, the international community has also appreciated

India's leadership in advocating for "pro-public health," in which government responsibility for providing critical healthcare services takes center stage (Leowski and Krishnan, 2009). And in 2001, the Indian government joined Brazil and other developing nations in establishing the Doha declaration for universal access to antiretroviral medications for the treatment of HIV/AIDS (Elliot Armijo, 2007). This rich history in global health partnerships generated incentives to maintain India's reputation as a cooperative nation committed to eradicating disease (Gómez, 2009).

After his election in 2004, Prime Minister Manmohan Singh (2004–14) vowed to strengthen India's diplomatic partnership and ties with other nations. Although India has historically been receptive to international assistance while working closely with other countries, the government has been perceived as a tough negotiator—it was difficult to appease and find consensus with Indian negotiators. Some observers claimed that the government's anti-imperialist stance toward the United States, fueled by the nonaligned movement, generated skepticism and anger toward other western powers, often leading to opposing views on international treaties (Grant, 2008; Kahn, 2009). Keen on positively transforming India's diplomatic image, Singh was committed to becoming less hostile and more cooperative, especially toward the United States (Kahn, 2009). Singh viewed diplomatic cooperation, consensus building, and support as vital to India's success in international diplomacy, but he also viewed India as a bridge between poor nations and the more industrialized nations (Kahn, 2009). Singh embraced US Secretary of State Hilary Clinton's promotion of "Smart Power"— in which a nation's international influence emerges not from physical prowess but from greater cooperation and diplomacy (Clinton, 2010). Singh viewed smart power as a necessary approach to bolstering India's international reputation and influence.

India has a long history of working with other nations, international organizations, and philanthropists to obtain funding for its development projects. India was one of the first developing nations to receive funding from the World Bank. In September 1958, the government received US$160 million in loans, disbursed in three phases, for the construction of a national railroad and electrical power system (Kapur, Lewis, and Webb, 1997). By the 1960s, India had become the World Bank's largest client, receiving loans for other initiatives such as the production of iron and steel as well as increasing its port capacity (Culpeper, 1997). But historically, the government has also been receptive to financial and technical assistance and support from philanthropists. In 1915, for example, the Rockefeller Foundation opened a country office in India to help local communities in their response to childhood and maternal diseases, while providing training for medical professionals (Bracken, 2009; Rockefeller Foundation, 2013). Provincial officials in states such as Uttar Pradesh also welcomed the support of the Red Cross in these endeavors (Bracken, 2009). After independence, the government would continue to welcome support from the international community to help achieve its economic and social policy objectives, especially in the area of health (Sridhar and Gómez, 2010).

With the arrival of HIV/AIDS several decades later, India's historical precedent of building its international reputation and working with the international community to help combat disease resurfaced, engendering similar types of reform incentives. The government followed in its own historical footsteps, viewing health policy reforms and loans from international lenders as a means to strengthen the government's international reputation and response to disease. Doing this again for HIV/AIDS led to a stronger national policy response.

Strengthening AIDS Policy Reforms

After the mid-2000s, international criticism and reputation-building pursuits led to a new level of parliamentary support for expanding India's national AIDS program. In this context, the parliament and MHFW increased their commitment to working with AIDS bureaucrats in NACO, providing additional funding while helping implement new prevention and treatment policies. Lieberman (2009) highlights a strong correlation between a spike in international pressure and a dramatic scale-up in the government's policy response to HIV/AIDS beginning in 2004. With regard to NACO, moreover, a firmer commitment emerged to provide additional funding while training national and subnational SACS officials on issues such as financial management and technical assistance (UN General Assembly, 2010). Indeed, a central theme of the third NACP (2007–12; commonly known as India's Phase III response) was a renewed commitment to "strengthen the infrastructure, systems, and human resources in prevention, care, support and treatment programmes at the District, State and National levels" (India, NACO, 2010). The plan also vowed to increase financial and technical assistance to SACSs, as well as providing technical training (UN General Assembly, 2010).

With regard to prevention, several targeted and innovative programs emerged. For example, in 2007, in cooperation with the Rajiv Gandhi Foundation and the Ministry of Rails, NACO cosponsored an awareness campaign, the "Red Ribbon Express"—bustling along in a locomotive, covering 9,000 kilometers, entering approximately 43,200 villages, and disseminating prevention information, condoms, and HIV testing. Given India's vast and hard-to-reach rural areas, the Red Ribbon Express is critical for increasing awareness and understanding of HIV/AIDS transmission and prevention (*Hindu*, 2009a; *Hindustan Times*, 2008). And in 2010, NACO launched an aggressive new Condom Social Marketing Programme, targeting sales of 47 crore (a crore is 10 million) condoms across 370 districts, especially in hard-to-reach rural areas (*Thaindian News*, 2010). Finally, Phase III maintains funding for a host of prevention programs geared toward groups at high risk, such as commercial sex workers, IDUs, and gay men (UN General Assembly, 2010).

In 2004, the government also launched a more progressive ARV treatment policy. Previously, NACO provided ARV medications only for pregnant women to prevent parent-to-child transmission. Since 2004, however, drugs have been provided to HIV-positive parents, infected children under the age of 15, and patients registered in public hospitals and at treatment centers in the highest prevalence states, such as Tamil Nadu, Andhra Pradesh, Maharashtra, Karnataka, Manipur, and Nagaland, and the capital city, Delhi (Lieberman, 2009). Yet the great irony—or perhaps, more appropriately, the ongoing tragedy—is that while India is home to one of the world's largest, most talented pharmaceutical industries (Shao, 2013), the government exports most of its generic medications rather than working with the MHFW to guarantee universal access to medicine in India (Gómez, 2009; Lieberman, 2009). This paints a sharp contrast to the case of Brazil, where the key purpose for developing a vibrant pharmaceutical industry has been to guarantee universal distribution of ARVs in Brazil (Flynn, 2008).

Nevertheless, more recently, the government of Prime Minister Narendra Modi has been praised for passing national legislation protecting the rights of individuals with HIV/AIDS while deepening the government's commitment to providing medical treatment. In March 2017, parliament approved the HIV and AIDS (Prevention and Control) Bill, which protects people living with HIV/AIDS from any form of government, corporate, or social discrimination; it also includes penal provisions for any discrimination toward them and protects them from any breach of confidentiality. Furthermore, this bill now makes ARV treatment a "legal right" for all in need of access to medication, guaranteed by the central and state governments (Deyl, 2017).

Thus, a stronger policy response to HIV/AIDS eventually emerged, triggered by international criticism and pressure and by India's reputation-building interests. Over time, these interests also motivated the government to help other nations combat AIDS in order to further enhance its international reputation. In 2001, India joined Brazil in helping establish the 2001 Doha agreement, which facilitated nations' access to ARVs by allowing them to manufacture and produce generic medications in periods of health crisis (Watt, Gómez, and McKee, 2014). By the turn of the twenty-first century, the government's primary agency responsible for providing foreign aid, the Ministry of External Affairs (MEA) (Nigam, 2015), not only helped to fund HIV prevention programs in several African nations (Morrison and Kates, 2006) but also provided ARVs to nations such as Mozambique and Angola—thus building on its success in becoming one of the world's largest producers of generic ARV medications (Ruger and Ng, 2010). Officials working in the Indian Technical and Economic Cooperation Programme, formed in 1964, also partnered with India's private pharmaceutical sector to help several African nations create pharmaceutical labs for the production of ARVs (Morrison and Kates, 2006; Ruger and Ng, 2010). The MEA also provided HIV test kits and policy lessons in AIDS prevention to several Southeast Asian, Caribbean, and African nations (Chaturvedi, 2015). Building on global recognition for its successful healthcare human resource training, management, and technology in HIV/AIDS, the government established the Global Political Advocacy Initiative, which sought to encourage other nations to engage in these activities while raising awareness and support for HIV research (Ruger and Ng, 2010).

In addition to HIV/AIDS, the government expanded its technical assistance to broader areas in healthcare, providing regional neighbors and several African nations with essential medicines, ambulances, and funding for hospital infrastructure. The MEA has also sent teams of medical doctors to Angola, Mozambique, and elsewhere to provide training, establish medical camps, and recruit and provide scholarships for students to attend Indian medical universities (Chaturvedi, 2015). Impressively, in 2009, supported by an MEA grant of US$17 million, the ministry also created the Pan-African e-Network project, which provides telemedicine training from elite Indian hospitals and universities to their counterparts in 53 African Union partnering countries (De Bruyn, 2013). Scholars have emphasized the government's efforts to enhance its international reputation as an emerging power dedicated to helping other developing nations overcome HIV/AIDS and establish effective public health systems (De Bruyn, 2013; Ruger and Ng, 2010). Despite these efforts, when compared with Brazil, India's prime ministers were not as committed to aggressively marketing the government's domestic AIDS policy achievements at international venues.

Despite India's long tradition of working with other nations to fight disease, it had no such long-term reputation for providing foreign aid in health. This partly reflected the fact that for most of its history, especially in the area of public health, the government had been accustomed to being a receiver rather than provider of foreign aid assistance (De Bruyn, 2013). This lack of historical engagement in foreign aid and global health diplomacy also reflected the government's low level of priority for healthcare during the 1990s (Dréze and Sen, 2013) and, consequently, its apathy toward using and marketing India's achievements in healthcare at the international level. The government's limited commitment to foreign policy in health became even more evident with its decision to refrain from participating in the Foreign Policy and Global Health Initiative in 2008. This initiative was organized by the WHO and health ministers from several countries, through the 2007 Oslo Ministerial Declaration at the UN General Assembly meeting in New York. Representatives from Brazil, France, Indonesia, Norway, Senegal, South Africa, and Thailand convened in Geneva, June 12–13, 2008, to establish an international normative consensus "toward a more sustainable relationship between foreign policy and health" (Ruger and Ng, 2010).

India's government nevertheless had several motivations for providing bilateral assistance in HIV/AIDS and other developmental endeavors. While bolstering its international reputation in health was certainly one of them, it also viewed this assistance as a means to enhance its broader image as an emerging global power, capable of influencing policy debate and international donor assistance (De Bruyn, 2013; Price, 2011). By increasing foreign aid, government officials sought to supplant, in the eyes of the international community, India's ongoing issues of domestic poverty and inequality with its new role as an advanced, emerging economy, positioning itself to help other developing nations address health and other social welfare issues (Kragelund, 2010). This assistance was also perceived as an effective geopolitical strategy: by helping neighboring nations such as Bhutan, Nepal, Sri Lanka, and Cambodia, India could strengthen its regional allies amid growing hostilities with Pakistan and China, while gaining more support for India's election to the UN Security Council

(Bijoy, 2010; De Bruyn, 2013). The government also saw providing bilateral assistance to Africa as a way to increase its access to new markets and especially natural resources (Bijoy, 2010; Nigam, 2015). For all of these reasons, India's foreign aid assistance has become a key aspect of its foreign policy strategy.

Did the government's newfound interest in building its domestic AIDS program while helping other nations eradicate HIV/AIDS contribute to ongoing support for the MHFW and NACO's prevention and treatment programs, ultimately leading to a centrist policy response? And has NACO provided state-level SACSs with adequate financial resources, training, and technical support?

Unfortunately, parliamentary funding commitments have not continued to increase since 2014. Government spending for NACO, as well as its total spending for the national AIDS programs, has decreased, due mainly to the government's efforts to reduce fiscal spending and budgetary deficits (Rajshekhar, 2015; Rochan, 2014; Sharma, 2015). NACO has become increasingly reliant on state governments to fund AIDS programs (Kalra and Siddiqui, 2015). In 2014, as a consequence of parliament's decision to reduce the overall healthcare budget, the AIDS program lost approximately 30% of its budget (Rajshekhar, 2015; Rochan, 2014). In 2015, parliament decided to slash the AIDS budget by a fifth, while asking state governments to fund approximately 50% of all AIDS projects, with the central government providing the rest (Kalra, 2015; Mascarenhas, 2015). When questioned about this decrease in funding, the Union health minister, J. P. Nadda, stated that "AIDS was a concern 10 years back" (quoted in Rajshekhar, 2015, 1), reflecting his belief that because of the government's increased reform efforts several years earlier, the number of HIV/AIDS cases had stabilized and no longer posed a threat. This perception generated a considerable amount of criticism and pressure from activists and state governments, essentially forcing the central government to promise to restore previous funding levels—which has yet to be achieved (Rajshekhar, 2015). These financial challenges are further compounded by the recent decision of major philanthropic organizations, such as the Bill and Melinda Gates Foundation, to reduce their financial contributions to India for HIV/AIDS programs and shift more funding to other diseases such as TB and to family planning (Deyl, 2015).

At the same time, there was a lack of coordination and an inconsistency in central government support between NACO and the SACSs, which complicated collaborative policymaking efforts (Chandrasekaran et al., 2006). Even after the government's renewed commitment to combating HIV/AIDS, the

SACSs continued to be in need of technical, managerial, and, especially, financial assistance (Sharma, 2015). Also, hospitals and rural health clinics continued to lack adequate funding, equipment, and medical personnel for HIV/AIDS (Mitra, Haté, and Schaffer, 2007).

As in Brazil, India's healthcare decentralization, which began in 1993 (Mitra, Haté, and Schaffer, 2007), has reinforced the country's inequalities in healthcare services among the states. That is, states with a higher level of economic development and therefore greater infrastructural, medical, and technical capacity (mainly the southern states of Tamil Nadu, Karnataka, Andhra Pradesh, and Maharashtra) have been more adept at responding to HIV/AIDS than the poorer states (Mitra, Haté, and Schaffer, 2007). This has some analysts convinced that the push for healthcare decentralization poses an ongoing formidable challenge to responding to the HIV/AIDS epidemic (Baruagh, 2008). In contrast to what we saw in Brazil, NACO has fallen short of adequately intervening to address the shortcomings of decentralization.

Indeed, to my knowledge, NACO has not tried to surmount such shortcomings by introducing conditional fiscal transfer programs as a policy strategy to induce compliance with NACO's policy recommendations. In fact, if anything, there has been a shortage of fiscal transfers to the states (Rajshekhar, 2015). This has provided few incentives for SACSs and municipal health officials to adequately implement policy. Furthermore, NACO has not contracted with NGOs to monitor SACSs' and local health departments' implementation of prevention and treatment policies. As we saw for Brazil, this type of contractual partnership between national AIDS bureaucrats and NGOs is vital for increasing subnational accountability to the center and the electorate.

Thus, in sum, while the government eventually pursued a stronger policy response to HIV/AIDS after the rise of international criticisms and pressures, it never joined Brazil in achieving a *centrist policy response*. As I explained in chapter 1, a centrist policy response requires three components: the creation and ongoing financial and administrative expansion of federal agencies, the development of effective prevention and treatment programs (particularly, universal access to medicines), and formal and informal strategies to increase the central government's policy influence in a context of healthcare decentralization. In India, however, the parliament has not continued to increase NACO spending and administrative expansion, no universal ARV treatment program was ever introduced, and NACO has neglected to formally increase its centralized policy influence by providing conditional fiscal grant assistance while informally contracting NGOs to monitor and hold local governments accountable for policy implementation.

Given the government's positive geopolitical positioning and stronger policy response to HIV/AIDS, why has it recently backtracked on its policy efforts and not engaged in a centrist policy response? What is the missing link in India's ability to achieve this?

The Absence of Strong Bureaucratic-Civil Societal Partnerships

In essence, in India, it is the absence of strong bureaucratic–civil societal partnerships in public health that has hampered the government's ability to achieve a centrist policy response. As we saw in Brazil, establishing these partnerships is important for increasing AIDS bureaucrats' influence and legitimacy when striving to solicit and obtain ongoing financial and political support. Unlike in Brazil, social health movements in India did not, historically, create well-organized, globally integrated movements that pressured the national government for an immediate policy response to a health epidemic. This was mainly because a centralized administrative response to public health issues was already in place during the British Raj and, later, under the newly independent Indian state (Mushtaq, 2009). Consequently, the few social movements that did exist often worked in isolation from the federal government and were focused on either antipoverty or general social welfare issues, not on public health (Andharia, 2009).

Furthermore, there was no long tradition of ministry of health bureaucrats and civil society working together to combat disease (Misra, 2013), so the bureaucracy did not have any interest in strategically finding and using AIDS NGOs to expand their federal programs (Gómez and Harris, 2015; Misra, 2013). Indeed, since the second NACP was introduced in 1999, NACO bureaucrats have refrained from strategically engaging in partnerships with the multitude of AIDS NGOs that emerged during the 1990s in order to justify ongoing parliamentary funding and thus a continued expansion of the national AIDS program (Gómez and Harris, 2015; Misra, 2013; Schaffer and Mitra, 2004). Instead, since 1999, NACO bureaucrats have relied entirely on state-level SACSs to contract with NGOs to provide prevention and treatment services (Lo et al., 2005; Rajshekhar, 2015; Subramanian, 2013). Problematically, this has led to the emergence of *subnational* rather than national bureaucratic–civil societal partnerships for policy implementation. As evidenced in Brazil, however, constructing a partnership between *national* bureaucrats and NGOs is needed to provide these bureaucrats with the legitimacy and influence necessary to obtain ongoing funding and political support.

To further complicate matters, in 2008 NACO decertified approximately 350 NGOs, based upon the results of a NACO survey and an external evaluation report by the World Bank in 2007, which concluded that these NGOs were nonexistent, corrupt, or ineffective in using domestic and international funding (John, 2008; Nambiar, 2012; Shrivastava, 2008). Because of this, analysts note, NACO has had a difficult time trusting AIDS NGOs (Global Fund, 2009a; Misra, 2013), and the government has shown distrust in organizations that receive financial support from western agencies and organizations (Jayaram, 2015). While the SACSs continue to work with NGOs, NACO seems to have backtracked from developing closer ties with them (Gómez and Harris, 2015), failing to reach out to activists and community healthcare workers for important consultation on prevention and treatment programs (Deb, 2014).

The recent merger of NACO into the MHFW provides even further insight into the government's weakening partnership with NGOs. In 2014, as part of Prime Minister Modi's effort to strive for "minimum government, maximum governance" (Nandan Jha, 2014, 1), NACO came under the auspices of the MHFW. This process entailed not only removal of NACO's director but also a loss of bureaucratic and funding autonomy (Nandan Jha, 2014). Throughout this restructuring effort, not one NGO was consulted about the consolidation process (Sachan, 2014), notwithstanding NGOs' historical reliance on NACO for funding (Gwalani, 2014). This decision upset the activist community (V. Krishnan, 2014; Sachan, 2014), as it revealed that the government was becoming increasingly apathetic to their needs. Worse still, NGO leaders such as Anandi Yuvaraj, a member of the International Community of Women with HIV, argued that the "decision [to merge] will push back all the progress made on HIV prevention and care, but also tarnish India's global image as a leader in this area" (quoted in V. Krishnan, 2014, 1).

Activists were also worried that NACO's merger would lead to fewer potential opportunities to work with AIDS bureaucrats. According to Shaleen Rakesh, director of technology support for the India HIV/AIDS Alliance, the merger "will likely cut down on human resources, which are essential for collaboration with civil society of the size and scale of our country" (quoted in Sachan, 2014, 842).

To complicate matters even more, in April 2016, Prime Minister Modi ordered that several of NACO's consultants with linkages to international funders and NGOs be relieved of their duties. And in 2016, of the 112 consultants financed by international donors and NGOs such as the Gates Foundation, 45 were ordered to resign (Kalra, 2016). These were individuals who played a critical role in formulating AIDS prevention and treatment programs. Analysts speculate that Prime Minister Modi ordered this downsizing to reduce the influence of NGOs—especially those from the West—over AIDS policy. The prime minister's decision further revealed the government's lack of trust in individuals with linkages to NGOs (Kalra, 2016).

There has also been a general decline in NACO's support for NGO activities. Those NGOs working to serve high-risk groups and to provide counseling and HIV testing have seen a dramatic decrease in funding since 2014 (Gwalani, 2014; Rajshekhar, 2015). This has occurred even in those states with the highest prevalence of HIV/AIDS cases, such as Nagaland, Maharashtra, and Mizoram, located on the India-Myanmar border. This decline in federal funding is mainly the result of NACO's decision in 2014 to begin bypassing NGOs and sending funds directly to state health departments, which in turn transferred funds to state-level SACSs (Gwalani, 2014; Kalra and Siddiqui, 2015; Rajshekhar, 2015). The upshot is that in Mizoram, for example, state finance officials redirected NACO funding to other social welfare programs before transferring funds to Mizoram's SACSs and NGOs. Mizoram's state finance ministry ended up transferring only 40% of the total allocated from NACO to Mizoram's SACSs and NGOs (Rajshekhar, 2015). Add to this the bureaucratic delays involved in this new federal funding process and we can see that NGOs have paid the price. In Maharashtra and Mizoram, NGO workers have had to borrow money from families and friends for the travel necessary to provide prevention and treatment services (Gwalani, 2014; Rajshekhar, 2015). Not only has this situation led to a downsizing of NGO staff in several states (Kalra and Siddiqui, 2015; Mascarenhas, 2015), but it has also damaged NGOs' trust in NACO and weakened their partnership all the more.

The outcome of all this is that unlike the national AIDS program in Brazil, India's NACO bureaucrats now have even fewer NGO allies to work with and to use to increase their legitimacy, influence, and justification for obtaining ongoing financial support from parliament (Kalra and Siddiqui, 2015; Mascarenhas, 2015). Furthermore, within a challenging decentralized context, NACO has refrained from increasing its policy influence by either contracting with NGOs to monitor SACSs' performance or implementing conditional fiscal transfer programs that could incentivize local governments to work more closely with SACSs. As we saw in Brazil, this kind of centrist policy response could help encourage local governments to implement policies more effectively.

In sum, India resembled Brazil in its delayed and initially underwhelming response to HIV/AIDS, then its stronger policy response after the emergence of international criticism and pressure. The government responded at that point so as to foster its international reputation as a modern state capable of eradicating disease while establishing close partnerships with the international donor community such as the World Bank to achieve these objectives. India's positive geopolitical positioning, fueled by a long history of foreign policy commitments to international reputation building, nonalignment, and multilateral cooperation, thus generated incentives to engage in a stronger policy response to HIV/AIDS. In contrast to what we saw in Brazil, however, India's national AIDS bureaucrats never sought to strengthen their partnership with NGOs after the government sought to increase its international reputation. Without strong bureaucratic–civil societal partnerships, the government could never achieve a centrist policy response.

Responding to Obesity

HIV/AIDS is not the only epidemic to emerge in India in recent decades. For a more complete picture of the government's commitment to meeting public health needs, it is instructive to analyze another of India's recent epidemics: new public health threats that are neither "flash epidemics" nor slow-moving chronic health conditions. Obesity poses one such challenge.

The old adage "India is a nation of contrasts" certainly rings true. While India is home to millions of people who suffer from malnourishment, hunger, and poverty, it is also home to thousands of people who are struggling with obesity—a product of economic modernity and economic growth. Within the last two decades, India has witnessed the rise of what scholars refer to as the "dual nutrition transition": burgeoning malnourishment and escalating cases of overweight and obesity among adults and, more recently, children (Gaiha, Jha, and Kulkarni, 2010; Gouda and Prusty, 2014; Shetty, 2002; Youfa Wang et al., 2009).[1] The rapid rise of the middle- and high-income classes, with an increasing demand for and consumption of unhealthy foods and drinks; technological developments that encourage sedentary lifestyles; the entry of women into the labor force, which contributed to their spending less time at home helping prepare nutritious meals and the consequent replacement of these meals with processed, high-caloric foods; a general lack of awareness about health and

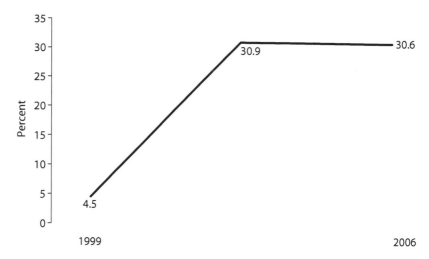

Figure 3.2. Obesity cases in India, defined as BMI >25 (percentage of population), 1999–2006. Source: WHO, Global Infobase, 2012.

nutrition; and a steady decline in physical activity—all have been perceived as contributing factors to the rise of India's obesity epidemic (*BBC News*, 2001a; Bishwajit, 2015; Gaiha, Jha, and Kulkarni, 2010; Gulati and Misra, 2014; Potarazu, 2015; Tharkar and Viswanathan, 2009). Figure 3.2 shows the increase in obesity nationwide from 1999 to 2006.

Cultural factors have also played a role. In a context where, historically, most individuals have suffered from malnourishment and stunting, for many families, gaining weight is viewed as a sign of health and prosperity (Ghosh, 2013). According to Dr. Anoop Misra, an endocrinologist specializing in childhood obesity in India, "If the child is overweight [the mothers] consider them healthy rather than fat." Misra went on to comment that "it has been handed down by grandmothers over the centuries . . . Once [their infants and children] became fat they were considered healthy" (quoted in Ghosh, 2013, 1). In fact, some studies claim that family members do not consider their children's excess weight to be a hindrance unless it hampers their daily activities (Patil et al., 2016). The consumption of sugary drinks and foods, such as Coca-Cola, Pepsi, and Nestlé products, has also become fashionable among the youth, often leading to peer pressure and children's incessant nagging of parents to purchase these foods. Parents also sometimes prefer to provide their children with prepackaged, high-caloric foods and soft drinks rather than meals sold at restaurants, mainly because of their fear that poor sanitary conditions in restaurants will make their children sick (Gulati and Misra, 2014).

In India, the rise in obesity first emerged among the privileged upper classes in major urban centers. When measured in terms of a body mass index (BMI) greater than 30, the percentage of obese adults in major cities increased between 1998 and 1999 to 9.2% in New Delhi, 3.8% in Kerala, 2.7% in Tamil Nadu, 4.3% in Goa, and 4.4% in Gujarat. For 2005–6, this percentage was 7.8% in New Delhi, 5.0% in Kerala, 5.1% in Tamil Nadu, 4.8% in Goa, and 4.6% in Gujarat (Youfa Wang et al., 2009). By 2010, the obesity rate had increased to approximately 58% of the total urban population (Gaiha, Jha, and Kulkarni, 2010).

Over time, obesity also began to emerge in poorer, rural areas, which were the historical epicenters of malnourishment and famine (Khandelwal and Reddy, 2013; Little et al., 2016; Madurai, 2016; Patil et al., 2016; Ranjani et al., 2014). This epidemiological transition was attributable to several factors, such as the arrival of sugary carbonated drinks and fatty foods, carried throughout India's vast highway system and making their way into shops in rural communities; increased access to transportation (such as motorcycles, cars, and buses) and reduced walking; and the emergence of televisions and computers, along with an increase in sedentary lifestyles (Gaiha, Jha, and Kulkarni, 2010; Unnikrishnan, Kalra, and Garg, 2012). In addition to a rise in obesity among poor rural adults, especially women (Srivastava and Rukmini, 2016), adolescents and teens also began to gain considerable weight. For example, in the state of Gujarat, in the rural city of Surat, researchers found that the number of overweight and obese adolescents exceeded the number found in Gujarat's wealthier urban centers (Kowsalya and Parimalavalli, 2014). Jiwane and Wadhva (2014) also found an 8.5% prevalence of obesity among children in rural areas of Maharashtra, and others discovered a gradual increase in childhood obesity in the rural Kochi district of Kerala (Jacob, 2014). Within the past decade, then, obesity has evolved from a condition more common among the wealthier upper classes in urban settings to one now prevalent in poorer, rural communities.

By the late 1990s, the challenge of childhood obesity also began to emerge, in tandem with the arrival of new fast food restaurants, sugary drinks, and high-caloric snacks in major cities (Rani, 2013). For example, in India's largest metropolitan city, New Delhi, researchers found that childhood overweight and obesity increased from 16% in 2002 to 24% in 2006–7 (Irwin, 2010; *Times of India*, 2007). According to the All India Institute of Medical Sciences, by 2010, obesity between the ages of 14 and 18 reached 17% for a randomized, select sample of schoolchildren in New Delhi (Dey, 2010). The number of obese children continues to increase in urban and rural areas (Madurai, 2016), with more cases being reported among poor children in urban slums and rural areas (Ranjani et al., 2014). At the same time, the number of teens between the ages of 13 and 18 who are obese increased from 16% in 2010 to 29% in 2015 (George, 2016). Studies also suggest that since 2011, approximately 22% of India's children aged between 5 and 19 are obese (Deyl, 2016).

The latest national survey results obtained from the fourth National Family Health Survey (NFHS-4, conducted in 2014–15), which was distributed by the MHFW in 13 states,[2] suggest that India's obesity epidemic has worsened (Pandey, 2016). According to this survey, from 2005 to 2015, the number of obese individuals doubled (*Pioneer*, 2016), which has earned India the title of third-most obese nation in the world (after the United States and China)—with 61 million reported cases (Anugu, 2015). The NFHS-4 survey revealed that women's obesity rates increased from 13.92% of the sampled population in 2005 to 19.56% in 2015, while men saw an increase from 10.35% to 18.04% for the same period (Srivastava and Rukmini, 2016).

Nevertheless, and as we saw with HIV/AIDS, the government did not immediately respond to the obesity epidemic. Although overweight and obesity issues were increasing throughout the 1990s, the office of the prime minister and the MHFW did not view the issue as an urgent public health threat, for several reasons. For years, public health officials were fixated on eradicating undernutrition, childhood malnourishment, and poverty (Irwin, 2010; Shukdev, 2008). By 2010, it was reported that more than 180 million chronically malnourished children lived in India, and 55% of preschool children were underweight (*Economic Times*, 2010). With Prime Minister Manmohan Singh (2004–14) publicly stating that malnutrition was India's biggest public shame (Khandelwal and Reddy, 2013), it is no wonder that India's most senior politicians and ministry of health officials placed most of their focus on eradicating malnutrition and poverty. This was reflected in an increased level of government spending to address this issue—a focus that made it nearly impossible for MHFW officials to immediately respond to obesity (Irwin, 2010).

Obesity was perceived by most senior government and health officials as a class-based issue, confined to the rich and the growing middle class (Irwin, 2010; Shukdev, 2008), who were deemed perfectly capable of taking care of themselves. Furthermore, as mentioned earlier, in a historical context of malnourishment and poverty, being overweight was considered to be a good thing: "In a country with so many undernourished people, those who could afford it wanted their children to look plump and healthy, not realizing that plump and pink children become plump and pink adults who die by the time they hit 40," commented Prema Ramachandran, director of the Nutrition Foundation of India (quoted in Brown-Polaris, 2004, 2). Some observers note that this perspective created few incentives for the prime minister and parliament to enact national legislation (Reddy et al., 2005; Shukdev, 2008). Moreover, obesity was still not on the international agenda, as the WHO and other organizations were primarily focused on addressing HIV/AIDS and tobacco-related illnesses in India (*BBC News*, 2001b). When combined with a dearth of national surveys and data (Irwin, 2010; Reddy et al., 2005), these factors convinced the government that there was no need for an immediate response to obesity.

Constructing an MHFW agency focused exclusively on obesity, while providing financial and technical assistance to the states, was deemed highly unlikely. A lack of parliamentary funding for those agencies attempting to create obesity awareness and prevention campaigns exacerbated the situation (Reddy, 2003; Reddy et al., 2005). At the same time, state health departments and hospitals did not have the resources needed to address obesity and its associated ailments, such as type 2 diabetes, high blood pressure, and heart disease (*BBC News*, 2001b). The absence of federal financial support imposed a constricting burden on state health departments (Reddy et al., 2005). In short, the parliament failed to provide both national and subnational support to combat the burgeoning obesity epidemic (Reddy, 2003; Reddy et al., 2005).

International Criticism, Pressure, and Reputation Building

A flurry of international criticism and pressure emerged in reaction to the government's lackluster policy response. In 2001, the BBC published an article claiming that for a nation troubled by malnourishment and poverty, it was perplexing to see the depth of India's obesity problems (*BBC News*, 2001a). The article went on to state that if the government did not engage in a stronger policy response, obesity rates would triple by 2025.

The brunt of international criticism and pressure emerged in 2004 with release of the WHO report *Global Strategy on Diet, Physical Activity, and Health*. In this report, WHO officials singled out India as having one of the worst cases of obesity, especially among children, and gave it the embarrassing designation of a country with the world's largest number of diabetes cases (Varshney, 2006). The *Global Strategy* of 2004 urged India to adopt the WHO's recommendations for a dramatic reduction of sugary content in foods, better food labeling and nutrition standards, more regulation, and even the imposition of a "snack tax" (Varshney, 2006; S. Rao, 2004). At the end of 2004, the WHO released yet another report claiming that India had failed to adhere to several of its recommendations, especially with regard to working with the private sector, NGOs, and other government agencies (S. Rao, 2004). Adding further criticism were research articles in the *Lancet* and *Nature Medicine* in 2005 and 2006 claiming that India and China had the greatest number of obesity and diabetes cases in the world and that if policy did not change, India would outpace the United States in the total number of deaths attributable to obesity and its related ailments (Reddy et al., 2005; Yach, Stuckler, and Brownell, 2006). Additionally, in 2006, the WHO singled out India as being the perfect "test lab" for experimenting with anti-obesity programs (Varshney, 2006). Within just six years, then, from 2001 to 2006, India's government confronted a mass of international criticism and pressure for a more aggressive policy response.

As with its response to HIV/AIDS, the government of India had several reasons for positively responding to this international criticism and improving its international reputation. For the same geopolitical reasons of passing muster as an effective emerging nation with international clout and influence (Bhava, 2007; Jabeen, 2010), the government was targeting the advanced industrialized western nations, international organizations such as the WHO and the World Bank, and western academic researchers and the media. Indeed, India wanted to show the West that it had the technical and infrastructural capacity needed to curb the spread of obesity and, in the process, would demonstrate that the MHFW could overcome this health threat and prosper. In February 2000, for example, the government worked with researchers in Mumbai to hold India's first international conference on obesity. According to the *Times of India* (2000), this was the largest obesity conference ever held in Asia. Researchers and health officials from several Asian countries, as well as the United States, Britain, and other European nations, attended. At this conference, Indian health officials and researchers had an opportunity to display their research and policy initiatives for reducing the number of obesity cases in urban centers, while addressing the causes of obesity and myths about how obesity spreads. This conference was India's first attempt to unveil to the world its research capabilities and commitment to addressing the epidemic (*Times of India*, 2000).

When it came to combating chronic illnesses, especially nutritional issues, India had a rich tradition of responding quickly to these problems since the 1950s. In fact, in 1957, it was the first nation to work with and warn the World Health Assembly of an inevitable future epidemic of chronic disease in the developing world, such as cancer, high blood pressure, and diabetes (S. Rao, 2004). Similarly, after the UN World Summit for Children in 1990 and the World Declaration and Plan of Action for Nutrition in 1992, Indian health officials worked with UN colleagues to develop India's first National Nutrition Policy in 1993, thus revealing the government's proactive commitment to working with the UN to address nutritional disorders among children. At that time, however, overweight and obesity were not a government priority (Khandelwal and Reddy, 2013). And as had occurred in the past with India's warnings to the World Health Assembly about the growing tide of noncommunicable diseases, in 2004 India's health officials were once again eager to work with the WHO in helping draft its *Global Strategy*. In the process, they worked closely with other nations to share knowledge and ideas about how to tackle obesity and several different types of noncommunicable diseases (Irwin, 2010). In 2006, shortly after India adopted the WHO's 2004 guidelines, MHFW officials, nutritionists, and activists invited members of the Global Alliance for the Prevention of Obesity and Related Chronic Disease to India to explore how the government could go about implementing the *Global Strategy*'s guidelines (Varshney, 2006). Thus, in sum, as in the AIDS epidemic, the government maintained its foreign policy tradition of working closely with other nations to contain a new public health threat—a key element of the government's positive geopolitical positioning.

The government did not take other nations' criticism and pressure lightly. Despite contributing to its initial drafting, India's prime minister and the MHFW did not immediately agree with the WHO's 2004 *Global Strategy*. The notion that foods high in sugary content should be scaled back did not comport with the government's belief that thousands of manual day laborers needed these sugary foods for extra energy to work; that the WHO's recommendation of a "snack tax" would make food too costly for the poor; and that regulating fast food would impinge on individual liberties (India, Government, 2004; S. Rao, 2004).

As international criticism mounted, however—including the special WHO report of 2004 stating that India had failed to create a multisectoral response to diet and obesity (S. Rao, 2004) and similar criticisms in a special issue of the *Lancet* in 2005 (Reddy et al., 2005)—the MHFW began to respond. In the spring of 2006, the ministry started to work with other health agencies to create a more aggressive policy response (Irwin, 2010; Reddy et al., 2005). The MHFW also started to collaborate with the private sector, nutritionists, and activists to devise a coordinated national strategy for noncommunicable diseases, which adopted most of the WHO's 2004 *Global Strategy* recommendations (Irwin, 2010; Reddy et al., 2005). MHFW officials also started to work with medical doctors and academics to devise new prevention policies that could be adopted by state governments (Varshney, 2006). And in 2006, the government released a report stating that it was wholeheartedly committed to creating an effective national response, focused on monitoring at-risk groups and prevention (India, Government, 2006). In fact, to expedite policy reforms, the report claimed that the MHFW should lead on this issue, with state governments eventually following suit—tailoring each response to India's unique cultural and economic contexts (India, Government, 2006). In 2007, the MHFW began meeting with health officials from the United States and the United Kingdom to learn from them how it could strengthen its response to obesity (*Hindu*, 2007).

In 2007, the MHFW also created policies to enhance its ability to monitor overweight and obese individuals. In that year, two major national surveillance programs were piloted by the MHFW: the WHO–Indian Council of Medical Research noncommunicable disease risk factor surveillance study and the Integrated Disease Surveillance Project (2007–8). These programs conducted surveys in several states, revealing the increased prevalence of hypertension, diabetes, and obesity in urban and rural areas (Khandelwal and Reddy, 2013). Furthermore, in 2008, in response to the 2004 *Global Strategy* and a 2006 follow-up conference in Geneva, the MHFW reformulated its BMI indices based on its own population's unique genetic profile. India's medical community maintained that, biologically, the typical Indian was more prone to creating and storing fat than were western Caucasians and East Asians (iGovernment, 2008). Because of this, Indian health scientists questioned the accuracy of the WHO's obesity guidelines, which stated that a BMI of 25–30 indicated overweight, and a BMI above 30 indicated obesity (Mudur, 2008). MHFW officials believed that these rates inaccurately measured the Indian population, as most of the health complications associated with overweight and obesity were seen at lower BMIs (*Lancet*, 2004). Consequently, MHFW officials reformulated their BMI index to state that overweight fell between a BMI of 23 and 25, with anyone having a BMI over 25 considered obese (Mudur, 2008). Given its importance to more accurately monitoring and anticipating obesity-related illnesses, "this revision has been long overdue," commented Dr. Anoop Misra, head of the diabetes and metabolic diseases division of the Fortis Hospital in New Delhi (quoted in Mudur, 2008, 1).

In 2008, new national prevention programs were created. The Ministry of Women and Children's Development, for example, introduced a nutritional program focused on diet and better exercise. This ministry also started devising new guidelines for better diets in schools (Parth, 2008). And in an effort to better monitor and control diseases directly associated with obesity, in January 2008 the MHFW piloted the National Program for the Prevention and Control of Diabetes, Cardiovascular Disease, and Stroke (NPCDCS) (Khandelwal and Reddy, 2013; WHO, 2009b).

The NPCDCS was designated as the primary federal program working on preventing overweight and obesity as health risks for diabetes, cardiovascular disease, and stroke (Bloom et al., 2014; Salve, 2014). The NPCDCS was designed as a vertical program, mainly managed, financed, and implemented by the MHFW, working through the National Rural Health Mission's decentralized approach to public health provision (i.e., taking advantage of the large network of the mission's primary healthcare workers at the local level), and in full cooperation with the state health departments (Bloom et al., 2014). The NPCDCS was focused on achieving several outcomes: early diagnosis and management of noncommunicable diseases; prevention and control of such diseases through the promotion of behavioral lifestyle changes; strengthening of health systems' capacity; additional training for healthcare personnel, especially primary care workers and nurses; and proactive detection and treatment of noncommunicable disease risk factors, such as overweight and obesity (Bloom et al., 2014).

In 2010, the MHFW also wrote affidavits to the New Delhi High Court stating that junk food causes health problems, including heart disease. Through the federal courts, the MHFW asked state chief ministers (i.e., the governors) to impose new nutrition guidelines in all schools, while requesting university administrators to withdraw all junk foods and carbonated drinks from cafeterias (Indo-Asian New Service, 2011). This was the first time that the central government had requested the chief ministers to proactively increase their attention and response to obesity.

In 2011, the MHFW decided to expand the NPCDCS program to all of the states as part of the Twelfth Five-Year Plan (2012–17) (Bloom et al., 2014). Expanding this program also reflected the government's desire to be in compliance with the WHO's 2011 High Level Meeting on Non-Communicable Diseases, thus underscoring the government's commitment to working with the WHO and solidifying India's reputation for upholding the organization's policy recommendations. Still managed and mainly financed by the MHFM in New Delhi, the NPCDCS is currently being implemented in 20,000 subnational health centers and 700 community health centers in 100 districts across 15 states. Approximately 32,000 healthcare personnel will be trained to provide screening and diagnosis of noncommunicable diseases and their risk factors, including overweight and obesity (Bloom et al., 2014).

Reinvigorated and ready to tackle childhood obesity, in 2014, Prime Minister Modi's governing BJP proclaimed its commitment to increasing regulation of the fast food industry and improving children's health. In accordance with the 2004 *Global Strategy* guidelines, the prime minister considered introducing a ban on the sale of junk food in schools, an increase in the price of sugary drinks, and a proposed 40% "sin tax" on sodas (Deyl, 2016; Prasad, 2014). In 2015, following an injunction filed by the Uday Foundation in 2010 and the Supreme Court of India's subsequent upholding of it, the Court ordered the Food Safety and Standards Authority of India (a government agency) to draft guidelines ensuring the availability of wholesome and nutritious foods in schools and to decrease the consumption of fatty foods (Khandelwal and Reddy, 2013; *Pioneer*, 2016). Once these guidelines were received, in 2015 the Supreme Court ordered the Central Board of Secondary Education to consider issuing directions to schools for implementing these guidelines (Menon, 2016). Some of the guideline's stipulations were to restrict the sale of high-fat, salty, and sugary foods (e.g., pizzas, chips, sodas, and chocolate bars) within 50 meters of a school's premises; prohibit the marketing of these foods to children on television; prohibit the appearance of sports and television stars in junk food commercials; and provide more informative nutritional content on product labels (Thekaekara, 2015). These Food Safety and Standards Authority guidelines were followed up with recommendations from the Ministry of Women and Children's Development in 2015 requiring that vendors within a 200-meter radius of schools refrain from selling junk food to children in uniforms (*TakePart*, 2015).

In contrast to what we saw with HIV/AIDS, the government was not committed to building on its stronger policy response to obesity by providing multilateral and/or bilateral aid in the area of obesity prevention in order to enhance its international reputation. To date, the MHFW has not introduced any foreign aid efforts to help developing nations combat the rising tide of childhood and adult obesity or the health ailments associated with it. As in Brazil, the only related foreign policy endeavor has been India's effort to help other nations in ensuring food security through investments in agricultural production, farming, and overall improvements in nutrition (Sridharan, 2014).

Were international criticism, pressure, and reputation building the main reasons that the government finally decided to increase its policy response to obesity? Several other factors could have contributed to this outcome. First, the Congress (I) Party, eager to regain political power in 2004, could have proactively campaigned on obesity. In fact, by the mid-1990s, obesity, especially childhood obesity, was of increased interest and concern among families throughout India (Joshi, 1995). However, the Congress (I) never referred to obesity during its electoral campaign. The campaign was instead focused on poverty alleviation, economic growth, and a return to secularism in politics (Kronstadt, 2004). Second, perhaps it was the government's realization during the early to mid-2000s of a burgeoning obesity epidemic that motivated its response. But this explanation does not hold either, as the MHFW and researchers in New Delhi had been reporting to parliament and the international community for several years on the nation's escalating overweight and obesity problem (Gaiha, Jha and Kulkarni, 2010). Finally, perhaps it was the increasing obesity among the influential upper- and middle-income classes in urban centers that triggered fears and a government response. Among all the possibilities, this seems the most likely, given that in India, the highest urban obesity rates are found among the upper-income classes. But there is very little evidence supporting this notion. As I discuss in more detail shortly, there were no well-organized obesity NGOs or civil societal organizations led by these individuals that consistently pressured parliament for policy reforms, nor was there a close partnership between NGOs and parliament (S. Rao, 2004). Most NGOs in India are composed of public health and nutrition experts, not wealthy, influential, obese individuals (Brown-Polaris, 2004).

Notwithstanding the government's new policy efforts, several challenges remain. Decentralization and its accompanying resource limitations have again emerged to limit state governments' ability to introduce innovative obesity prevention programs (Reddy et al., 2005). There is an ongoing lack of sufficient financial and infrastructural resources at the local level to keep up with the heightened demand for hospital treatments for obesity-related illnesses such as hypertension, coronary heart disease, and type 2 diabetes, and the states vary considerably in their ability to fund healthcare programs (Gómez, 2015b; Leowski and Krishnan, 2009). The lack of federal assistance to the states to help overcome these challenges is further compounded by national interagency fragmentation and conflict over which agency should be responsible for creating and implementing obesity prevention programs (Irwin, 2010). In addition, researchers question whether the MHFW and state health departments have the commitment necessary to enforce the program's policy regulations, effectively use federal funding, and coordinate with all of the states to achieve full implementation (Bloom et al., 2014; Sengupta, 2013).

Indeed, while the Modi government is verbally committed to reducing obesity, especially among children, pundits claim that few concrete efforts have been made to finance and to work with the states in implementing the national surveillance and prevention programs described above—highlighting a general lack of political will (Gulati and Misra, 2014). While MHFW officials did request that chief ministers and state health departments pursue certain policies, such as banning fatty foods in schools (which comports with 2011 WHO policy recommendations), there were no subsequent efforts to ensure that these policies were enforced (Khandelwal and Reddy, 2013). Moreover, neither the government's fiscal policy suggestions, such as a 40% tax on sugary products, nor the Food Safety and Standards Authority of India guidelines and Ministry of Women and Children's Development suggestions for banning the sale of junk foods to children in school uniforms have been enforced (*Takepart*, 2015). What's more, most policies focused on prevention, especially for children, have been created as pilot programs introduced by local school districts, with essentially no financial and administrative guidance from the MHFW. In contrast to what we saw in Brazil, there have been few if any MHFW-administered and -financed childhood obesity prevention programs (Ranjani et al., 2014).

Finally, the MHFW was never able to secure sufficient funding for its national obesity prevention programs (Reddy et al., 2005). Parliamentary support has been marginal at best, ranging from an allocated budget of Rs 292.5 million (rupees crores) for the 2014–15 budgetary year, decreasing to Rs 235 million (rupees crores) for 2015–16, then slightly increasing to Rs 300.00 million (rupees crores) for the 2016–17 year (India, Ministry of Health and Family Welfare, 2016). Moreover, most of the money allocated for the NPCDCS, the primary agency responsible for obesity and noncommunicable disease prevention, is allocated for other specific diseases. For example, approximately 40% of the funds for the Twelfth Five-Year Plan (2012–17) was allocated to cancer (Bloom et al., 2014). In a context where the MHFW has agreed to a cost-sharing arrangement with state health departments of 80% to 20%, respectively, for funding implementation of the NPCDCS (Bloom et al., 2014), securing federal funding is a priority. And yet, the parliament and MHFW have been inconsistent in this regard, providing insufficient funds to meet growing policy needs at the state level.

And finally, despite the challenges associated with healthcare decentralization and the need to work with state health departments to ensure effective policy implementation, MHFW bureaucrats never strove to work closely with NGOs to achieve this objective. This resulted in the MHFW's inability to leverage those organizations to exercise and maintain some authority over the states. According to several NGO leaders that I interviewed, MHFW bureaucrats never tried to contract with them to monitor what local governments were doing in response to obesity (Jagannivas, 2013; D. Krishnan, 2013; Singh, 2013). This monitoring strategy could have helped to increase state health departments' accountability to the MSFW, thus facilitating policy implementation. Given the high level of fiscal dependence of state health departments on the MHFW for financing specific public health programs designed at the national level (India, Ministry of Health and Family Welfare, 2005), this kind of accountability process could have created further incentives for state health departments to respond to obesity more aggressively.

In sum, as we saw with HIV/AIDS, the government was never capable of achieving a centrist policy response to obesity. Parliamentary funding and administrative expansion for the MHFW's obesity programs has been minimal, limited national prevention programs have been pursued, and no effort has been made to formally increase MHFW's influence over state health departments to ensure effective policy implementation either through conditional fiscal grant transfers or by contracting NGOs to monitor policy and hold state health departments accountable.

Why did the government fail to achieve a centrist policy response? Given its positive geopolitical positioning and its consequent interest in international reputation building while working closely with the international community, shouldn't these factors have been sufficient for such a response? As we saw with the government's response to HIV/AIDS, however, these conditions on their own were insufficient for engendering a centrist policy response. What is also needed is the presence of strong bureaucratic–civil societal partnerships.

The Absence of Strong Bureaucratic–Civil Societal Partnerships

Beginning in 2001, several NGOs were created in India to focus explicitly on obesity and its related illnesses. These organizations included the All India Association for Advancing Research on Obesity (2008), the Obesity Foundation of India (*Hindu*, 2007), the Nutrition Foundation of India (Brown-Polaris, 2004), the Association for the Study of Obesity (HealthJockey, 2007), and the Centre for Science and the Environment (Centre for Science and Environment, 2017). All of these organizations are focused on increasing awareness, conducting research, and working with the government, private sector, and other NGOs while organizing social events, creating websites for online dating, and aggressively picketing fast food restaurants and companies—the Obesity Foundation's well-known "human chaining" efforts in front of the Pepsi and Coca-Cola headquarters in New Delhi provides a good example (*Hindu*, 2009b). Several beauty and nutrition centers, such as Vandana Luthra Curls and Curves Center, which combines beautician studies with nutrition, exercise, and women's empowerment, emerged throughout the country (*New Indian Express*, 2010). In 2009, Vandana Luthra Curls and Curves Center worked with NGOs and the private sector to establish November 26 as India's official "anti-obesity day" (Sagar, 2001). Other NGOs have focused on diseases associated with obesity, such as the Diabetes Foundation and the National Diabetes, Obesity, and Cholesterol Foundation; these have been proactive in organizing international conferences (Diabetes Foundation, 2010; *Mail Today*, 2010).

Despite this vibrant civil societal response, several problems emerged. MHFW officials working on obesity made no effort to cultivate a closer partnership with these NGOs (*Mail Today*, 2011; S. Rao, 2004). While the NGOs and the nutritional scientific community tried to approach the MHFW about being more proactive in working with them for a policy response, nutrition experts claimed that they could not get health officials' attention or obtain resources (Khandelwal and Reddy, 2013). Consequently, these NGOs were left to work on their own, mainly with local schools, to help increase awareness, provide healthy eating suggestions, and promote physical fitness (*Mail Today*, 2011). At no point have MHFW bureaucrats tried to work closely with NGOs to achieve these objectives or partner with them to monitor policy implementation at the local level, as mentioned earlier. The MHFW's commitment to working with NGOs, families, and schools and carefully meeting their needs is questionable, considering the extent to which the ministry is negatively influenced by countervailing private sector interests.

For example, the MHFW recently created the Reproductive, Maternal, Newborn and Child Health Coalition (RMNCH), a network of health officials, NGOs, activists, university researchers, media, and representatives of international donors and UN agencies (Prasad, 2014). The RMNCH's mandate is to advocate for policy programs and achieve improved outcomes for the coalition—one outcome, of course, being improved nutrition (WHO, 2012). However, the government knows full well that the children's rights NGO in charge of managing the RMNCH, Save the Children, is funded by private corporations such as Pepsi, Coca-Cola, Britannia, and several pharmaceutical companies (WHO, 2012). It is well known that Coca-Cola has vehemently opposed the introduction of a proposed "sin tax" on its products, claiming that this will hinder its production process as well as its ability to hire local workers, while potentially disincentivizing future foreign investment (Chilkoti, 2014). This, of course, poses a considerable conflict of interest, given the private sector's desire to avoid potential regulatory and fiscal policies that are against their interests, and further questions the government's commitment to truly representing the needs of society.

We should also consider the fact that patronage politics may be accounting for parliament's unwillingness to increase spending for national obesity programs. It may be the case, for example, that the powerful corporate interest groups are pressuring committees in parliament not to increase spending for initiatives such as a soda tax or the regulation of the fast food industry. Though not the focus of this chapter, this issue certainly warrants further investigation.

Further complicating matters is the fact that, in India, none of the obesity NGOs have historical predecessors—that is, social health movements and/or civic organizations in the past that were dedicated to working closely with national health bureaucrats, proffering ideas for immediate, centralized bureaucratic policy responses to weight-related issues. Instead, and as we saw with the response to HIV/AIDS, the civic organizations of the past, focused on combating poverty and malnourishment, worked from an isolated, community-based, grassroots perspective (Andharia, 2009). The upshot to this historical context is that NGOs working on obesity did not have the experience and successful track record needed to legitimize MHFW bureaucrats and to work with them to improve the bureaucrats' ability to secure ongoing funding from parliament. This may be why MHFW bureaucrats were unwilling to partner with these NGOs.

Obesity in India has now emerged as a serious public health issue. As we saw with the government's response to HIV/AIDS, for a variety of reasons—ranging from the fight to tackle malnourishment to the absence of credible and convincing epidemiological data and preexisting government commitments to healthcare decentralization—the central government did not immediately respond to the obesity epidemic. Nevertheless, the rise of international criticism and pressure beginning in 2004, as well as the government's interest in collaborating with the WHO in addressing its own and other nations' obesity challenges, prompted a stronger policy response in obesity prevention. This marked an important advantage associated with India's positive geopolitical positioning. For the time being, obesity appears to occupy a prominent position on the national agenda.

Nevertheless, and, again, as we saw with HIV/AIDS, the parliament has not been sufficiently committed to increasing funding for the MHFW's obesity programs and initiatives to allow a centrist policy response. It seems that one of the reasons that this has occurred is the unwillingness of MHFW bureaucrats to establish strong partnerships with NGOs after the government strove to increase its international reputation through a stronger policy response. While NGOs and other civic and private sector organizations have recently emerged to draw attention to obesity and its associated ailments, they are too few in number and lack collective influence. Without a strong partnership with NGOs, MHFW bureaucrats have not been able to introduce innovative programs, induce state health departments to comply with national policies, or work with NGOs to monitor policy implementation and hold state governments accountable—the ingredients of a strong centrist policy response.

Conclusion

In response to increased international criticism and pressure, India's political leaders instituted a stronger policy response to HIV/AIDS and obesity in order to improve the government's international reputation in health. To facilitate the reform process, these leaders pursued international financial and technical assistance, eventually providing foreign aid to help other nations combat HIV/AIDS while enhancing the government's international reputation. Influenced by a deep foreign policy tradition of sensitivity to world opinion, reputation building, and peaceful multilateral partnerships with other nations, these efforts reflected the government's positive geopolitical positioning. However, and in contrast to what we saw in Brazil, in the absence of a strong partnership with NGOs working on HIV/AIDS and obesity, MHFW bureaucrats have not proved capable of creating a centrist policy response. This has limited the MHFW's ability to ensure that prevention and treatment policies were effectively implemented, especially in a context of healthcare decentralization processes.

NOTES

1. While the number of obese children in India has increased, we must keep in mind that more than one-third of the world's malnourished children live in India (Varadharajan, Thomas, and Kurpad, 2013).

2. The surveyed states were Andhra Pradesh, Bihar, Goa, Haryana, Karnataka, Madhya Pradesh, Meghalaya, Sikkim, Tamil Nadu, Telangana, Tripura, Uttarakhand, West Bengal, and the two Union Territories of Andaman and Nicobarese Islands and Puducherry.

4

China's Response to HIV/AIDS and Obesity

In the late 1980s, while making efforts to strengthen its economy and political institutions, China joined Brazil and India in confronting the HIV/AIDS and obesity epidemics. Like the governments of Brazil and India, China's government did not immediately engage in a strong policy response; China would only achieve this after the arrival of criticism and pressure from influential international institutions such as the WHO and the UN. Building on a foreign policy tradition of striving to build the government's international reputation and peaceful partnerships with other nations, the governing elites eventually pursued a stronger policy response to HIV/AIDS and obesity in order to enhance China's international reputation as a modern state capable of eradicating disease and of developing. These reputation-building interests would later incentivize the government to provide foreign aid assistance for HIV/AIDS programs in other developing nations. The government's positive geopolitical positioning therefore mattered considerably, fostering not only stronger policy reforms and global health diplomacy but also the pursuit of financial and technical assistance from the World Bank to sustain China's domestic reform efforts.

Nevertheless, the government was not capable of pursuing a centrist policy response for HIV/AIDS and obesity. This reflects the absence of a strong bureaucratic–civil societal partnership and thus the bureaucracy's inability to garner support for innovative programs and initiatives that would augment its capacity to ensure effective policy implementation at the provincial government level. While the government eventually sought to use NGOs as effective "arms of the state," that is, in helping the central and provincial governments provide prevention and treatment services in hard-to-reach (mainly rural) areas and among at-risk groups, beyond this, there never emerged an ongoing effort by AIDS bureaucrats to develop a strong sense of solidarity and cooperation with NGOs (especially with those not affiliated with the government) and to strategically use this partnership to advance the bureaucracy's position within government.

Responding to HIV/AIDS

The first reported case of HIV/AIDS in China emerged in 1985, when a tourist from Argentina was diagnosed in northern China. The first indigenous cases were found among IDUs in 1989, in the province of Yennan, nestled along the Mayaram border. By the mid-1990s, AIDS had spread to hundreds of poor farmers in central China through contaminated blood supplies, as indigent farmers often sold their blood plasma and then required reinjection of blood (N. Li et al., 2010; Wu, Rou, and Cui, 2004). Because of poor surveillance, politicians' cover-up of the epidemic, and the black market for transfusable blood—mainly due to the central government's 1988 drug importation ban (Lei and Wu-Kui, 2008)—the virus spread quickly among blood transfusion recipients in rural areas. By the late 1990s, infection through heterosexual sex also began to rise, while cases among gay men and sex workers rose in the 2000s (Lei and Wu-Kui, 2008; L. Wang, 2007; Wu, Rou, and Cui, 2004). The trajectory of HIV/AIDS in China is shown in figure 4.1.

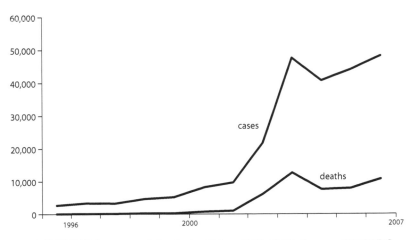

Figure 4.1. HIV/AIDS cases and deaths in China, 1997–2007. Source: UNAIDS, 2008. *2008 Update. China. Epidemiological Fact Sheet on HIV and AIDS.*

The government's initial response was divided. The premier, president, and MOH officials believed that HIV/AIDS was a foreign disease, transferred from immoral, capitalist, foreign travelers (Y. Huang, 2006; Kaufman, 2010; Knutsen, 2012; Wu et al., 2004). Once word got out that the virus was spreading through extramarital sex and drug use, Party and senior MOH officials claimed there was simply no way AIDS could have come from China. The cultural revolution of the 1960s, government leaders held, had cleansed Chinese society of such atrocious, immoral acts. It was also believed that Confucian conservatism, especially in the realm of sexual activity, safeguarded China from AIDS (Knutsen, 2012; H. Zhang, 2004). The government therefore initially viewed people living with HIV/AIDS as "social deviants," "immoral sinners," the naughty and disgusting "other them," partakers of forbidden western vices. The virus was often referred to as *AIZibing*, the "loving capitalist disease" (*People's Daily Online*, 2009). Those afflicted with *AIZibing* were perceived not only as social deviants but as traitors to communist China, having acquiesced to the sinful nature of western capitalist ways (Y. Huang, 2006). This was a public and social manifestation of the conservative moral tenets that shaped the rise of elite perceptions within the Communist Party. This initial stance toward HIV/AIDS shaped the government's first policy response to the epidemic: to test all foreign travelers planning to stay in China for more than one year, quarantine people living with HIV/AIDS, and deny and cover up the problem (Y. Huang, 2006; Kaufman, 2010; Knutsen, 2012).

MOH officials also believed there simply was not enough credible epidemiological evidence to warrant an immediate government response. By the late 1980s, only a handful of AIDS cases had been reported throughout China, and most were located in the hinterland, among the rural poor. HIV/AIDS was quickly classified as a type B infectious disease and, in a context of multiple diseases and health challenges, was not seen as a serious national threat (Y. Huang, 2006). Furthermore, there was little evidence suggesting that AIDS was affecting the military (D. Thompson, 2003).

All of these attitudes conflicted with the views of several concerned MOH officials. Though marginalized and often ignored, like their counterparts in Brazil and India, these officials viewed the epidemic as urgent and worthy of an immediate policy response (Y. Huang, 2006; Kaufman, 2010). They pushed the envelope to propose not only several prevention and awareness campaigns but also the creation of a centralized AIDS bureaucracy. For instance, in 1989, Minister of Health Chen Minzhang submitted a report to the State Council asking for the creation of a national AIDS organization to coordinate the government's response (Y. Huang, 2006). The State Council rejected the proposal on the grounds that only 260 HIV infections had been reported in the country (Y. Huang, 2006). The MOH reformers also brushed aside their moral reservations and tried to work closely with high-risk groups, striving to provide prevention and treatment in any way they could. By 1991, they had succeeded in creating China's first National AIDS Counseling Center in Beijing. But once the State Council found out that its director, Wan Yanhai, was trying to reach out to the gay community by establishing telephone hotlines, she was fired and the center was shut down (Y. Huang, 2006).

By the early 1990s, MOH reformers realized they were not going to get the support they needed. Providing adequate fiscal and technical support to the provinces was simply out of the question, given the emphasis on decentralized public health provision (Kaufman, Kleinman, and Saich, 2006; Y. Liu and Kaufman, 2006). In fact, and as we saw in Brazil and India, the provinces were initially left to respond to HIV/AIDS on their own. State government politicians were nevertheless just as discriminatory and repressive as their central government counterparts. And provincial health officials received essentially no financial or technical assistance from Beijing (Kaufman, Kleinman, and Saich, 2006; Y. Liu and Kaufman, 2006). Within this politically contested and divisive context, MOH officials' ability to secure government funding was even less, and consensus building and timely implementation of policies were essentially impossible (Y. Huang, 2006).

Despite these challenges, there was a national policy response, but it was shaped more by the State Council and its provincial policy views than by reform-minded MOH bureaucrats. Indeed, as early as 1986, the State Council created a phalanx of national committees, laws, regulations, and stipulations. It was a time of aggressive state building through the enactment of laws and regulations, seemingly done to manage the HIV/AIDS situation through top-down monitoring, control, and condemnation.

In 1986, for example, the State Council created its own Working Group on the Prevention of AIDS, within the MOH, cosponsored with the China Academy of Preventive Medicine (Knutsen, 2012). In 1988, the council created the Regulations Concerning the Monitoring and Control of AIDS, and in 1989, the People's Representative Committee passed the Law on Infectious Diseases, Priority and Control—which essentially quarantined individuals with AIDS (Wu, Rou, and Cui, 2004). In 1990, the council created the National

Expert Committee on HIV/AIDS Prevention and Control (Knutsen, 2012), followed in 1991 by the National AIDS Counseling Center, through the MOH (Y. Huang, 2006). In 1995, it also devised the Recommendations on Strengthening AIDS Prevention and Control, which essentially developed new laws and regulations for policy enforcement (Wu, Rou, and Cui, 2004). And in 1996, while creating the Responsibilities of Ministries and Departments of State in AIDS Control, the council also created the State Council on AIDS/STD Prevention Coordinating Committee (Y. Huang, 2006; Wu, Rou, and Cui, 2004), which sought to increase interagency coordination. This was followed in the same year by the State Council's Mid- to Long-Term Plan for AIDS Control, which emphasized blood safety, education, behavioral intervention, and care; the vice premier's AIDS Coordinating Committee; and the council and MOH's Principles for AIDS Education and Prevention Messages. These were followed in 2001 by the Plan of Action for Containment and Control of AIDS (2001–5) (Wu, Rou, and Cui, 2004).

In sum, there was a myriad of national regulations, laws, coordination committees, and official plans to administer a top-down eradication of HIV/AIDS. Nevertheless, and in sharp contrast to what we saw in Brazil and India, no single, autonomous, national AIDS bureaucracy was created within the MOH to coordinate all of these endeavors. Moreover, this slew of institutional initiatives revealed that much "discussion," "advising," and "planning" were going on but little concrete action (Y. Huang, 2006; Knutsen, 2012; Wu, Rou, and Cui, 2004), convincing some that China's institutional and policy initiatives were "hollow" (Knutsen, 2012).

The State Council's lack of attention to prevention and treatment further revealed its intent of giving the impression that it was effectively responding to HIV/AIDS, when in reality it was not. By 1991, the government had closed down China's first National AIDS Counseling Center (Y. Huang, 2006). No national program for the distribution of condoms or needle syringes was introduced, save for two brief experimental trial programs—one for condom distribution in 1997 and another for clean needle exchange in 1999 (Knutsen, 2012; Wu, Rou, and Cui, 2004). Commercial programs on condom use were introduced in 1999, but were banned that same year because of the State Council's view that this was inappropriate (Kaufman, 2010). An experimental program provided sex and AIDS education for all college freshmen—sponsored and controlled by the 1995 Recommendations on Strengthening AIDS Prevention and Control—but no national program for sex and AIDS education in high schools was provided (Lei and Wu-Kui, 2008). And finally, there was no national program to provide universal ARV treatment or care for families. Though the Medium- to Long-Term Plan recommended this, the government's first attempt to provide ARVs was in the following year, and even then it was "fee for service" care, not freely provided (Dechamp and Couzin, 2006; Y. Liu and Kaufman, 2006).

International Pressure and Positive Geopolitical Positioning

The government's lackluster response to HIV/AIDS eventually garnered much of the international community's attention. By the early 1990s, international views on China's response became rather critical. In 1994, for example, Michael Merson, then executive director of the WHO's Global AIDS Program, stated that China needed to hasten its response to AIDS, emphasizing the need for greater sex education and condom use (Y. Huang, 2006). By the late 1990s, Kofi Annan, then UN secretary general, was also reported to have raised the AIDS issue every time he met with Jiang Zemin (Knutsen, 2012). In 2001, the UNAIDS office in Beijing released a report titled *China's Titanic Peril*, projecting that more than one million people were likely to be infected with AIDS and that 10 million might be infected by 2010 (Wu et al., 2007). MOH officials immediately rejected the report, claiming that China would never see such numbers by 2010 (Y. Huang, 2006, 2010a). The report, of course, caused "an uproar in other parts of China's government" (Kaufman, 2010, 74). As if that were not enough, the next year the US National Intelligence Council published *The Next Wave of HIV/AIDS: Nigeria, Ethiopia, Russia, India, and China*, highlighting these nations' poor policy responses to AIDS (Kaufman, 2010).

China's leaders were very sensitive to all of this international criticism. As a former senior Chinese foreign minister claimed: "China is history's most self-conscious rising power" (J. Lee, 2009, 1). China was incessantly worried about its government's image, viewing international reputation building as a key to its domestic development and geopolitical importance (Goldstein, 2001; J. Zhang and Cameron, 2002). Like Brazil and India, China was concerned with maintaining a good reputation with the West, particularly with international institutions such as the WHO, World Bank, and UN—organizations that Beijing was striving to work with to facilitate the modernization of its economy, such as through financial loans and technical assistance (Finch, 2007). In the 1990s, China was also aspiring to win favor with the West during its application to join the WTO, which came to pass in 2001. Moreover, striving to build an attractive, thriving market after delayed market reforms following the Tiananmen massacre and the collapse of the Soviet Empire in 1991, Beijing was also concerned with gaining the trust and confidence of investment bankers and the business community in the United States and Europe (Bremmer, 2010). It feared that a poor reputation in health would be of concern to investors and thus deter investments (Y. Huang, 2013).

Where did China's interest in international reputation building and its cooperative relationship with the international community—in other words, its positive geopolitical positioning—come from? As in Brazil and India, China's interest in these endeavors had a long historical precedent.

China's history depicts a government that has always been concerned about solidifying its international reputation in foreign affairs. Since the imperial period, scholars note, Chinese rulers had been committed to portraying China as a peaceful, prosperous nation, the center of Confucianism, steeped in rich Asian culture (Hongying Wang, 2003; Yiwei Wang, 2008). After a brief period of withdrawal from the international community during the 1950s and 1960s (Fook and Chong, 2010; Yiwei Wang, 2008), by the late 1970s, as part of the government's drive for economic modernity, China reintegrated itself into the global sphere. In 1971, it rejoined the UN and the WHO (WHO, 2004a). By the early 1980s, an important aspect of the government's foreign policy goals had become global reintegration and rejuvenation of China's international reputation as a prosperous state, capable of achieving economic growth and social welfare, while establishing relations with other nations through harmonious partnerships and multilateral cooperation (Goldstein, 2001; Yiwei Wang, 2008; X. Zhang, 2008). Some observers viewed international reputation building as an important aspect of China's revitalized foreign policy endeavors (Goldstein, 2001).

To gain a sense of how important international reputation has been for China's foreign policies, we can just follow the institutional trails. A concern about how other nations perceived China's prosperity and capacity prompted the government to create federal agencies focused on international propaganda and the marketing of China. The Central Foreign Propaganda Agency was created in 1980 and closed in 1988, but the State Council reauthorized the agency in 1990 and renamed it the Central Foreign Propaganda Office—which was renamed again in 1993 as the Information Office of the State Council (X. Zhang, 2008). In 1990, the State Council created the Overseas Propaganda Department, and in 1991, a new Information Officer (Hongying Wang, 2003). By

2004, the Ministry of Foreign Affairs took the extra step of creating a special Division of Public Diplomacy (X. Zhang, 2008). Furthermore, under Deng Xiaoping, state leaders often hired prestigious marketing firms and consultants to learn how China could better market its government in the international sphere (J. Zhang and Cameron, 2003). And finally, China increased its image-building capacity by creating national television stations, such as China Central Television and China Xinhua News Network Corp., which broadcast the nation's economic, social, and cultural accomplishments (X. Zhang, Wasserman, and Mano, 2016). As China's former president Jiang Zemin (1993–2003) once stated: "We should . . . establish a publicity capacity to exert an influence on world opinion that is as strong as China's international standing" (quoted in X. Zhang, Wasserman, and Mano, 2016, 7).

China also used country visits as a strategy to build its international reputation. Since the 1980s, countless government agencies, individuals, and cultural groups—such as dance companies—have traveled throughout the United States and Europe to promote China's cultural richness (J. Zhang and Cameron, 2003). China has strengthened this information sharing by establishing Confucius Institutes in other nations (Chung Dawson, 2010). When it came to HIV/AIDS, China's MOH sponsored medical visits to Australia and the United States to learn from best practices. This endeavor gave the impression that the government wanted to enhance its international reputation as a responsible and cooperative global partner in the fight against HIV/AIDS (Wu et al., 2007).

Through these international reputation-building institutions and endeavors, China has been committed to marketing its government as culturally rich, prosperous, peaceful, and cooperative, as always striving to join others in partnership rather than leading the international community through force. In essence this highlights one of China's "soft power" strategies, in which winning the hearts and minds of citizens in other nations through the promotion of Chinese culture and cooperation has been the key to increasing China's reputation and importance (Y. Huang and Ding, 2006).

China also has a long history of cooperating with other nations in response to disease. Beginning in the 1930s, China's MOH dispatched scores of medical doctors and healthcare workers to Africa. This was done to show good will and support for other nations troubled by poor health. In the 1960s, however, in an effort to spread his revolutionary spirit and engage in health diplomacy, Chairman Mao increased the number of medical teams sent to nations such as

Algeria, which was striving for liberation from France, and several African nations. These medical teams essentially acted as the "Peace Corps" of China and were managed not by the MOH but by the Ministry of Foreign Affairs and the Ministry of Economics and Trade (Y. Huang, 2010b). Between 1963 and 1982, approximately 6,500 Chinese health workers joined the medical teams and served a total of 70 million people in 42 countries (Y. Huang, 2010b).

Shortly after China rejoined the UN in 1971, the government began to collaborate closely with the UN on several health initiatives. In 1972, the government signed an agreement with the United Nations Development Program (UNDP) to allow the latter to fund projects addressing human resource development, medical information, traditional medicine, and primary care. Moreover, in 1978, China signed a memorandum of understanding with the WHO to create 41 WHO research centers throughout China (Y. Huang, 2012).

China also had a long history of cooperating with international donors and receiving their financial and technical assistance. Since the formation of the World Bank and the IMF in 1944, China had worked closely with these institutions to receive financial and technical assistance. Beijing's relationship with the World Bank heightened during the early 1990s, with the organization of several conferences and World Bank studies on China's economic potential. Shortly thereafter, China became one of the bank's largest loan and technical assistance recipients for instituting several economic, social welfare (including health systems reform), and institutional policies. China's political leadership also had a long track record of obtaining technical assistance from the IMF, with the goal of strengthening macroeconomic and fiscal adjustment programs under Premier Deng Xiaoping (Bottelier, 2006).

In this context, China's long history of building its international reputation and engaging in multilateral partnerships in foreign policy and health shaped how the government positioned itself in relation to the international community. These historical precedents eventually engendered a government that became highly sensitive about any kind of international criticism and pressure concerning its policy response to HIV/AIDS, while maintaining its rich tradition of seeking international financial and technical assistance for its response to disease. This positive geopolitical positioning would incentivize the government to strengthen its institutional and policy response to the epidemic.

Because China had positioned itself as an emerging power seeking to bolster its international reputation in health, when it came to HIV/AIDS, the international criticism and pressure had a positive effect on the State Council's reform interests. By the late 1990s, not only did Chinese officials begin to address HIV/AIDS in public, but the State Council decided to ramp up funding for the MOH's AIDS program (Gill, Chang, and Palmer, 2002). In 1998, the MOH worked closely with the World Bank to receive a loan package for a project titled "Health 9," worth US$25 million, to help construct provincial facilities unifying HIV and STI (sexually transmitted infection) prevention and treatment services, to fund implementation of the Medium- to Long-Term AIDS Control Plan, and to receive suggestions from the World Bank on how to improve public awareness campaigns (Jiang et al., 2011).

With regard to HIV/AIDS, no other year stands out as much as 2003. That spring, the SARS epidemic emerged. As it spread rapidly throughout the mainland and especially in concentrated urban centers such as Hong Kong, the government was soon accused by the international community of covering up the epidemic (Y. Huang, 2006; Kaufman, 2010). SARS not only unmasked government denial and apathy toward health surveillance and human safety but also revealed China's poor public health system (L.-H. Chan, Chen, and Xu, 2010; Y. Huang, 2006; Kaufman, 2010). And the timing could not have been worse. As one scholar put it: "SARS occurred when China had made great strides in improving its international image" (Y. Huang, 2010b, 115). The international media, governments, and the WHO began to criticize the Chinese government for covering up the SARS epidemic (Y. Huang, 2010b), for ignoring Taiwan's struggles with it, and for the MOH's failure to provide timely and adequate information. MOH officials quickly denied everything (E. Zhang and Benoit, 2009). In the midst of these criticisms, government officials once again became concerned with their international reputation: "the health and security of the people, overall state of reform, development, and stability, and China's national interest and international image are at stake," commented Premier Wen Jiabao, when responding to these international accusations (quoted in Y. Huang, 2010b, 116).

But more importantly, SARS further magnified China's poor response to HIV/AIDS. SARS and the flurry of international criticisms it instigated not only opened the Chinese leadership's eyes to the importance of public health—up to that point, public health had not been a government priority (Y. Huang, 2013)—but also made it much more attentive to HIV/AIDS, as officials feared that SARS would further reveal China's HIV/AIDS situation and undermine the government's international reputation. In fact, some argue that SARS "radically changed the Chinese government's attitude toward, and response to, public health issues" (Zunyou and Sullivan, 2006, 76). Others claim that "after the outbreak of severe acute respiratory syndrome (SARS), the government abruptly changed course, launching aggressive measures against AIDS" (Gill and Okie, 2007, 1801). Yet others maintain that because of SARS, "image restoration" became a key government concern (E. Zhang and Benoit, 2009). Analysts indeed note that "China's leaders understand that a part of its international image and prestige will be judged by how it handles domestic challenges including environmental quality, HIV/AIDS, tuberculosis, and avian influenza" and that "China's growing reputation concerns could potentially contribute to a reassessment of its internal approaches to matters such as health" (Gill, Morrison, and Lu, 2007, 16).

Thus, while international pressure and criticism, beginning in the mid-1990s, certainly helped in putting HIV/AIDS on the national agenda (Y. Huang, 2010a; Kaufman, 2010), many claim that international pressure from SARS was the turning point in China's response to HIV/AIDS (L.-H. Chan, Chen, and Xu, 2010; Y. Huang, 2006, 2013; Knutsen, 2012; Wu et al., 2007). As Joan Kaufman (2010, 76) put it, "China learned a hard lesson that not responding to infectious disease threats can undermine economic growth and tarnish its global image." China's leadership reasoned that it was time to show the world that China had the political will, commitment, infrastructural capacity, and resources needed to combat HIV/AIDS and, moreover, was fully committed to providing public health as a human right. SARS not only helped put AIDS squarely back on the national agenda, but it also fostered wider commitments to strengthening China's overall healthcare system and human security (L.-H. Chan, Chen, and Xu, 2010; Yu, 2015).

By 2004, then, the government appeared more firmly committed to strengthening its policy response to HIV/AIDS. The premier and State Council by this point viewed an aggressive response to the epidemic as a means to rejuvenate China's international reputation in health. More than ever, the State Council and the premier were committed to expanding the national AIDS bureaucracy, funding new prevention and treatment programs, and signaling to provincial governments that a stronger policy response was needed (Y. Huang, 2006; Kaufman, 2010).

As we saw in Brazil and India, in an effort to further strengthen its international reputation, China's AIDS officials also started to host conferences and meetings to reveal the government's AIDS policy commitments. Some claim that this process began as early as 1997, when AIDS officials invited UNAIDS director Emile Fox to attend domestic AIDS workshops in China and discuss the government's policies (Chinese Society for the Study of Sexual Minorities, 1997). In 2001, the government sponsored its first international AIDS conference. Representatives from more than 20 nations were present. This conference provided an opportunity for the government to display several of its policy initiatives (Rubin, 2002). AIDS officials organized another major international AIDS conference in 2003, while at the same time hosting US President Bill Clinton for a discussion about the epidemic (Yardley, 2003). Over time, AIDs officials would continue to show off their "best practices" in AIDS policy interventions by organizing study tours for foreign delegations in China, while also sharing their successful experiences at international conferences (Yan Wang, 2011).

But was international reputation building the only factor motivating the government to strengthen its policy response? Several other factors could also have been important. First, politicians at the national level may have used their response to the HIV/AIDS epidemic as a means to win office or stay in power. This thesis does not hold, however. There are no national elections in China and, consequently, no need for State Council members to campaign on health or any other social welfare issue. Second, perhaps it was the accelerated growth of AIDS cases by the late 1990s and early 2000s that startled the premier, State Council members, and the MOH and motivated them to respond. But this argument is equally problematic, as the central government had known for some time that AIDS rates were accelerating, and it already had many plans and strategies to curb the spread (Y. Huang, 2006; Kaufman, 2010). Finally, perhaps the spread of HIV/AIDS among famous politicians, movie actors, or activists prompted them to mobilize and pressure the government for a response. This rationale also does not apply in China. The AIDS epidemic was mainly present among the poor, sex workers, IDUs, and farmers in rural areas (N. Li et al., 2010; Wu, Rou, and Cui, 2004). Moreover, AIDS was so stigmatized during this period that upper- and middle-income individuals would have little interest in disclosing their HIV/AIDS status (Kuhn, 2009; UNAIDS, 2002).

Others have argued that China's central government is unique in its provision of social welfare policies. That is, there is a general perception, both within and outside government, that the center should guarantee basic social welfare benefits and that doing so helps to build social stability, solidarity, and government legitimacy and long-term survival (Bingqin, 2012; X. Huang,

2013); in this context, citizens expect that, regardless of the presence of electoral institutions and accountability, the central government will take care of their needs, which include a wide array of social welfare benefits (X. Huang, 2013; O'Brien, 2013). The government's failure to do this can lead to what O'Brien (2013) refers to as "rightful resistance," that is, citizens' protest of the government's unwillingness to comply with their social welfare commitments. Thus, it could very well be the case that when it came to HIV/AIDS, the central government was motivated more by its preexisting commitment to providing public healthcare than by international criticism and pressure. However, this assertion is questionable. If this indeed were the case, then the central government would have engaged in a stronger policy response to HIV/AIDS before the emergence of international criticism and pressure; and yet, as noted earlier, this never occurred.

In a context in which China's positive geopolitical positioning appeared to matter most in accounting for its eventual stronger policy response to AIDS, the previously marginalized AIDS bureaucrats who had initially sought this outcome took note of the government's renewed policy commitment. As Kaufman (2010, 76) claimed: "Waiting in the wings after the SARS crisis died down, China's AIDS advocates from the government, civil society, academia and their international partners grabbed the opportunity to push forward greater action on AIDS . . . the resulting transformation led to the open admission of the AIDS problem and the initiation of a set of pragmatic policy responses."

A host of bureaucratic and policy reforms followed, leading to a stronger policy response to the epidemic. Y. Huang (2006) explains that, in 2003, after years of applying pressure to the government for a centralized response, AIDS bureaucrats took advantage of the government response to SARS to promote institutional and program change. In November 2003, Zeng Yi proposed the establishment of a national HIV/AIDS headquarters, similar to that for SARS, to mobilize local governments while effectively improving epidemic surveillance and public awareness. His advice did not fall on deaf ears. Several months later, a new State Council HIV/AIDS Working Committee was established (Y. Huang 2006). This consisted of 23 MOH health ministers and 7 provincial leaders, with a committee formed by these local leaders (DFID, 2005), thus deepening coordination between the center and local governments. The premier and State Council delegated considerable autonomy to the working committee and allowed it to meet frequently and regularly (Zunyou and

Sullivan, 2006). In addition to promoting condom use and increasing clean needle exchange in the provinces, the working committee mandated that state and local governments develop plans and guidelines for increased assessment and accountability. Through these endeavors, the center would now hold local governments more accountable for AIDS policies (Kaufman, Kleinman, and Saich, 2006; Zunyou and Sullivan, 2006). In total, after 2003, 30 new government policies were issued at the national and provincial levels, clearly stipulating the objectives, responsibilities, and legal framework for the rights of people afflicted with AIDS. The State Council authorized an increase in federal spending for the MOH's AIDS program, from 100 million yuan in 2002, to 390 million yuan in 2003, and 810 million yuan in 2004 (Zunyou and Sullivan, 2006). This money would also be used to help local governments finance central policy mandates.

In 2006, the State Council also implemented the Regulations of Prevention and Treatment of HIV/AIDS. These regulations encouraged voluntary testing for HIV, created antidiscrimination laws and legal protection for the rights of people living with HIV/AIDS, and outlined the roles and responsibilities of all federal agencies involved in the formulation and implementation of AIDS policies (Lu and Gill, 2007; UNAIDS, 2015; L. Wang, 2007). And finally, that same year, the State Council created its Second Five-Year Plan (2006–10), which built on the first plan's policy goals and ambitions (Wu et al., 2007).

The government, with the assistance of the 1998 "Health 9" loan from the World Bank (World Bank, 2009), also substantially increased its infrastructural commitment for surveillance and HIV screening. For example, the number of national sentinel surveillance sites increased from 194 in 2003, to 247 in 2004, and 295 in 2005. More than 400 surveillance sites were established at the provincial level. Voluntary counseling and testing services also increased, from services in 365 counties/districts in 15 provinces in 2002 to services in 1,973 counties/districts in all 31 provinces by 2005 (Zunyou and Sullivan, 2006).

By far the most progressive policy response was the Comprehensive AIDS Response (CARES) program, implemented in 2003. Through the CARES program's "Four Frees, One Care" initiative, for the first time the MOH provided free ARV medications for two primary AIDS-affected communities: indigent city residents and people living with HIV/AIDS in the hinterland (F. Zhang et al., 2006). The program also provided free counseling and testing services, free treatment for HIV-positive pregnant women and babies, payment of school fees for children with AIDS, and financial support for affected families (Kaufman, 2010; F. Zhang et al., 2006). In his speech at the UN General Assembly meeting at the end of 2003, Gao Qiang, then executive vice minister of health, boasted about China's new commitment to providing ARVs for patients experiencing financial difficulties. The CARES program, however, was not as universal as claimed, since it targeted indigent at-risk groups. Nevertheless, since AIDS is primarily concentrated among the urban and especially the rural poor, this program has been important in increasing access to ARV medicines (F. Zhang et al., 2006).

The MOH also put forth several new treatment programs. In 2004 and 2005, it broke from its prior views—mainly rooted in conservative moral tenets—to fund the creation of several methadone maintenance and treatment sites in cities with high HIV prevalence (Gill and Okie, 2007; Wu et al., 2007). The MOH also worked with Australia's Agency for International Development to expand needle exchange programs (Halter, n.d.). Although drug use is still illegal in China and the government has not condoned the use of free needle exchanges as a preventive measure, it has overlooked the fact that clean needles are sold and at times distributed.

Regarding prevention, since 2003 the MOH has worked with local governments to implement sex and AIDS education programs in high schools, though not yet at the primary and secondary school levels (Lei and Wu-Kui, 2008; Wu et al., 2007). In 2003–4, the MOH also lifted the ban on commercial advertisements for condoms on television, and it sponsored new AIDS awareness campaigns on television, the Internet, and billboards and in train stations (Lei and Wu-Kui, 2008). In 2008, recognizing an increase in AIDS among men who have sex with men (MSM), the MOH created the MSM AIDS Comprehensive Prevention and Control Pilot Program. Although established as a pilot and managed by provincial offices of the Chinese Center for Disease Control and Prevention (CCDC), this was the first comprehensive effort to establish awareness programs, HIV testing, counseling services, prevention education about safe sex provided by gay peers, organizational development, implementation of policies for the MSM group, and increased funding (UNDP, 2015). Beginning in 2013, in an effort to curb the burgeoning growth of HIV among college-age students, the MOH and other local governments placed free condom dispensing machines on college campuses—to the dismay of conservative groups and churches that saw this as encouraging promiscuous sex (Grimm, 2015).

But a closer look at China's stronger policy response suggests that these reforms have been challenging, for there were several ongoing institutional and policy shortcomings centered mainly on the effectiveness of national institutions, federalism and decentralization, and a scarcity of human resources.

With regard to federal funding for the MOH's AIDS programs, though this gradually increased, it consistently fell short of providing AIDS bureaucrats with what they needed (Gómez, 2009; Y. Liu and Kaufman, 2006). Federal funding increased over time, from 2.42 billion yuan in 2011, to 2.95 billion yuan in 2013, and 4.64 billion yuan in 2014, targeted especially to at-risk groups such as the gay community and college-age students (China, National Health and Family Planning Commission [NHFPC], 2014, 2015; Yinan and Xiaodong, 2014). But this is still perceived as insufficient, considering the growing number of HIV-positive individuals (Marchant, 2015).

While the CARES and 2006 Regulations of Prevention and Treatment of HIV/AIDS legislation called for greater interagency collaboration, analysts note that the MOH response to HIV/AIDS was too vertical in nature, failing to incorporate the advice of several related agencies such as education and justice (Lu and Gill, 2007; Saich, 2006). This is especially perplexing given that since the late 1990s, as mentioned earlier, several national committees had been created to increase interagency coordination. Finally, despite the introduction of the 2006 regulations that safeguard people with HIV/AIDS from discrimination and social intolerance and ensure rights to care, recent UNAIDS reports claim that the federal and provincial governments have been negligent in their efforts to enforce these regulations (UNAIDS, 2015). Consequently, social fears and discrimination continue to fuel the epidemic: fewer HIV-positive individuals seek treatment and care, especially sex workers and members of the gay community, while hospitals continue to neglect the treatment of these individuals (Marchant, 2015; UNAIDS, 2015).

The government also continues to fall short in providing effective public awareness and educational campaigns (Tatlow, 2015). Although the MOH has worked with universities in Beijing to increase sex education and AIDS awareness (*Economic Times*, 2015), and the National Health and Family Planning department issued a circular in 2015 requiring that students in middle and high schools attend six to four hours of HIV/AIDS prevention classes (Abkowitz and Xin, 2015), most of these initiatives are still funded and managed by provincial governments, with little assistance from the central government (China, NHFPC, 2015; Jingxi, 2015). Moreover, recent studies question the government's commitment to implementing the requirements in the new circular, while teachers have recently encountered strong resistance from conservative groups striving to safeguard a moral foundation for children (Burki, 2016). Additionally, the government still has not created any federal programs mandating sex education for young gay men in schools (Jiaying, 2015), a problem that reflects the persistence of conservative cultural beliefs within government and society.

Decentralization has also presented problems. Despite impressive strides to decentralize fiscal and economic activity in order to foster economic development and growth, for social welfare—especially public health—the imposition of federal mandates without adequate financial and infrastructural resources abounds. CARES and other AIDS programs, for example, were imposed on states and townships—especially in rural areas—that did not have the human, financial, or institutional resources to adequately implement such policy (Y. Liu and Kaufman, 2006; Lu and Gill, 2007; Saich, 2006; F. Zhang et al., 2006). Some claim that this led to wide variation in subnational implementation of CARES and other preventive programs recommended by the national CCDC and donor institutions (Global Business Council, 2008; Y. Huang, 2013). At the same time, the MOH has made no effort to create formal procedures that resolve conflicting interests and policy initiatives between the central and provincial governments. This has often motivated provincial governments to reinterpret and implement central government policy to their liking, or to blatantly ignore national policies without fear of repercussion (UNAIDS, 2015).

In addition to the poor implementation of decentralization programs, other analysts note that China's large geographic size makes it difficult for the government to monitor subnational governments' compliance to national policies (Gill and Okie, 2007; *Lancet*, 2009; J. Parry, 2008). This problem has motivated state and municipal health departments to shirk their policy responsibilities (Y. Huang, 2013). In a context where the national government provided inadequate financial and technical support, local politicians had few incentives to adhere to the center's policy requests and, consequently, few incentives to implement them effectively (Y. Liu and Kaufman, 2006; Wu et al., 2007). And because of this, there has been little subnational accountability to the national CCDC and central government in general (Y. Huang, 2013; Y. Liu and Kaufman, 2006). Until this accountability level increases, the MOH can pass all the regulations and policies it wants but will still fall short of ensuring their implementation at the local level.

Finally, human resource constraints pose an ongoing problem. State and local governments continue to have inadequate numbers of AIDS-trained medical doctors and nurses to examine and treat patients with HIV/AIDS. As expected, this problem is far worse in rural areas (China, NHFPC, 2014; Lu and Gill, 2007; Wu et al., 2007). In 2006, there were only 200 clinicians in Yunnan province who had AIDS training, serving an estimated 80,000 HIV-infected people (Zunyou and Sullivan, 2006). Because local governments do not have enough funding, they have not been able to motivate medically trained personnel to work on HIV/AIDS in remote areas. There is consequently a consistent scarcity of medical personnel, as well as lab technicians that can properly administer HIV tests and examine blood results (China, NHFPC, 2015; Kaufman, Kleinman, and Saich, 2006; Wu et al., 2007). Given that the HIV/AIDS epidemic is still mainly concentrated in rural areas, these human resource shortcomings suggest that the central government is still not entirely committed to ensuring an improved response to HIV/AIDS.

In addition, there was and continues to be a dire need, not only to increase federal financial, technical, and human resource commitments, but also to incentivize local governments to adhere to national policy mandates. However, the CCDC and NAP have not pursued any effort to supplement and enhance healthcare decentralization through the creation of new discretionary fiscal transfer programs, which could incentivize provincial governments to comply with national policy mandates. As we saw in chapter 2, Brazil's success at implementing a centrist policy response to HIV/AIDS was attributable to the MOH's creation of the Fundo-a-Fundo program, which provides supplemental cash transfers for prevention, treatment, and antidiscriminatory AIDS policies. But to qualify, states must periodically provide information showing that they are in full compliance with national policy guidelines. China has not made this kind of innovative policy response. Although having a historically strong central government presence in the area of public health (Y. Huang, 2013)—in contrast to Brazil, but similar to India—China has relied entirely on decentralization to guide the bulk of its policy response.

Furthermore, the MOH has not introduced efforts to informally increase its policy authority over the provinces by working with NGOs to monitor provincial government performance in order to increase accountability to the NAP—a key aspect of building a centrist policy response. In a context of increased decentralization and scarcity in rural areas, the usage of NGOs in this regard is much needed (Y. Huang, 2013). And yet, the institutional conditions are propitious, as most AIDS NGOs are already used to acting in coordination with, or, more accurately, being manipulated by, the central government (Y. Huang, 2013; Keping, 2009). But because the national CCDC and AIDS program do not have a close partnership with NGOs—an issue that I will return to shortly—these accountability mechanisms have not been introduced.

Others have called for integrating the subnational healthcare civil service into the national MOH system (Y. Liu and Kaufman, 2006). State health officials would then be increasingly accountable to the center, as the latter pays their salaries and determines standards for promotion. And finally, analysts have argued that the national MOH and CCDC need to better coordinate with state-level branches of the CCDC and rural public hospitals (Y. Huang, 2013; Kaufman and Meyers, 2006). This would help provide the information that the national level needs to provide an adequate supply of resources and to improve policy. Thus, in contrast to what we saw in Brazil, China's government has not been able to achieve a centrist policy response.

Nevertheless, since 2012 the government has pursued new policy reforms that clearly signal an increased commitment to combating HIV/AIDS, showing that it has gradually been able to achieve a stronger policy response. For example, consistent with the government's historical track record of building institutional and program initiatives, in 2012 the State Council published the Twelfth Five-Year Action Plan for the Containment and Prevention of HIV/AIDS, which established the China Action Plan to Prevent and Control HIV/AIDS. This plan called for an immediate increase in access to affordable ARV medications, while addressing intellectual property issues such as the potential to issue compulsory licenses and the improved domestic production of ARVs (UNDP, 2015). Premier Li Keqiang has recently promised to further increase federal funding for AIDS prevention, with a focus on the most vulnerable groups in society such as the gay community (*China Daily*, 2014).

At the same time, several new programs have been created. The MOH and Ministry of Civil Affair's Notice on Granting Subsistence Allowance to Children Living with HIV provides monthly stipends for food to approximately 7,000 HIV-infected children nationwide. A Ministry of Education program pays education fees for children with HIV/AIDS. The 2014 official Notice on Overall Establishment of Temporary Assistance System provides funding for HIV/AIDS-affected families undergoing financial hardship. And the program Strengthening the Work of Medical Services for People Living with HIV/

AIDS in essence provides more funding and support for healthcare services for people living with HIV/AIDS (China, NHFPC, 2014, 2015). The MOH also continues to work with provincial health departments in opening methadone treatment clinics, needle exchange projects, and clinics providing ARV treatment (China, NHFPC, 2015). Finally, the MOH has recently worked with an NGO, the All-China Federation of Industry and Commerce, to cooperate with a hundred or so universities to distribute Red Ribbon Health Packages to nonlocal migrant workers in approximately a thousand business enterprises (China, NHFPC, 2015).

In 2013, the State Council created a new working group, the AIDS Working Committee, later renamed the State Council AIDS Working Committee Office (SCAWCO), which consists of 25 departments and 11 provincial government representatives. Vice Premier Liu Yandong serves as SCAWCO's director. SCAWCO has organized yearly meetings to evaluate the impact of the government's AIDS programs. To match rhetoric with action, in 2014 the government proposed a further increase in the federal budget for HIV/AIDS, for all federal ministries involved, from 3.5 billion yuan to 4.42 billion yuan (China, NHFPC, 2015).

And finally, as yet another component of China's positive geopolitical positioning, which entailed the government's pursuit of a stronger policy response to improve its international reputation while seeking the assistance of international donors, the government also provided foreign aid assistance to further enhance its international reputation in the health arena (Y. Huang, 2010b). However, in contrast to what we saw in Brazil, China's provision of foreign aid for HIV/AIDS has been limited (Grépin et al., 2014; Y. Huang, 2012), with the government placing more emphasis on helping developing nations strengthen their broader health systems capacity (Grépin et al., 2014). Following historical precedent, most of this bilateral support has gone to the African region, followed by Oceania and Latin America (J. Wang et al., 2013). Since the 1960s, China has supplied several African nations with medical teams providing primary care services (Y. Huang, 2013; P. Liu et al., 2014). Since 1963, the government has sent approximately 23,000 medical personnel to 66 nations, with the majority sent to Africa (P. Liu et al., 2014). Over time, China extended its bilateral assistance to provide funding for the construction of hospitals and clinics and for drugs, equipment, and health worker training throughout Africa, Asia, and Latin America (P. Liu et al., 2014; J. Wang et al., 2013). The government has also built pharmaceutical factories in nations such as Mali,

Tanzania, and Ethiopia (Bräutigam, 2011). China has sustained its commitment to helping several African nations fund anti-malaria programs (Bräutigam, 2011; Wang et al., 2013). At the 2006 Sino-African Summit, for example, President Hu pledged to provide US$ 37.5 million in grants to provide the anti-malaria drug artemisinin and to construct 30 malaria prevention and treatment centers (Y. Huang, 2010b).

In the 1990s, China began to provide bilateral assistance for strengthening other nations' response to HIV/AIDS (Zou, McPake, and Wei, 2014). The MOH has, for example, conducted training courses for HIV/AIDS professionals in Africa and helped to establish pilot programs in cross-border areas of China, Myanmar, Laos, and Vietnam (Y. Wang, 2011). During the third summit of the Forum of China and Africa Cooperation in 2006, Beijing announced plans to provide training courses in HIV/AIDS prevention for healthcare workers throughout Africa (J. Wang et al., 2013). And in 2015, China provided Kenya's Ministry of Health and Education with training in HIV/AID prevention, care, and management (Xinhua, 2015). However, as noted above, China's bilateral assistance for HIV/AIDS has not been as extensive as its commitment to strengthening other nations' healthcare systems (Grépin et al., 2014). Indeed, from 1978 to 2008, China provided only two projects to help fund HIV/AIDS prevention, both of them to Papua New Guinea in 2005 (J. Wang et al., 2013). At the multilateral level, however, China has continued to increase its financial contributions to the Global Fund to Fight AIDS, Tuberculosis, and Malaria, from a yearly provision of US$2 million beginning in 2003 to US$4.6 million beginning in 2010 (Dickinson, 2010).

China's bilateral support for HIV/AIDS has been less prevalent for several reasons. First, China realized that traditional international donors, primarily from the West, such as the World Bank, and other international NGOs and philanthropists, have already contributed a large amount of funding to HIV/AIDS. Consequently, Beijing has seen no need to increase its foreign aid assistance in this area. Second, since the 1960s, China's aid has been shaped by the principles of noninterference in the domestic politics of aid recipients, as well as sovereignty and mutual economic benefit (J. Wang et al., 2013). The political and cultural sensitivities surrounding HIV/AIDS programs, as well as the fear of upsetting important trade partners (Y. Huang, 2010b), also may explain why China has refrained from investing more in bilateral HIV/AIDS assistance.

There have been several motives behind China's foreign aid in health. Despite the minimal role of aid for HIV/AIDS in this process, foreign aid in strengthening other nations' healthcare systems has been used to enhance the government's international reputation as having an effective healthcare system and providing technical assistance and policy advice to other nations (Xinhua, 2015). Aid in health has also enhanced China's reputation as a nation that is powerful, influential, responsible, and benevolent in helping lesser-developed nations overcome disease and develop (Y. Huang, 2010b; P. Liu et al., 2014; Naidu, 2009; J. Wang et al., 2013). Furthermore, these endeavors have facilitated China's ability to expand its network of geopolitical allies in Africa and Latin America (Lum et al., 2009), which, in turn, has helped to advance its position within international organizations such as the UN (Y. Huang, 2010b). And finally, as several scholars emphasize, China has accrued economic benefits through its foreign aid assistance, such as increased trade, access to natural resources, and opportunities for business investment in those nations, particularly in Africa, that it helps (Y. Huang, 2010b; Naidu, 2009; J. Wang et al., 2013).

In sum, despite the government's stronger policy response and foreign aid endeavors, it never proved capable of creating a centrist policy response for HIV/AIDS. As we recall from chapter 1, a centrist policy response requires three components: the creation and ongoing financial and administrative expansion of federal agencies, the development of effective prevention and treatment programs (particularly, universal access to medicines), and formal and informal strategies to increase the central government's policy influence in a context of healthcare decentralization. In China, however, central government funding for the MOH's HIV/AIDS programs has continuously proved to be insufficient, no effort has been made to establish an effective universal ARV treatment program, and there have been limited prevention programs—especially for at-risk groups. Moreover, in a context of decentralization, the MOH has not tried to formally influence policies at the provincial level by creating grant conditionalities while informally sustaining its influence by working closely with NGOs to monitor provincial health departments and hold them accountable for policy implementation. But why was this the case? In essence, China's AIDS bureaucrats were missing a necessary condition for an ongoing centrist policy response: strong bureaucratic–civil societal partnerships.

The Absence of Strong Bureaucratic-Civil Societal Partnerships

Historically, China's government, like India's, was never fully committed to establishing a strong partnership with healthcare activists in the area of public health. To understand why, one must first understand the nation's culture and political environment throughout the early twentieth century. Culturally, perhaps more so than any other nation discussed in this book, conservative moral beliefs deeply penetrated the fabric of Chinese politics and society. These Confucian moral tenets espoused self-sacrifice of one's individual rights, communitarianism, and respect and obedience as values that all good citizens should strive for (Pye, 1996). In short, excellence in moral citizenship was based on self-less dedication to communities and to the state. Many civic associations were present during the early twentieth century, such as lineage societies, benevolent associations (providing food, water control, public works, health services, women's groups, and schools), trade guilds, and landsman halls (where members of a community came together to discuss matters). These organizations— reinforced and circumscribed by imperial laws and regulations (a type of top-down control of civic associational life that reemerged later)—beginning in 1908, under the Qing government (Keping, 2009), were designed to enhance self-identity and security, not to collectively pursue a new political agenda or confront and pressure the government for policy reform. Concerned members of society and physicians were viewed as a compliant, supportive ally of the state. But more importantly, the notion of someone and/or some group of individuals creating a new reformist agenda, and associations supporting that agenda, was an alien concept (Pye, 1996). There was no room or expectation for ideational creativity, interest group mobilization, or pressure for policy reform. And even if citizens had problems with the government, passivity and respect were culturally expected (Yang Da-hua, 2004). In the early twentieth century, then, there were vibrant networks of civic organizations—enriching China's culture, engendering a sense of collective identity and security, but acquiescing to government interests and policy goals (Yang Da-hua, 2004). In this context (and in sharp contrast to what we saw in Brazil), despite the need to respond aggressively to many diseases, no new civic movements or organizations emerged that would both confront the government for a stronger response to epidemics and work closely with bureaucratic officials to create centralized institutions and policies.

China's Confucian style of associational life took a downturn with the rise of the Communist Party in 1949. Seeking to control all sources of power while instilling new ideas and beliefs, the Communist Party made it a point to completely eradicate all civic associations that thrived under the previous Kuomintang regime (Keping, 2009). To help ensure political stability, the Party sought to replace these groups with its own brand of civic associations and groups working on a host of cultural, educational, and scientific topics.

Civic activism, quelled and suppressed for roughly three decades, did not regain its vibrancy until the emergence of Deng Xioping as Party leader in 1979 and his decision to introduce China to free markets (Béja, 2006; Keping, 2009). Gradual liberalization in markets, ideas, and culture, as well as the emergence of highly esteemed, well-published intellectuals who organized conferences, workshops, or what scholars refer to as informal "salons," fostered renewed interest in civic life and freedom of expression and movement. But this was an elite-driven process, confined to highly educated, respected individuals within the Party, and without any formal linkages to activists and concerned individuals in society. Civic *abertura*, if you will, was therefore a gradual, top-down process. Over time, while associational life slowly began to develop in society, these reformist elites also started to organize conferences, unofficial journals such as *Beijing zhi chun*, and newsletters that incorporated concerned individual outside the state into policy discussions (Béja, 2006). These movements further intensified after the 1989 Tiananmen incident, when a decline in government legitimacy and civic unrest further encouraged and propelled civic action (Béja, 2006; Keping, 2009).

But because civic activism had reemerged so recently (under Deng in 1979), and because this was an elite-driven process, when HIV/AIDS arrived there was no rich history of civic movements and resources in health and individual rights that activists could use for effective lobbying and pressure for policy reform (Cai, 2006). In contrast to what we saw in Brazil, fear and harassment thwarted any interest in the gay community in collectivizing to form organizations or even to pressure the government. In fact, the first official AIDS NGO to emerge, the Chinese Foundation for HIV/AIDS Control and Prevention, was a government-organized NGO (called a GONGO), with its leadership and management entirely controlled by the MOH (N. Li et al., 2010). To receive funding and support from the government, NGOs had to register with the State Council, a requirement that became law in 1996 (N. Li et al., 2010). However, the requirements for official registration with the government were quite high. For example, to qualify, organizations needed to have 100,000 yuan in an established checking account and to have a "management unit" linked to the MOH or another agency (N. Li et al., 2010; Saich, 2006). This, of course, severely limited the participation of civic organizations and created few incentives to mobilize (Gómez and Harris, 2015; N. Li et al., 2010; Saich, 2006). Some scholars estimate a very high level of unregistered NGOs working on AIDS, mostly lacking adequate financial support or resources—often instigating competition rather than cooperation between groups—and lacking managerial expertise (Kaufman, 2009). Nevertheless, these organizations, by the mid-1990s, received the backing of international donors and philanthropists such as the Ford Foundation and the Asia Foundation (N. Li et al., 2010).

In the mid-1990s, with the 1996 Regulations of Prevention and Treatment of HIV/AIDS and the Action Plan for the Containment and Prevention of HIV/AIDS (2006–10), the State Council began to recognize the need for a government partnership with AIDS NGOs. In fact, both initiatives stipulated that local governments should work with AIDS NGOs to implement policies (N. Li et al., 2010). In a context of increased decentralization and the presence of hard-to-reach, at-risk groups in rural areas, the central government soon recognized the advantages of working with and using NGOs to reach this population. AIDS NGOs were therefore viewed as increasingly important arms of the state, as well as being instrumental in providing prevention information in a health systems context emphasizing preventive care (Kaufman, 2009; Y. Liu and Kaufman, 2006; Xu, Zeng, and Anderson, 2005). Moreover, because intravenous drug use, prostitution, and gay sex were illegal, the central government and especially local governments found it advantageous to work with AIDS NGOs.

Despite the challenges of having to meet rigorous registration requirements and a general lack of resources, both official and unofficial AIDS NGOs have flourished in the past 20 years (H. Chen et al., 2015; Gómez and Harris, 2015; N. Li et al., 2010). As Nana Taona Kuo Li and colleagues (2010) report, during the 1990s several organizations emerged, including the Chinese Association of STD/AIDS Prevention and Control, the China Red Cross, and AiZHi Action, and by 2006 the China HIV/AIDS directory reported 100 domestic AIDS NGOs working in the field. Another estimate followed: in 2007, the State Council Working Group on AIDS and the UN Theme Group on AIDS estimated that there were 400 community-based organizations (N. Li et al., 2010). More recent estimates suggest that in three provinces alone, Yunnan, Beijing, and Guangdong, 263 AIDS NGOs were at work (H. Chen et al., 2015). AIDS NGOs have provided a host of services such as prevention and awareness through classroom education, pamphlets, movies, and the media, HIV testing, and outreach to youth, while enlisting the support of movie stars (H. Chen et al., 2015; Ru, 2006; Xinhua, 2016; Xu, Zeng, and Anderson, 2005). In addition, they have been important for protecting the rights of harassed at-risk groups such as the gay community and IDUs and providing educational and legal services, home care, and treatment (H. Chen et al., 2015; N. Li et al., 2010). As a result of their efforts, some observers maintain, adherence to ARV medication regimens has increased in areas where NGOs, especially unofficial NGOs, have provided home care and treatment services (N. Li et al., 2010). Many unregistered AIDS NGOs in China have also worked closely with the international community, attending many conferences, partnering with human rights groups, and receiving funding from international NGOs such as the Red Cross of Australia, UNAIDS, and Save the Children (H. Chen et al., 2015). Thus, by providing key health services where the state has been absent, most notably in rural areas, AIDS NGOs have been vital for keeping the spread of HIV/AIDS in check.

But there are several challenges that may limit the effectiveness of HIV/AIDS NGOs. Because there are so many unofficial AIDS NGOs, and because many have links to foreign (often western) organizations, and because they are autonomous and unlikely to strictly adhere to government policy, local governments often do not trust them and will avoid working with unregistered organizations as much as possible (H. Chen et al., 2015). Analysts claim, moreover, that the government is still committed to clamping down on social movements and NGOs that are raising public awareness about HIV/AIDS, thus contributing to volunteers' skepticism about their organization's efficacy (Marchant, 2015). Regardless of the central government's verbal commitment to working with AIDS NGOs, there is still very much a climate of distrust toward them (L.-H. Chan, Chen, and Xu, 2010; H. Chen et al., 2015).

The incident of the Global Fund election in 2005 provides a good example of this. Analysts note that the elections held that year for the Country Coordinating Mechanism were initially rigged, leading to the selection of government officials and representatives from government-sponsored GONGOs. The Global Fund discredited the election and asked for another, this time carefully monitored. The new vote led to the election of several representatives from non-government-sponsored AIDS NGOs, activists, and people living with HIV/AIDS. This result forced the government to become more transparent in its relations with activists and people living with HIV/AIDS (Kaufman, 2009, 2010). The event nevertheless underscored that despite the State Council's public commitment to working with NGOs, it still did not trust them, nor was the government entirely committed to integrating them into the policymaking process. This problem is often reinforced by local and central government views that the AIDS NGOs providing treatment services are competing with the government's CARES program, implying that CARES is ineffective. Therefore the government's general view of NGOs is one of self-interest and distrust: they are allowed to operate as long as they are not tied to questionable western donors and do not interfere with state policies (L.-H. Chan, Chen, and Xu, 2010; Gómez and Harris, 2015).

As seen in India, moreover, the vast numbers of unregistered AIDS NGOs lack sufficient funding and technical and managerial support (H. Chen et al., 2015; N. Li et al., 2010). While many do receive funding from international donors, it is often on a short-term basis, without adequate funding to continue their work after donors have left (China, NHFPC, 2015; N. Li et al., 2010). This situation will—and has—left many organizations in need, without the opportunity or incentive to turn to the government for help. If NGOs manage to get registered, they are then subject to the government's selection of their staff and governing board; this undermines organizational autonomy, capacity, and policy interests (Keping, 2009).

In this context, and in contrast to what we saw in Brazil, reform-minded AIDS bureaucrats have not been able to establish and strategically use close ties with NGOs to increase bureaucrats' legitimacy in garnering more federal attention and support for their agency and policies (Gómez and Harris, 2015; Kaufman, 2010). While partnerships have recently been formed between select state-level CCDC branches and NGOs working with at-risk groups such as gay men, these bureaucratic–civil societal partnerships are found only at the subnational level (Kaufman, 2009, 2010). As a report from China's NHFPC (2014, 28) states, such partnership is lacking at the national level: "Also, the mechanism for information communication between relevant government departments and social organizations is still not well-established and there is inconsistency in the support of social organizations participating in AIDS response work." Yet, as we saw in Brazil, if national AIDS bureaucrats are to succeed in finding additional funding for provincial CCDC branches and for hospitals lacking the resources and personnel needed to provide treatment—especially in rural areas—then they must develop closer ties with AIDS NGOs, especially non-government-sponsored AIDS NGOs. To this day, however, no such bureaucratic–civil societal partnership has emerged.

Recent allegations of human rights violations and crackdowns on AIDS NGOs in select cities lend credence to the notion that the bureaucracy's partnership with NGOs may not be as fruitful as once claimed. Notwithstanding the central government's verbal commitments to working with AIDS NGOs, as well as the federal regulations mandating this, many AIDS NGOs have reported being harassed by local officials and in some instances forced to close their operations—such as in the province of Henan (Human Rights Watch, 2007). Some analysts note that while, on paper, China supports AIDS activists, in practice it is an entirely different matter (Amon, 2010).

In sum, although China joined Brazil and India in demonstrating positive geopolitical positioning by immediately responding to international criticism and pressure through a stronger policy response in order to improve the government's international reputation while seeking the assistance of the international donor community, China's AIDS bureaucrats, unlike Brazil's, never strove to establish a strong partnership with NGOs after these reputation-building interests and policy reforms ensued. Consequently, the bureaucracy could never achieve a centrist policy response.

Responding to Obesity

How did the Chinese government respond to a different type of public health challenge: the obesity epidemic? Because of its burgeoning economy and significant increase in consumption, within the past two decades China has seen a surge in the number of obesity cases. Was the government more interested and successful in its response to this new public health challenge?

As in Brazil and India, this challenge presented a new public health paradox: the rise of adult and childhood obesity amid ongoing malnourishment and poverty. Many blame modernity. Since the opening up of China's economy in the 1980s, society has experienced what some refer to as a "wealth deficit"—a heightened level of economic growth and modernization within a relatively short period of time. This has led to the introduction of both a bustling fast food industry and an increased availability of consumer goods that foster more sedentary lifestyles—all of this landing in the laps of citizens who for years were deprived of such amenities due to communist isolation (French and Crabbe, 2010). Figure 4.2 shows the increase in obesity nationwide.

There are several reasons for the emergence of obesity in China. First, China, like India, went through a nutrition transition. The traditional staples of the Chinese diet, such as grains, wheat, rice, vegetables, and fruit, were gradually replaced with meats, oils, and fatty foods, facilitated through increased trade

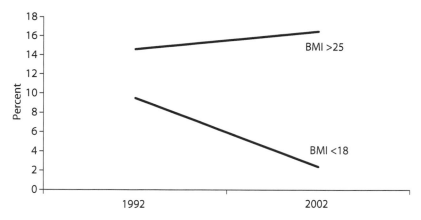

Figure 4.2. Obesity cases in China, defined as BMI >25 (percentage of population), 1992–2002. Source: WHO, Global Infobase, 2012.

and consumerism since the early 1980s (T. Cheng, 2003, 2007; Du et al., 2002; French and Crabbe, 2010; Zhai et al., 2007). In addition, the burgeoning growth of supermarkets, from 1 in 1990 to an estimated 53,000 by 2002, and of snack bars and corner markets facilitated the introduction of unhealthy foods (Hawkes, 2007). Perhaps more so than in any other country in Asia, the fast food industry opened shop throughout China. The number of McDonald's and Kentucky Fried Chicken restaurants increased at an alarming speed—allegedly at a growth rate of 13% a year, as opposed to just 2.9% in the United States. There were 560 Pizza Huts, 1,200 McDonald's, and 3,000 Kentucky Fried Chickens in China as of 2010 (Scarlatelli, 2010). Eating at McDonald's was and still is viewed as "stylish," increasing one's social status and suggesting prosperity and the ability to afford western foods (T. Cheng, 2003; *Health & Place*, 2004). Others claim that McDonald's and other western fast food chains are seen as cleaner, more orderly establishments with higher standards, and thus more enticing than less-regulated local establishments (Bardsley, 2011).

While partaking of fatty goods, over the past three decades China also saw a change in lifestyle, which mimicked western trends. Due to the purchase of cars and motorcycles and many new desk jobs, physical exercise declined (Popkin, 2006; *Renmin Ribao*, 2010b; H. Wang and Zhai, 2013). Computers, video games, and television sales burgeoned—by 2006, an estimated 91% of households had color televisions, as opposed to 63% in 1989 (Popkin, 2006). Cities often lack playgrounds or parks where adults can exercise (Bristow, 2010). Much like attitudes toward AIDS, some believed that the evils of the western lifestyles had once again emerged, causing obesity, stress, and discrimination to rise (Fan, 2007). Also, obese individuals often complained about job and social discrimination, forcing parents to enroll their children in costly weight loss clinics, while paying higher health insurance premiums (Xinhua, 2010a).

Yet another problem was—and continues to be—an ongoing cultural misperception that being overweight is a good thing. Ever since the food famine of the late 1950s, when thousands died due to starvation, overweight in adults and especially in children has been viewed as an indication of good health and prosperity (French and Crabbe, 2010; Gordon, 2010). To this day, every Chinese New Year, posters (*nianhua*) of chubby kids riding on top of plump fish are freely distributed—to connote good health, wealth, and prosperity (French and Crabbe, 2010). Conversely, to be thin in China was for years seen not only as a sign of financial impoverishment and physical illness but, worse still, as a sign of spiritual deficiency, immorality, an indication that an individual has been "sucked dry from within by demons" (Gordon, 2010).

Many blamed the government for the obesity problem: specifically, the government's one child policy. Since implementation in 1979, though supposedly helping China avoid a population crisis, this policy probably contributed to the emergence of what the Chinese referred to as "Little Princes" (*BMJ*, 2006; *Renmin Ribao*, 2010b). These "princes" were single children in middle- and upper-income families who were spoiled and constantly being fed by parents and grandparents.

But the nutrition transition, modernization, and the government's one child policy mainly affected urban areas (Bekedam, 2008; Du et al., 2002). As in Brazil and India, obesity was initially perceived as a problem of luxury, confined to the upper- and middle-income classes in growing urban centers and rarely seen among the poor in rural areas (Balfour, 2010; French and Crabbe, 2010). While obesity cases escalated in the cities, millions of children in rural areas continued to suffer from malnourishment and poverty (Xinhua, 2008b). Only recently has obesity started to emerge among poor rural children, the product of several factors, such as children's preferences for western foods that are high in fat or sugar (e.g., soft drinks), less physical exercise, and the lack of adequate knowledge about good nutrition and healthy food habits (Whitten, 2016).

Obesity was rare during the 1980s. In 1982, only 3.5% of adults 20–45 years of age had a BMI above 25, and only 0.2% were classified as obese. These rates had increased to 14.1% and 1.3%, respectively, by 1997. By 1992, more than

40% of urban residents in Beijing were overweight or obese (Du et al., 2002). These trends continued throughout the 1990s, and by 2002, the prevalence of obesity reached 2.6% of the total population (*BMJ*, 2006). By 2010, there were an estimated 100–120 million obese people in China, and about half of them were children (French and Crabbe, 2010). By 2014, China had overtaken the United States to become "the world's fattest nation" (Xiaodong, 2016).

But nowhere did the epidemic hit as hard as among children. Increased television viewing, computer games, and a decline in physical activity were commonly named as causal factors (Balfour, 2010; *BMJ*, 2006). Elementary and high schools were not emphasizing physical education, and cities often lacked safe playgrounds (M. Li et al., 2007). While an emphasis on rigorous educational standards and test scores has certainly been instrumental in creating a highly educated populace and strong economy, physical and nutritional education in schools has been a neglected issue, with severe consequences—so much so that China reached out to US universities to learn how to incorporate physical activity into school curricula (Stein, 2009).

The rate of obesity among children saw an 8% yearly increase by 2010; an estimated 40% of children in major urban centers such as Beijing were reported to be overweight or obese in that year (Balfour, 2010). In urban areas, where the epidemic was initially concentrated, the prevalence of obesity increased from 1.5% in 1989 to 12.6% in 1997, and the prevalence of overweight increased from 14.6% to 28.9% over the same period (*Health & Place*, 2004; Lou, 2002). The Chinese National Surveillance on Students' Constitution and Health found that the prevalence of overweight and obesity in children aged 7–17 increased from 5.2% in 1991 to 13.2% in 2006 (H. Wang and Zhai, 2013). More recent studies suggest that 23% of boys and 14% of girls under the age of 20 are overweight or obese (Ng et al., 2014).

Little is known about how the government initially perceived the obesity epidemic. What is known is that in society, and thus presumably within government as well, the rising rate of obesity in the 1980s was not perceived as a serious public health threat; rather, and especially among the older generation, it was viewed as a sign of prosperity and good health (French and Crabbe, 2010). At no point did the idea of responding to a "national obesity epidemic" enter into the minds of Central Party members or MOH bureaucrats. Some claim that this lack of attention was also attributable to the increased domestic and international pressure for a response to HIV/AIDS and SARS, which forced the government to overlook what were arguably much more serious chronic diseases (Bekedam, 2008).

This lack of response to obesity is surprising, given that the government was fully aware of rising levels of overweight and obesity in the 1990s (*Obesity Reviews*, 2008). In fact, the Ministry of Education had been conducting extensive yearly surveys since 1985, reporting an increase in childhood overweight and obesity in urban areas (Xinhua, 2006b). By the late 1990s, however, MOH bureaucrats became increasingly concerned with rising prevalence rates in the cities and the potential healthcare costs involved (Frederik, 2010). As more studies in China and the WHO emphasized these rising trends, MOH experts snagged the attention of senior health officials. However, no immediate consensus was reached on the need to pursue a stronger policy response.

Indeed, during the 1980s and 1990s, the government's response was anything but stellar, relegated mainly to limited prevention efforts and funding (Yang et al., 2008). The most concrete policy action taken was the introduction of national guidelines and laws requiring that children spend one hour a day on playgrounds, while the MOH urged schools to add more time for physical education. Federal funding was also provided to help build playgrounds in schools (Xinhua, 2006a). A series of federal regulations on food safety such as labeling and nutritional content were implemented in 2003 through the Special Nutrient Food Labeling Law, and in 1994 legislation on advertising was passed with the goal of protecting the health of minors by regulating false advertising (Hawkes, 2007). And in 2003, the CCDC promulgated Guidelines for Prevention and Control of Overweight and Obesity of Chinese Adults, which appeared to focus mainly on improvements in monitoring and measuring BMI for the Chinese population rather than providing effective prevention efforts (H. Wang and Zhai, 2013).

During this period, the MOH did not provide funding or technical assistance to the provinces for awareness and prevention programs. As was the case with HIV/AIDS, in a time of increased fiscal and health policy decentralization, the states were expected to respond to obesity on their own. Consequently, most provincial responses were isolated and occurred in the more affluent urban centers, where resources and hospital capacity were more ample. In the city of Shanghai, for example, in response to increasing overweight and obesity trends among bureaucratic officials, the local government authorized a special budget to encourage officials to obtain gym memberships (Watts,

2005). And in the city of Hangzhou, the provincial government worked with its CCDC branch officials to publish a report and policy plan for addressing obesity among adults, as well as other chronic diseases. In 2004, the CCDC followed suit with the Hangzhou CCDC prevention and treatment programs for hypertension, diabetes, cancers, and other noncommunicable diseases, including obesity among adults (Lim et al., 2010).

International Pressure and Positive Geopolitical Positioning

Throughout the 1980s and 1990s, the international community knew little about China's escalating obesity problem. This motivated a team of physicians and nutritional experts from the WHO to visit China in 1999 with the intent of learning more about the epidemic. Led by W. P. T. James (2007) and Chunming Chen, the WHO team organized a workshop in Hong Kong to better understand the factors contributing to obesity and its forecasted health and economic costs. By 2001, workshops organized by foreign and Chinese academics in the cities of Shanghai, Beijing, and Guangzhou predicted that there would be approximately 200 million obese people in China in the coming decade (Xinhua, 2001). Not long afterward, the international community began to criticize China for its lackluster policy response.

Indeed, by 2004, the WHO's *Global Strategy on Diet, Physical Activity, and Health* singled out China as leading the developing world in terms of poor nutrition, increased consumption of fatty foods, decline in physical activity, and, consequently, obesity (WHO, 2004b). By 2006, the WHO began to urge China to "step up its commitments to fight the country's top killer—chronic diseases [obesity being one of them]—warning that millions of lives will be lost if rapid action is not taken." The WHO further warned that obesity was a "growing problem" and that "these risk factors will cause an unacceptable number of people to die prematurely" (Agence France-Presse, 2006, 1).

The media also joined in the criticism. In 2004, the BBC published an article stating that China's obesity rates had increased by 97% (*BBC News*, 2004). In 2005, the *Guardian* of London reported that China faced a severe obesity epidemic, with 200 million people projected to be dangerously overweight in the next 10 years (Watts, 2005). Media pundits brushed up against academic researchers proffering similar forecasts (P. James, 2003).

China's response to these criticisms was in large part positive and predictable. With regard to the WHO's 2004 *Global Strategy*, China was far from resistant to its recommendations (S. Rao, 2004). Chinese officials asked to carefully review the report, provided comments, then quickly agreed with its findings. Apparently the only concern that Chinese officials had was that not enough attention was paid to a well-balanced diet, which meant a variety of foods, including fats and oils. It quickly became apparent that China wanted to work with the international community on curbing the spread of obesity (Fleck, 2004; Rao, S. 2004), as seen in the past with HIV/AIDS and other diseases.

Again, as we saw with HIV/AIDS, heightened international criticism and pressure motivated the government to improve its international reputation by pursuing a stronger policy response, while working cooperatively with the international community. However, the timing of this international pressure and the policy expectations were different for HIV/AIDS and obesity. Pressure for an HIV/AIDS response emerged in the mid-1990s versus the mid-2000s for obesity, resulting in earlier national political and policy responses for HIV/AIDS than for obesity. Nevertheless, when striving to build its international reputation for obesity prevention (and for the same reasons), the government once again focused on western institutions and countries, such as the WHO, the United States, and western European nations, from which essentially all of the criticism was emanating.

But were international pressure and reputation building the only reasons that the government began to respond? Perhaps it was politicians' incentives to campaign on the obesity issue that triggered a response. This cannot be the case, however, as there are no national elections in China, let alone efforts to campaign on the obesity issue (Bekedam, 2008; French and Crabbe, 2010). Or, perhaps obesity rates were growing at such an alarming pace that by the early 2000s government officials had no choice but to respond. But again, this cannot be the case. The MOH had already reported on the burgeoning obesity epidemic in major urban centers. Throughout the 1990s, the MOH was clearly aware of the epidemic, expressed its concern, and was reporting the situation to the State Council (Frederik, 2010). Finally, perhaps it was the rise of obesity among the upper- and middle-income classes and their relationship with politicians and bureaucrats that got the government's attention. This argument has two problems. First, while obesity and overweight certainly developed among the upper- and middle-income classes, by the early 2000s it was becoming increasingly prevalent among the lower-income classes and in the suburbs (Reynolds et al., 2007). It was therefore viewed as a shared, collective problem, providing little incentive for the upper- and middle-income classes to use their status as leverage for pressuring friends in government for policy reform. Second, there was no organized civil societal movement for obesity and, consequently, no established venue and funding through which the more affluent classes could lobby the government.

In an effort to bolster its government's international reputation for being capable of effectively responding to obesity, China began to host international conferences and sponsor public speeches. In 2001, the MOH hosted the 2001 China International Conference on Traditional Eating Patterns. At this conference, MOH officials and scientists demonstrated their knowledge of the factors that contribute to obesity, such as supplanting traditional foods with processed foods, while discussing the government's concern and actions to combat this epidemic (*People's Daily*, 2001). Next, in 2006, the director of the CCDC, Wang Wu, worked with the WHO to hold a conference titled "Obesity and Related Disease Control in China." At this conference, not only did Wang acknowledge China's rising noncommunicable disease and obesity problem, but he also highlighted the CCDC's commitment to tackling this issue through, as he claimed, "strong government action" (WHO, 2006, 1). Wang went on to claim that the MOH had been developing the Medium- and Long-Term High Level National Plan for Chronic Disease Control and Prevention and how this helped reduce the burden of obesity and related diseases. Wang closed his speech to the WHO by stating that the CCDC was unwaveringly committed to prevention policy and to eradicating obesity and other noncommunicable diseases (WHO, 2006). Finally, in November 2008, the MOH authorized the International Conference on Childhood Obesity, which was held in Hong Kong (Chinese University of Hong Kong, 2008). At the conference, organized by the Department of Sports Science and Physical Education at the Chinese University of Hong Kong, academics, scientists, and health officials presented their research on the causes and prevention of childhood obesity in China and the MOH's policy commitments to addressing the issue.

In response to heightened pressure emanating from the WHO's 2004 *Global Strategy on Diet, Physical Activity, and Health* report, in 2005 the MOH announced plans to create laws and regulations for improved public nutrition, emphasizing children and the elderly (Xinhua, 2005). The director of China's Public Nutrition and Development Center, Yu Xiaodong, was quoted as stating: "The nutrition level is an important indicator of a nation's overall strength. However, in the current Chinese laws, little attention is paid to public nutrition . . . it is time to make supporting laws now" (Xinhua, 2006b, 2). The laws and regulations would focus not only on avoiding overweight and obesity but also on malnourishment and anemia.

This discussion led to a reform of the preexisting National Plan of Action for Nutrition implemented in 1997. Through this revised program, the government provided a framework for establishing food policies that was focused on improved nutrition, such as promoting healthy diets and lifestyles and providing fiscal incentives for agricultural producers of healthy foods (T. Cheng, 2007). In 2006, the government also explored the possibility of working with community-based organizations to share its policy recommendations and to increase civic participation in promoting healthy lifestyles (French, 2015).

In December 2006, the State Council authorized passage of the Sunshine Physical Education Policy, which required that students master two types of basic physical skills in physical education classes and take part in one hour of physical education each day. China State Counselor Chen Zhili also called on all prevention-education departments and schools to embark on concrete measures to improve physical education and change teachers' and parents' conventional ideas about nutrition (Xinhua, 2006a).

National funding for provincial governments was also provided. In an effort to help curb the spread of obesity among Chinese youth, the central government spent 20 million yuan (US$2.5 million) on bodybuilding equipment for 681 rural primary schools and invested 6 million yuan (US$750,000) in other physical fitness machines. Provincial governments followed suit: that year, the Beijing municipal governments invested more than 700 million yuan to renovate 300 pieces of playground equipment, while the province of Jiangsu funded the hiring of 2,500 new physical education teachers (Xinhua, 2006a).

In 2007, the MOH further strengthened its policy response. It created the Healthy Action Strategy of Ten Thousand Steps a Day: The Balance of Eating and Activity and a Healthy Life. This government program encouraged overweight and obese individuals to adopt a good diet and incorporate a moderate level of exercise into their daily routine. The program also required that the MOH disseminate and promote healthy lifestyle concepts, promote technical and educational tools, and fulfill national health plans (H. Wang and Zhai, 2013). Moreover, in that year the Central Committee of the Communist Party and the State Council issued a circular "urging" more efforts to develop physical education classes and strengthen children's health. The circular emphasized that "if the problems cannot be effectively solved, the health of Chinese youngsters will be seriously affected, and the future of China and Chinese people will be affected" (Xinhua, 2007a, 1). For the first time, the government drew a connection between children's health and the health of the nation. The circular went on to require one hour of physical education each day in primary and middle schools and two sports days each week, and it required middle schools and universities to take entrance fitness exams seriously. Furthermore, in 2008 the CCDC released its official Guidelines on Snacks for Chinese Children and Adolescents (H. Wang and Zhai, 2013)—the first of its kind in China and based on the advice of nutrition scientists from the United States and Hong Kong. The guidelines warned that children should not be eating foods and consuming drinks with excessive fat, sugar, and salt, such as instant noodles, candies, and canned foods, which the report claimed led to obesity and diabetes. The Chinese state news agency alleged that parents started to take the official snack guidelines as a reference when shopping for their children (Xinhua, 2007b).

In 2008, the government also became a bit more aggressive in its policy response. It produced yet another national guideline for children's obesity while planning for the creation of a new Medium- and Long-Term High Level National Plan for Chronic Disease Control and Prevention (Bekedam, 2007). And the Ministry of Education, in a somewhat supercilious, centralized manner, mandated that all schools force children to run every day during the winter season, between October 26, 2008, and April 1, 2009, through its National School Running Campaign (Xinhua, 2008a). Parents quickly expressed their discontent, claiming that this was a violation of their children's freedoms and would take away time from study. The government directive further specified that primary school children should run 1 kilometer per day, junior high school students 1.5 kilometers, and senior high school and college students 2 kilometers. The government's position was that these brisk winter runs could help "improve children's endurance and team spirit" and help them lose weight and stay in shape (Xinhua, 2008a). In 2011, the Department of Education expanded this initiative by establishing a national policy that required an hour of physical activity in schools every day (H. Wang and Zhai, 2013).

In 2010, more federal guidelines were issued to address the prevention of obesity among adults: the Chinese Adults' Physical Activity Guidelines (H. Wang and Zhai, 2013). Through the Regulation to Improve Nutrition, the MOH established a national monitoring system for nutrition-related diseases and the effects of improved nutrition on citizens' diets (*Renmin Ribao,*

2010a). The MOH vowed to periodically publish a report on the nutritional status of Chinese citizens, with a focus on nutritional deficiencies and excessive nutrition. The goal of the monitoring system was to enhance national surveillance of food intake, changes in dietary status, macro- and micronutrient intake, overweight and obesity, anemia, calcium deficiency, lack of vitamin A, and other nutrition-related conditions (*Renmin Ribao*, 2010a). The MOH followed up in 2010 with the release of the Nutrition Improvement Work Management Approach, which sought to enhance nutritional surveillance, education, guidance, and intervention programs (H. Wang and Zhai, 2013).

Also in 2010, the government implemented additional educational programs focused on avoiding obesity and living a more active lifestyle. Through the MOH's endorsement of Chronic Disease Comprehensive Prevention and Control Demonstrations Areas, the central government worked with provincial governments to encourage civil societal participation and collaboration with the government to control obesity and other chronic diseases and to reduce individual risk. More specifically, through this initiative, local communities worked with health officials to increase health education and promotion, early detection and treatment, and standardized management to reduce the prevalence and economic burden of obesity and other noncommunicable diseases. By 2013, this initiative had been adopted by 140 counties in 30 provinces (H. Wang and Zhai, 2013).

In 2012, the MOH took further steps to increase its policy commitment to obesity and other noncommunicable diseases through the National Plan for NCD Prevention and Treatment (2012–15). Through this initiative, the MOH outlined a series of policy goals aimed at preventing overweight and obesity and other ailments related to noncommunicable diseases, with a focus on the following: ensuring that the Ministry of Education worked with schools to provide nutrition and physical education classes; strengthening primary healthcare systems, with a focus on monitoring and detecting ailments in individuals most at risk; usage of the media to increase social awareness of good nutrition and exercise; promoting the production and sale of healthy foods; and ensuring the sharing of resources between the central government and provinces to implement programs and monitor noncommunicable diseases (China, Ministry of Health, 2012).

In contrast to what we saw with HIV/AIDS, the government has yet to provide aid to other developing nations striving to reduce obesity. While the MOH has provided aid assistance in farming and agricultural production to several

African nations, with the intent of improving its international reputation as a benevolent state committed to eradicating global hunger and poverty (De Bruyn 2013; Sun, 2011), it has yet to achieve this in the area of obesity prevention. This may change as the government strives to improve its domestic response to obesity.

Despite China's strengthening of its policy response to obesity, several challenges remain, highlighting the need for ongoing political and financial investments. First and foremost is that, in contrast to HIV/AIDS, not one explicitly obesity-focused national agency or even sub-agency within the MOH was created. Obesity policy either has dovetailed with preexisting programs and agencies, often intertwined with efforts to address broader nutritional concerns and noncommunicable diseases, or has taken the form of national guidelines and laws. Consequently, to this day there is no separate line-item budget for obesity prevention programs. The upshot is that this has led to irregularities in federal financial assistance and physical resources to schools and communities. In this context, the initiative and entrepreneurship of cities has been important for stimulating any kind of federal assistance—as seen with local government funding for gym facilities (Xinhua, 2006a) and intervention studies providing information on the different types of prevention programs that can work (H. Wang and Zhai, 2013).

In this situation, scholars claim that there is a need for a heightened government commitment to building national institutions, a clear policy vision, and a national strategy (Xinhua, 2010b). The government's response to obesity has certainly improved but is still far from complete. For example, there are still no federal laws regulating the fast food industry or regulating television and other media advertising of fast food, no adequate warning labels, and insufficient funding for children's sports programs in schools (French, 2015). Moreover, there has been no effort to explore different types of fiscal incentives for reducing the consumption of sugary drinks, such as a soda tax, or for increasing consumption of healthier foods. In contrast to what we saw in Brazil and India, there has been no government effort to regulate consumption in public schools and hospitals (H. Wang and Zhai, 2013). While the government has engaged in a series of policy regulations and initiatives, with the most recent advice coming from the NHFPC's new dietary guidelines suggesting that citizens drastically cut back on meat and egg consumption (E. Henderson, 2016), federal funding still has not matched this heightened policy attention (French, 2015). Meanwhile, the 2008 and 2011 MOH regulations requiring schools to engage their students in more physical exercise have in many instances been ignored by provincial schools and governments, mainly due to strong parental resistance because of time taken away from study. Employers have also resisted recent government recommendations for more exercise in the workplace (French, 2015).

Finally, in contrast to what we saw in Brazil, the State Council and MOH are still not fully committed to providing more funding to the provinces to create and implement obesity prevention programs (Altherton, 2016; French, 2015). And in even starker contrast to Brazil, despite the State Council's voicing its commitment to improving the food supply and nutrition in rural areas in 2011, it has not worked with the MOH to help isolated, poorer rural governments implement these kinds of programs—even with the well-known spike in obesity cases in these areas (Altherton, 2016), increasing from an estimated 0.5% in 1985 to 30.7% in 2014 (Y. Zhang et al., 2016). Even a highly regarded government official, Dr. Ying-Xiu Zhang of the Shandong branch of the CCDC, recently commented that "rural areas of China have been largely ignored in strategies to reduce childhood obesity . . . [and that] this is a wake-up call for policymakers that rural China should not be neglected in obesity interventions" (quoted in Altherton, 2016, 1).

Therefore, as we saw with HIV/AIDS, while the government was capable of achieving a stronger policy response to obesity, it never achieved a centralized policy response. It has fallen short of creating a national agency—or even sub-agency—explicitly focused on obesity prevention, provided only limited prevention programs with no ongoing federal assistance to provincial governments, and made no efforts to increase the MOH's policy influence over the provinces through conditional fiscal transfers or by working with NGOs to monitor local policy implementation. But why has this occurred? As we saw in India, what was missing was a strong bureaucratic–civil societal partnership, due to the absence of NGOs that MOH bureaucrats could work with.

The Absence of Strong Bureaucratic-Civil Societal Partnerships

Perhaps the weakest link in China's national response to obesity is the role of civil society. There is no history of civic mobilization or of civil society's proffering of new ideas for a policy response to obesity and overweight. In fact, if anything, the opposite health challenge has garnered more attention: malnourishment and underweight, the product of historically high levels of poverty and inequality. Malnourishment and underweight were historically addressed through civic associations at the community level (Pye, 1996), but these efforts dissipated over time and were relegated to isolated community responses in poor rural areas (Yang Da-hua, 2004). With the resurgence of civic mobilization in the 1980s, there was no civic movement addressing overweight and obesity and their associated ailments such as high blood pressure and type 2 diabetes (Ji, 2015). This in large part stems from the obesity epidemic being so recent and mainly found in urban areas and among more affluent socioeconomic classes, which do not feel the need to organize collectively to address the issue.

In fact, to my knowledge, not a single social health movement or NGO exists that focuses on obesity. While concerned citizens have periodically disseminated information promoting fat acceptance through cultural groups, such as the popular singing and dance group Qian Jin Zu, these efforts are poorly organized and funded and do not appear to have a strong relationship with government. Other associations have been organized by famous athletes—such as former Houston Rockets basketball star Yao Ming and his National Basketball Association Yao School in Beijing—to increase government action and social awareness about childhood obesity, while proposing to work with the government for the creation of fitness programs for youth (Barris, 2014). Scientific associations such as the Chinese Medical Doctor Association provide guidelines on how to lose and maintain weight (Xiaodong, 2016). None of these organizations, however, commit all of their time and resources to obesity, and consequently they have not been able to obtain the resources, political attention, or influence needed to affect local or even national legislation.

The only NGO in China that focuses on obesity is located outside the mainland: in Hong Kong. Hong Kong's Association for the Study of Obesity (HKASO) was formed in 2003 by medical scientists, nutritionists, pharmacists, and physical education experts. Through the HKASO, these individuals conduct research on obesity and its broader health and socioeconomic implications while providing policy suggestions (HKASO, 2016). The association worked with Hong Kong's Department of Health to improve school lunches through the city's Eat Smart campaign (HKASO, 2013), but the HKASO has been limited to working with local governments and schools and has not collaborated with NGOs on the mainland to propose and/or strengthen existing federal policies.

On the other hand, there are well-organized NGOs addressing ailments directly associated with obesity, such as type 2 diabetes. For example, the Chinese Diabetes Society is well organized, well funded, and committed to increasing awareness, prevention, and research on diabetes (Ji, 2010). The current vice president of the International Diabetes Federation, Dr. Linong Ji, is from China and is wholeheartedly committed to working with the government, academic institutions, nutritionists and activists to achieve these initiatives (Ji, 2015). Such efforts have been absent in the area of obesity. While newer NGOs such as the United States–China Joint Collaboration on Clean Energy in Shanghai have reached out to children and families to provide more information about how to cook and eat better—such as the collaboration's 2014 A New Way to Eat Initiative (Cerini, 2016)—they have not worked in close partnership with the central government.

In sum, although the benefits of positive geopolitical positioning also emerged for obesity, that is, the government immediately responded to international criticism and pressure by pursuing a stronger policy response in order to improve its international reputation, after this occurred, MOH bureaucrats did not have access to NGOs that they could work with to increase their legitimacy within government and to monitor provincial policy implementation. In contrast to what we saw in Brazil, because such a strong partnership never emerged, the MOH was hampered in its ability to achieve a centrist policy response. Despite the increased realization that activists need to be more proactive in helping government formulate policy (French, 2015; H. Parry, 2010), until civic associations organize better and focus explicitly on obesity prevention issues, achieving this type of policy outcome will be challenging.

Conclusion

In China, as in Brazil and India, positive geopolitical positioning eventually led to a stronger policy response to the HIV/AIDS and obesity epidemics. With the arrival of increased international criticism and pressure, political leaders were eager to improve the government's international reputation in health through a stronger policy response, in turn helping to secure investor confidence and support from international institutions. At the same time, to facilitate reforms, China's leadership pursued the help of international donor institutions, and later decided to provide foreign aid to nations striving to eradicate HIV/AIDS. These positive geopolitical endeavors built upon a foreign policy tradition and institutions that bolster the government's international reputation in development and health, while working in peaceful, collaborative partnership with other nations to eradicate disease. Nevertheless, in the context of the challenges presented by healthcare decentralization, China's MOH has not proved capable of introducing a centrist policy response. This limitation reflects the bureaucracy's unwillingness to establish a strong partnership with NGOs and thus its inability to secure the ongoing funding and political support needed to achieve a stronger policy outcome.

5

Responding to HIV/AIDS and Tuberculosis in Russia

While having a different history and political culture, by the 1980s Russia had joined Brazil, India, and China in confronting a series of public health threats, including HIV/AIDS and tuberculosis. In contrast to the other BRICS nations, however, Russia's negative geopolitical positioning generated few incentives for the government to pursue a stronger policy response to these epidemics when confronted with international criticism and pressure. Given the government's foreign policy legacy of positioning Russia as an independent geopolitical power and a leader in international diplomacy, it had little interest in using such a response to bolster its international reputation in health. In this context, the government would begin to address HIV/AIDS—though not TB—more concretely only after the disease began to pose a national security threat. Even then, recognition of this threat did not lead to a strengthening of policy response. Moreover, while the government joined its BRICS counterparts in providing foreign aid assistance to other nations for HIV/AIDS and TB, the goal was always to improve Russia's international image as an influential global leader rather than a government committed to disease eradication in Russia and elsewhere.

The government's ability to improve its policy response was further complicated by the absence of strong bureaucratic–civil societal partnerships. With a president suspicious of independent civil societal organizations that have linkages to international donors, the political environment has not been propitious for an improvement in these partnerships or, ultimately, the possibility of either a stronger or perhaps centrist policy response.

Responding to HIV/AIDS

Russia's initial response to HIV/AIDS was marked by government denial, inaction, and discrimination. Initially, a combination of conservative moral and social beliefs, government pride, and putting blame on other nations shaped the government's perceptions. When HIV emerged, toward the end of the Cold War, the Soviet government accused the United States of clandestinely planting the virus in Moscow (Williams, 1995). At the time, this made a lot of sense to the paranoid Soviet intelligence: HIV could easily have been a ploy to undermine the health of state officials. It took the government several years to realize that HIV/AIDS was not a CIA operation. The initial response underscored the deeply held belief, much as in China, that Russia's socialist, conservative, pious moral beliefs, permeating the government and certain segments of society, could not possibly have allowed the emergence of HIV (Williams, 1995).

Indeed, the historical infiltration of conservative moral beliefs within government helps to explain Russia's delayed response to HIV/AIDS. In this respect, Russia was perhaps most similar to China and India. A strong Orthodox Christian faith, institutionalized in the eighteenth century through the political appointment of individuals with such beliefs,[1] and the creation of federal laws and regulations based on these beliefs, engendered a state that was highly discriminatory toward acts of immorality and crime (Williams, 1995). Beginning with Stalin, a host of federal laws banned homosexual activity—punishable by years of imprisonment (Williams, 1995)—and intravenous drug use; such activities were deemed "morally defective" (W. E. Butler, 2003). While the Boris Yeltsin presidential administration (1991–99) successfully overturned the laws affecting the gay community, political and social discrimination persisted (Pape, 2014).

Russian health officials also believed that, when compared with the myriad of health threats the nation confronted, the small number of HIV/AIDS cases did not pose a serious national health threat (Brown, 2006; Wallander, 2005). There simply was not enough credible epidemiological evidence pointing to a public health crisis (Wallander, 2005). Moreover, Twigg (2007) notes that in the 1980s, AIDS paled in comparison with the health threats mainly affecting working-age men, such as heart disease, diabetes, and high blood pressure. With so many health problems, the scarcity of infrastructural and human resources, and the mysterious nature of the virus itself, there was little interest

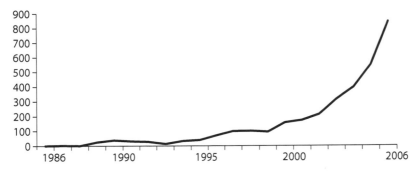

Figure 5.1. HIV/AIDS cases in Russia, 1986–2006 (thousands). Source: Demikhova and Karamov, 2011.

and incentive for the government to aggressively respond. The increase in HIV/AIDS in Russia since the mid-1980s is shown in figure 5.1.

Under the Soviet Union, the threat posed by HIV/AIDS to the military and thus to Russia's national security was also a nonissue. During the late 1980s and early 1990s, the number of enlistees denied admission to serve in the military was minimal at best, as the government was not testing enlistees or expecting them to test positive for HIV (Holacheck, 2006). AIDS was therefore not viewed as a national security issue (Holacheck, 2006; Sjostedt, 2008).

The government's historical commitment to decentralization also created few incentives for a response. In the late 1980s, in an effort to expedite economic development, the government accelerated its commitment to healthcare decentralization (Newsholme and Kingsbury, 1993; Tkatchenko-Schmidt et al., 2010). When AIDS emerged, the government therefore believed that the regional *oblast* governments should be primarily responsible for containing the epidemic's spread (Brown, 2006; Davis and Dickinson, 2005).

Thus, in the late 1980s, the Soviet government had no incentives to create strong federal institutions that would not only treat individuals with HIV/AIDS but also offer effective public awareness campaigns and services. As described by Pape (2014), what the government instead focused on was monitoring the spread of AIDS throughout the nation, quarantining people with AIDS, and deporting foreign nationals suspected as HIV carriers. The first federal legislation in response to the epidemic was enacted on August 25, 1987: the Decree Concerning Measures to Prevent Infection with the AIDS Virus. This decree required mandatory testing for blood donors, Russians who had traveled abroad, foreign visitors, and people in high-risk groups. For the state, an effective response could be contrived only through mass screening, forced isolation, deportation, monitoring, and control. A Federal AIDS Center was created within the MOH to facilitate these efforts, and the Russian Federal Scientific and Methodological Center for AIDS Prevention focused on surveillance. At no point did the government consider the creation of mass public awareness campaigns or of prevention programs such as sex education, condom distribution, or drug treatment.

Even after the fall of the Soviet Union in 1991, the president and the Duma (assembly) still had no interest in pursuing a stronger policy response. Powell (2000) notes that while President Boris Yeltsin had plans to construct a more effective national AIDS program superseding the Federal AIDS Center within the MOH, it was meant to be a temporary solution, lasting for approximately three years. At the time, the Federal AIDS Center was poorly staffed and did little to coordinate policy with the states. In response, a Coordinating Council on AIDS was created in 1994, which sought to bring the Federal AIDS Center, other ministries, state agencies, NGOs, and academics together to build a stronger, more cohesive policy response (Wallander, 2005). The Coordinating Council was ineffective, however, according to Wallander (2005), given the absence of high-level political officials serving on the council (Davis and Dickinson, 2005). Furthermore, Yeltsin made no effort to concentrate all prevention and treatment programs under either the Coordinating Council or the Federal AIDS Center. Twigg and Skolnik (2005, 14) write that at the time, the MOH was "divided into preventative (the State Committee for Sanitary and Epidemiological Surveillance) and curative (The Ministry of Health of the Russian Federation) branches; since then, separate structures for anti-AIDS work have co-existed in these two branches." Davis and Dickinson (2005) claim that this led to a lack of coordination between agencies working on AIDS, such as the Justice, Internal Affairs, and Defense departments. Also, the MOH during this period received little financial support for its programs (Davis and Dickinson, 2005; Specter, 1997). In 1995, for example, the MOH received approximately half of the money that the Duma authorized for its work on AIDS (Specter, 1997).

As we saw in Brazil, India, and China, Russia's government initially relied on a decentralized administrative and policy response to HIV/AIDS, with little coordination from the center (Twigg and Skolnik, 2005). What this essentially meant was that, as under the old Soviet system, health system responses were completely decentralized (Newsholme and Kingsbury, 1993) and run by local health clinics and AIDS centers, with wide variation in the financial resources and administrative capacity of regional governments to provide prevention and treatment services.

In the 1990s, neither the Boris Yeltsin nor the Vladimir Putin (2000–2008) administrations sought to rectify this situation by creating a central agency that could meet regional governments' needs while working with them to implement policy. State governments received very little if any financial and technical assistance to combat the epidemic (Kiselev, 2010; Twigg and Skolnik, 2005). Without federal assistance, subnational inequalities in access to HIV/AIDS prevention and treatment services resulted, as the only cities capable of providing such services were the larger, more affluent cities of Moscow and St. Petersburg.

When it came to prevention and treatment policy, there was a response, albeit limited. Although the MOH disseminated information about the spread of HIV/AIDS, no major prevention programs were created to enhance sex education on how to avoid acquiring the virus (Specter, 1997; Williams, 1995). In fact, Specter (1997) writes, the national Institute of Preventative Medicine stopped translating foreign-language AIDS information booklets in 1991, and essentially no money was being provided for increasing knowledge and prevention. It was not until 1997 that the MOH created a program geared toward increased sex education, information for IDUs, and training for healthcare workers (Veeken, 1998). Williams (1995) claims that conservative ideological beliefs rendered these policies essentially meaningless, however, and that there was no political commitment to enforcing sex education policies and awareness.

The Yeltsin administration was somewhat more effective at creating laws and regulations on providing healthcare services for people living with HIV/AIDS, testing, and antidiscrimination. In 1996, Yeltsin signed the Federal Anti-AIDS Law, which guaranteed the universal provision of ARV medications, prevention services, professional and specialized medical treatment services, social support, and the safeguarding of human rights (Gage, 2008). But in addition to continuing human rights violations, such as breaches of medical confidentiality and unauthorized AIDS testing, there was little funding for the ARV program, thus leaving many state and local clinics incapable of providing treatment (Kiselev, 2010; Pape, 2014). And despite the Federal Anti-AIDS Law's mandate on ARV provision, few people actually received the treatment they needed (Kiselev, 2010).

Finally, throughout the 1990s and the early years of the Putin administration (Putin served as president from 2000 to 2008 and as prime minister from 2008 to 2012, then was reelected as president in 2012, a position he continues to hold to the present day), the MOH did not provide any funding to regional governments to help IDUs through harm reduction, counseling, or support programs. This inaction was attributable to the Putin administration's conservative moral outlook and discrimination toward drug users (Gómez, 2006). Furthermore, the Russian Orthodox Church adamantly insisted that Putin and the Duma refrain from creating legislation providing harm reduction, as this would fuel the great "social evil" of addiction (*ITAR-TASS*, 2000a). With this lack of national political support, the Federal Anti-AIDS Law enacted by Yeltsin in 1996 was rendered essentially meaningless, and IDUs had to rely on city governments for help (W. E. Butler, 2003).

International Criticism and Pressure

The emergence of international criticism and pressure in response to Russia's lackluster response to HIV/AIDS was somewhat delayed compared with the other BRICS nations. The later emergence of HIV in Russia explains this difference in timing: HIV was first detected in Russia in 1987, compared with 1982 in Brazil, and had slowly spread from the gay to the IDU community by the 1990s. International criticism, pressure, and policy expectations therefore did not arise until the mid-1990s and did not intensify until the mid-2000s, compared with the late 1980s in Brazil and the early and mid-1990s in India and China, respectively.

Throughout the 1990s, Russia became the focal point of international health agencies such as the WHO, focused on a timely and effective policy response for high-risk groups such as the gay and IDU community (WHO, 2009b). Equally critical was a 2000 World Bank report claiming that if the government did not escalate its response, the epidemic would cause an estimated 4.5% slump in gross domestic product and a 5.5% downturn in investment (Ruhl, Pokrovsky, and Vinogradov, 2002).

Furthermore, in 2002, a CIA report titled *The Next Wave of HIV/AIDS* criticized Russia for its inadequate response to AIDS. The report also predicted that Russia would see approximately three to four million cases of AIDS by 2010 (CIA, 2002; Twigg, 2007). Moreover, that same year the WHO published statements from Russian officials that underscored the government's lack of focus and resolve in responding to AIDS. In the WHO's journal *Bulletin of the World Health Organization*, Dr. Vadim Pokrovsky, chief of the Russian Federal AIDS Center, stated in an interview with Robert Walgate of the *Bulletin* "that the government must be more active in prevention. . . . At the moment HIV/AIDS doesn't get enough attention from the government" (Pokrovsky quoted in Walgate, 2002, 686). In 2003, the World Bank's lead health specialist for Europe and Central Asia Olusoji Adeyi explained in the *Lancet* medical journal that after receiving a loan from the World Bank for TB and AIDS prevention and treatment programs, the Russian government needed to " 'move fast and decisively' to fight the compound epidemics through better planning, bolstered treatment, and prevention campaigns" (Webster, 2003, 1355).

Other international health agencies, such as UNAIDS, also began to criticize the Russian government directly. For example, in 2005, the executive director of UNAIDS Dr. Peter Piot made the following statement at a symposium in Moscow: "Rarely in the twenty-year history of response to the AIDS epidemic around the globe has there been such a clear-cut choice as the one that now faces this nation. The Russian Federation is on the verge of an HIV epidemic that will be very difficult to contain. Policy decisions and programme actions taken over the next year will determine whether the epidemic continues its explosive course or whether it is stabilized and its impact reduced" (quoted in Gerber and Mendelson, 2005, 28).

In the light of this international criticism and pressure, how did Russia respond? Did the government mimic Brazil, India, and China in pursuing stronger policy reforms in order to enhance its international reputation in health? The simple answer is no. In line with my negative geopolitical positioning framework, and as I explain shortly, Russia's political leadership ignored this criticism and pressure, preferring instead to determine its own strategies for financing, creating, and implementing AIDS policies, even when these policies flew in the face of countervailing international policy consensus, such as the importance of providing methadone treatment for drug addicts, harm reduction, condom distribution, and sex education—issues that we will return to shortly. Why did this occur? Understanding the historical precedents behind Russia's negative geopolitical positioning—that is, the government's foreign policy history and ambition in international relations and global health diplomacy—provides insight into this matter.

The Historical Precedents of Negative
Geopolitical Positioning

Since helping to establish the Peace of Westphalia in 1648, Russia's government has always taken an aggressive foreign policy stance aimed at securing its position as a world leader and global power. Beginning in the seventeenth century, the government was committed to proposing and signing international treaties to maintain the peace and to engaging in international economic trade and, at times, in military campaigns to expand Russia's territories (Ivanov, 2009). And even when Russia's generals lost their military campaigns, such as against the French in 1856 over the territory of Danube near the Black Sea, the government was committed to quickly recovering and "dressing up" its regional dominance—that is, boasting of its great power, securing its regional image, while secretly noting its military limitations (Hosking, 2001).

By the time the Soviet Union emerged, in 1917, the government's belief that it was a global leader and superpower shaped the Communist Party's mentality and foreign policy strategies (Ivanov, 2009). Ivanov (2009, 13–14) writes that this belief was passed on to the Russian democratic government in 1989: "one legacy bequeathed by Soviet foreign policy was a 'superpower mentality,' which induced post-Soviet Russia to participate in any and all significant international developments." He goes on to cite George Kennan's views on the matter: "Kennan attributed the foreign policy particularities of the Soviet period to an 'ideological super structure' that was 'superimposed' in 1917 onto the essentially unchanged foreign policy legacy of previous eras . . . Kennan identified this legacy with negative traits of Russian 'imperial' policy, such as a tendency towards territorial expansion, claims of 'ideological exclusivity,' deep mistrust towards the west and foreigners in general."

Russia also developed an interest in helping to lead the world in the fight against disease, establishing a reputation for being a provider rather than receiver of foreign aid assistance. In 1922, for example, through creation of the International Sanitary Commission, the government provided developing nations with technical assistance in response to a host of diseases (Balinska, 1995). Hepler (2012) notes that by the mid-1980s, the Soviet Union had allocated roughly US$25 billion a year to such kinds of foreign aid projects, which were seen as helping to achieve Russia's global influence and prominence. As discussed shortly, this foreign policy tradition would resurface with the HIV/AIDS epidemic.

Russia also displayed a great deal of leadership and foreign aid assistance when it came to eradicating the smallpox epidemic. In 1958, at a time when the WHO was not taking the eradication of smallpox seriously (due to perceived challenges in reaching distant rural populations with vaccines and funding limitations), Russia's deputy minister of health Victor Zhadanov adamantly lobbied the WHO to prioritize eradication (D. Henderson, 1988). By explaining Russia's ability to successfully devise and provide a vaccine, Zhadanov succeeded in prompting the WHO to take smallpox eradication more seriously. At the same time, he worked closely with WHO representatives from the United States to ensure the WHO's renewed commitment to smallpox eradication, which ultimately led to the World Health Assembly's passage of its new global smallpox eradication program in 1968. From that moment on, Russia joined the United States in providing the bulk of financial assistance to the WHO, staffing WHO field offices with epidemiologists trained in smallpox detection and eradication (D. Henderson, 1988). What's more, Russia's donation of 25 million vaccines greatly exceeded any other country's contributions—even the United States'; Russia supplemented these efforts with direct bilateral contributions of vaccines to other nations such as Afghanistan (D. Henderson, 1988). In short, it was during this time that Russia began establishing its role as a global leader and provider of foreign aid in health.

In 1976, at a WHO meeting in Geneva, Russia once again displayed global health leadership by taking the lead in proposing an international conference on primary health care. Dr. Dimitrios Venediktov, Russia's deputy health minister at the time, offered US$2 million to host the WHO conference in Moscow (WHO, 2008). Ultimately, however, the conference was held in Alma-Ata, Kazakhstan, and was the first WHO conference to establish an international agreement for governments to provide healthcare as a human right, building effective primary healthcare systems grounded in decentralization, community participation, and accountability (WHO, 2008). Russia's efforts nevertheless revealed its geopolitical ambitions: Moscow wanted to secure its position as the leading socialist power in the world, replacing China's influence throughout the developing world as a leader in providing primary healthcare innovation (WHO, 2008).

The fall of the Soviet Union and the emergence of a Russian democratic state led to new foreign policy interests, though the government's historical beliefs in and legacies of global leadership and being a superpower remained. The foreign policy objectives of General Secretary of the Communist Party

Mikhail Gorbachev (1985–91) were to build closer ties with the West and deepen international economic collaboration in order to develop Russia's new market-based economy, while maintaining the government's national interests and its hegemonic power over Eastern Europe. The Boris Yeltsin administration (1991–99) followed Gorbachev's path while confronting growing resistance from a conservative political wing seeking isolationism and fewer relations with the West. During this period, conflicting views and political interests, when combined with the increased role of the parliament and media, led to an identity crisis in Russian foreign policy (Curtis, 1996). After reasserting his constitutional right over all foreign policy matters, Yeltsin ordered his Ministry of Foreign Affairs to draft a new foreign policy strategy that the parliament could agree to. In April 1993, decades after any legislation on foreign policy had been ratified, a new Foreign Policy Concept emerged, approved by the Security Council, which among other goals explicitly emphasized "ensuring Russia an active role as a great power" (Curtis, 1996, 4).

These goals were clearly evident in the twentieth century. For instance, Russia took a proactive stance in signing peace treaties, working with others to form the UN, helping conclude wars (including the Second World War), signing the Helsinki Accord, and working with the United States to sign the Nuclear Non-Proliferation Treaty in 1970 and the Convention on Chemical Weapons in 1993 (Ivanov, 2009). This history gave strength to the government's belief that its involvement and leadership in international relations was essential for solving international problems (Curtis, 1996).

The government's belief in its superpower status and responsibility as a world leader has deepened. Following Russia's decline in economic and military prowess in the late 1990s due to an economic recession, President Vladimir Putin (2000–2008) made it a point to use foreign policy as a means to restore Russia's world power status (Katz, 2005). Wallander (2005, 142–43) claims that "the Putin leadership seeks economic growth to increase the country's wealth and power, and hence reestablish Russia as a great power on the global stage." In a public speech given to the Federal Assembly in 2003, as quoted by Katz (2005, 27), Putin made the following remarks: "All our actions must be subordinated to the goal of ensuring that Russia truly takes its place among the major powers." Katz (2005, 27) goes on to claim that Putin "wants Russia to be seen as a great power so that other countries—including the United States and the European Union—will accommodate its positions on issues it sees as important." Putin believed that Russia should be equal to the United States in terms of geopolitical power and influence (Blank, 1996). Despite their political differences, Russia's next elected president, Dmitry Medvedev (2008–12), shared Putin's concerns, believing that Russia had to reposition itself as a world power (Likhachev, 2010).

Both the Putin and the Medvedev administrations also engaged in several activities to uphold Russia's foreign policy objective of sustaining its superpower status. For example, many view the Putin administration's military engagement in Georgia in 2008 as a way to enhance Russia's regional power status. The many military training exercises during his administration have been conducted with the same intentions in mind (R. Allison, 2008). Moreover, Putin's efforts in 2014 to annex Crimea in the Ukraine through military force revealed his intentions to increase Russia's territorial presence and influence in the Ukraine, secure the Ukraine's subordination to Russia, limit the Ukraine's relationship with the West, and establish regional stability and Russia's ongoing influence (Menkiszak, Sadowski, and Zochowski, 2014). Similarly, some analysts view Russia's military involvement in Syria and its support of the allied Assad regime as yet another instance in which the government has used its military presence to secure its relationship with Syria, resist western (mainly US) influence over the ensuing conflict, and consolidate its influence in the Middle East (Tabachnik, 2016). Despite initial hopes that Russia's involvement in the effort to help restrain terrorist groups in Syria would lead to the United States dropping sanctions for Moscow's wrongdoing in Crimea, Putin's recent inability to comply with a ceasefire agreement with the United States has hampered the relationship between the United States and Russia (*BBC News*, 2016). All of these efforts have revealed Russia's ongoing interest in sustaining its superpower status by influencing politics beyond its boarders, securing its geopolitical interests, and expanding its international authority through military action.

The government has also maintained its tradition of engaging in international leadership. For instance, the government used its position on the UN Security Council and in the Group of Eight (G8) to strengthen its leadership and build coalitions on human rights and environmental issues (Kassianova, 2002). And in a move to modernize Russia's foreign policy stance, Medvedev tried to take the lead in working with other nations to reform international financial institutions such as the IMF and the World Bank to develop a sustainable system of energy security in Europe, and in peace building. Scholars emphasize that

Russia perceives itself and has been perceived by others as a key actor in solving the world's problems (Likhachev, 2010).

Finally, these military, security, and leadership activities create the perception within and outside Russia that not only is it a world power, like the United States, but it is also an independent, sovereign, all-powerful nation. Its increased military intervention in Eastern Europe, for example, has given the impression that Russia is what R. Allison (2008, 1171) describes as an "independent pole in a multilateral world." In fact, Allison writes, these activities have led to a "strategic independence," a position necessary for Russia's and others' perceptions of its world power status. Sjostedt (2008, 21) writes that "international identity constructions can help us to understand this resistance [to international influence], since Russia, according to one predominant discursive line, predicates itself as an important international power. Russia is predicated as active—not passive; a provider—not a receiver, and this is reflected in its reluctance to accept the suggestions of 'the West,' including advice from international organizations and nations."

When taken together, then, Russia's historical precedents of government leadership, power, and sovereignty in foreign policy and global health diplomacy ultimately contributed to the formation of a government that was apathetic toward international criticism and policy pressure. These historical precedents contributed to the emergence of the government's negative geopolitical positioning.

This positioning entailed serious consequences in responding to HIV/AIDS. For unlike in Brazil, India, and China, the rise of international criticism and pressure had essentially no impact on the Russian government's interest in reforming its bureaucratic institutions and policies while working with international organizations. Indeed, Wallander (2005, 143) claims that "the Russian leadership's policy of reestablishing its position as a global power has hampered effective engagement with the international community, which has a great deal of experience that could help Russia mount a more effective national response [to AIDS]." The MOH agreed to receive a loan from the World Bank in 1999 to fund TB and, eventually, HIV programs, but the loan was substantially delayed due to vehement political resistance and negotiations. The MOH was essentially forced to accept US$150 million in loans at the height of Russia's financial banking crisis (Sridhar and Gómez, 2010). At the peak of the HIV/AIDS epidemic in 2006, Hannah Brown (2006, 438) of the *Lancet* wrote that "until this year, Putin has seemed largely oblivious to the concerns of the scientists and international AIDS organizations about Russia's burgeoning HIV crisis."

Challenging National Security and Instituting Reforms

In this geopolitical context, what factors could have inspired Russia's government to respond, as it eventually did, to the HIV/AIDS crisis? The government did not begin to address the epidemic seriously until it was perceived as posing a national security threat (Pape, 2014; Sjostedt, 2008). International health organizations such as the WHO and UNAIDS had officially declared HIV/AIDS to be a national security threat as early as 2001, but as Sjostedt (2008) writes, Putin essentially ignored these warnings and instead decided to respond at his own time and pace.

By the early 2000s, Russian military statistics were revealing an escalating increase in the number of military enlistees testing positive for HIV; inadequate, poorly organized screening and prevention programs within the military were to blame (Holachek, 2006). In response, senior military and MOH officials started writing reports and warning the government that a national security crisis was at hand (Sjostedt, 2008). A startling report in a Russian newspaper in 2006 revealed that approximately 200,000 young enlistees were released from the army because of their positive HIV status (*Central Eurasia–OSC Report*, 2006). After reviewing the information himself, in April 2006 Putin for the first time began to describe HIV/AIDS as a national security threat. The only other time Putin had mentioned HIV/AIDS was during a speech in 1993 when discussing how intravenous drug use was contributing to the spread of HIV (Interfax, 2006). Faced with overwhelming statistical data and incessant pressure from military and health officials, Putin finally began to respond. He stated on April 21, 2006, in his opening speech to the Assembly of the Presidium of the State Council, that "this is a serious situation that requires us to take the appropriate action. We need more than words; we need action, and the whole of Russian Society must get involved" (quoted in Pape, 2014, 74). Putin perceived HIV/AIDS as a national security threat on two fronts: first, its significant contributions to an ongoing demographic decline, and second, as a threat to military capability (Interfax, 2006; Sjostedt, 2008). In June 2006, the fight against HIV/AIDS was declared a priority issue at the G8 summit in St. Petersburg, and a new government commission was organized in that year to explicitly deal with HIV/AIDS. These events motivated

UNAIDS representative Bertil Lindblad to describe Putin's speech as a "milestone in the fight against HIV/AIDS in Russia" (quoted in Pape, 2014, 74).

But was a national security threat the only factor motivating the government to respond? One could just as easily argue that by 2006 the number of HIV/AIDS cases had reached an apogee, that it was a grave situation in need of a response, and that the increase in cases in the military was merely coincidental and not a primary catalyst for reform. Under scrutiny, however, these arguments do not hold up. The MOH had known about the fast-paced growth of the epidemic prior to 2006. Gennady Onishchenko and other public health officials were warning the government and pressuring it for a response well before then (Davis and Dickinson, 2005; Sjostedt, 2008). Alternatively, perhaps politicians were sensitive to growing social hostilities and citizens' demands for a more aggressive response. This does not hold either, as the Yeltsin, Putin, and Medvedev administrations all campaigned on the HIV/AIDS issue (Gómez, 2015a). In fact, the biggest electoral constituent was, and still is, conservative segments of society attached to the Russian Orthodox Church, which maintains a discriminatory view toward the HIV/AIDS community (Pape, 2014). So, perhaps it was the ongoing pressure from AIDS NGOs, reinforced through partnerships with the international community, that prompted the government response. As discussed in more detail below, this argument falls short, too, due to the absence of a well-organized, politically influential NGO community that might have succeeded in garnering sufficient political attention and support, as well as vehement state resistance to those NGOs supported by highly suspect western organizations (Pape, 2014).

Instead, scholars emphasize that it was the government's national security concerns that prompted the Putin administration to increase its attention to HIV/AIDS (Pape, 2014; Sjostedt, 2008). In 2006, Putin called for an increase in federal spending for the Federal AIDS Center, which in 2004 had been integrated into the newly established Federal Service for Surveillance on Consumer Rights Protection and Human Well-being (Rospotrebnadzor) of the MOH; the funding totaled 3.1 billion rubles (US$47 million). At the same time, he publicly committed to putting HIV/AIDS on the national and international (G8) agenda (*ITAR-TASS*, 2006a; Pape, 2014; Sjostedt, 2008). That 3.1 billion rubles was double the amount provided in 2005; according to head MOH sanitary physician Gennady Onishchenko, "only 130 million rubles [US$1.9 million] were allocated for HIV/AIDS prevention and treatment in 2005 and in all the previous years" (*ITAR-TASS*, 2005, 1). Birch (2009, 1) claims that by 2009, federal spending for HIV/AIDS had increased by 33%, "making it a central part of an ambitious new national health care strategy." In 2009, HIV/AIDS officials claimed that the government planned to increase the federal budget from 8.9 billion rubles (US$135 million) to 13.4 billion rubles (US$204 million), and a further increase in spending of up to 19 billion rubles (US$290 million) was planned for 2011–12 (*ITAR-TASS*, 2009b).

In 2007, several other national prevention and treatment programs were implemented. As reported by the Global Business Council (2009), in 2007 the government created the federal program Prevention and Fight against Socially Significant Diseases, 2007–11, which led to the creation of the HIV Infection Subprogram. With an allocation of 9 billion rubles (US$379 million), the subprogram's goal was to reduce the number of new HIV infections, broaden the surveillance coverage of HIV-positive pregnant women under the mother-to-child transmission prevention program, and increase the share of Russian medicines produced/purchased for ARV treatment. In addition, on October 13, 2006, just months after Putin's public speech, the government authorized creation of the Government Commission on Prevention, Diagnosis, and Treatment of HIV/AIDS. The purpose of this commission was to increase coordination and cooperation between federal and regional health centers focusing on HIV/AIDS prevention and medical and social support for people living with HIV/AIDS.

In 2006, Putin also sided with other leaders and the MOH to propose the creation of Russia's first Subregional Center for AIDS Control (*ITAR-TASS*, 2006c). This organization was established to help the Federal AIDS Center coordinate the implementation of HIV/AIDS policies throughout its network of Regional AIDS Centers. In large part this initiative stemmed from Putin's growing realization that federalism and decentralization contributed to a lack of national and intergovernmental coordination in response to HIV/AIDS (*ITAR-TASS*, 2006b).

New efforts were also made to increase access to medical treatment. By 2006, the MOH was using the preexisting Regional AIDS Centers to dispense ARV medications, and in the following year, the MOH further increased its commitment to providing ARVs to anyone in need. Nevertheless, Vadim Pokrovsky, head of the Federal AIDS Center, noted that approximately 58,000 people were in need of treatment but only 18,000 were receiving it (Osadchuk, 2007)—a recurring problem that I return to shortly. Finally, in 2007, the Duma authorized the Decree Concerning Palliative Care to the HIV-Infected.

Through this decree, the government strove to enhance the quality of medical aid to persons with HIV who were undergoing palliative care (Pape, 2014).

During this period the government also decided to expand its renewed commitment to HIV/AIDS at the global level. In the mid-2000s, after a pause in providing foreign aid assistance to other nations due to Russia's precarious economic situation associated with the transition to democracy (Bakalova and Spanger, 2013), the Putin administration sought to revive the government's historical leadership role in global health. In the process, Russia would regain its geopolitical position as donor rather than receiver of foreign aid in health (Brezhneva and Ukhova, 2013; Hepler, 2012). From 2007 to 2010, funding for global health took up the lion's share of foreign aid assistance, reaching as much as 50%, followed by agricultural (food) security, environment and energy security, and education (Bakalova and Spanger, 2013; Troilo, 2012). Most of the government's contributions to global health went to the Global Fund to Fight AIDS, Tuberculosis, and Malaria (Bakalova and Spanger, 2013; Troilo, 2012) and to Gavi, the Vaccine Alliance (originally named Global Alliance for Vaccines and Immunization)—consistent with the government's ongoing focus on providing foreign aid through multilateral channels rather than bilaterally (Brezhneva and Ukhova, 2013; Hepler, 2012). Indeed, between 2002 and 2014, Russia contributed an estimated $US317 million to the Global Fund (Zaardiashvili, 2014). By 2012, as table 5.1 shows, Russia led the BRICS nations in total contributions to the Global Fund and Gavi, with US$297 million (Sridhar et al., 2013). Through the Global Fund, Russia contributed funding for HIV/AIDS and TB programs in Russia itself and in other countries.

Reflecting the Putin administration's negative geopolitical positioning, during the MOH's initial interaction with the Global Fund in 2003, the

Table 5.1.   BRICS' Contributions to Global Health Organizations (in US$ millions, 2012)

	Contributions to the Global Fund*	Contributions to Gavi, the Vaccine Alliance
Brazil	0.0	0.0
Russia	297.0	24.0
India	10.0	0.0
China	25.0	0.0
South Africa	10.3	6.0

Source: Sridhar et al., 2013.

*Global Fund to Fight AIDS, Tuberculosis, and Malaria.

administration resisted the idea of receiving financial assistance from the fund, preferring instead to remain autonomous in the timing and depth of government funding for HIV/AIDS. As Wolfe (2005, 2) explains, this "attitude [was] characteristic of [the government's] dislike of receiving handouts or advice from outsiders . . . [and it was] reluctant to be an applicant." In fact, Russia's first Global Fund grant proposal in 2003 came not from the government but from a consortium of NGOs, which lacked the requirement to form a Country Coordinating Mechanism panel consisting of government representatives, people living with HIV/AIDS, and activists (Wolfe, 2005). In an effort to further consolidate Russia's historical leadership role as a foreign aid donor and leader in global health, by 2010 the government pledged to repay all of the money it had received from the Global Fund to help Russian NGOs, while requesting other bilateral donors, such as USAID in 2012, to refrain from providing any more support (Hepler, 2012). While the government has authorized receiving limited funds for NGO activities related to democracy and the rule of law, as Bakalova and Spanger (2013, 8) explain, the "government has repeatedly stressed its discomfort around receiving them." To this day, Russia receives no bilateral or multilateral funding for HIV/AIDS or other diseases (Bakalova and Spanger, 2013).

Russia provided some direct bilateral assistance for HIV/AIDS and for health systems strengthening. In 2010, the Medvedev administration increased its bilateral assistance for combating HIV/AIDS in neighboring Central Asian states (Jack, 2011). Throughout Central Asia and Africa, the government helped to establish research centers on HIV/AIDS and provided technical assistance (Morazán et al., 2012). Between 2006 and 2009, Russia provided a multimillion-dollar grant package to help strengthen health systems in neighboring countries, mainly in response to the influenza pandemic (Provost, 2011). Nations in other regions of the world, such as Kyrgystan, Nicaragua, and Nauru, also received approximately US$50 million from Russia to help strengthen their health, education, and infrastructure sectors (Bakalova and Spanger, 2013). Russia has also sent physicians to several Eastern European and African nations to train their counterparts (Troilo, 2012), provided assistance in implementing medical support projects (Makarychev and Simão, 2014), and given direct support to help strengthen the human resource capacity of health systems and malaria control programs (Jordan, 2010).

Russia's ongoing leadership role in global health also extended to international agenda-setting efforts. For example, in 2006, Russia took advantage of its G8 presidency to propose specific health initiatives, such as placing infectious disease control and prevention firmly on the G8 agenda for the first time in its history (Hepler, 2012).

In sharp contrast to what we saw in Brazil and India, however, Russia's government never sought to increase its international reputation in health and/or its reputation as a geopolitical power by engaging in aggressive negotiations with pharmaceutical companies for greater access to ARV medications. This was so despite a context in which the government did not produce generic versions of ARVs (voiding the potential to issue compulsory licenses through the 2001 Doha declaration), thus making the price of such medicines excessive (Pape, 2014). In theory, this situation should have compelled Russia to join Brazil, India, and other developing nations in collectively bargaining for more affordable pharmaceutical prices, but Russia did not do so (Watt, Gómez, and McKee, 2014). I maintain that the government's unwillingness to bargain with pharmaceutical industries reflected a lack of political priority and commitment to ensure that it had sufficient medication to treat all those in need (Gómez, 2009). Pape (2014) concurs and adds that the MOH also lacked the proper diplomatic training to effectively bargain with pharmaceutical companies, while NGOs and people with HIV/AIDS were unable to mobilize and effectively pressure the government—which could have been facilitated through a strong partnership with health officials. Finally, Pape (2014) goes on to attribute these challenges to a high level of corruption among international suppliers and government health officials, thus making it easier for the suppliers to manipulate conditions to their advantage.

Hence, whereas Brazil, India, and China sought to provide bilateral and multilateral assistance in HIV/AIDS to further enhance their international reputation in health, Russia instead strove to use foreign aid in health as an opportunity to increase its international power, leadership, and influence (Bakalova and Spanger, 2013; Jack, 2011; Makarychev and Simão, 2014). Russia wanted to reclaim its historical position and status as a donor rather than receiver of foreign aid in health (Bakalova and Spanger, 2013; Brezhneva and Ukhova, 2013; Gómez, 2015a; Jack, 2011; Makarychev and Simão, 2014). NGO leaders note that the government's geopolitical beliefs and ambitions shaped its interest in helping other nations combat HIV/AIDS. Dr. Alexi Brobrik, former director of Moscow's Open Health Institute, stated that "Russia always tried to be an international power, to present itself like a donor country . . . We wanted to be among the leaders—to launch Sputnik, to put the first person in space, to help other developing nations. So basically the commitment of Russia to the Global Fund is in the same role" (*Frontline*, 2006, 1).

The only reputational issue that Russia's leadership has been concerned with is enhancing its global status as a sovereign power and becoming a force in a multipolar world (Bakalova and Spanger, 2013; Brezhneva and Ukhova, 2013; Jack, 2011). In fact, the notion of foreign aid securing "Russia's status of superpower" was listed as one of the four goals in the government's first and only official document discussing its foreign aid objectives: the *Concept on Russia's Participation in International Development Assistance* (Bakalova and Panger, 2013). In contrast to what we saw in China, Russia's aid assistance also is not primarily motivated by economic and financial gain, though efforts to facilitate access to agricultural markets have been pursued through the provision of food grains (Makarychev and Simão, 2014). In essence, it is the government's concern with Realpolitik—that is, ensuring that it can secure control and influence, especially within the former Soviet region—that has guided its interest in foreign aid assistance (Brezhneva and Ukhova, 2013).

The government has been criticized for assuming this kind of donor leadership role at a time when it needs to invest more in its domestic HIV/AIDS programs. In an opinion survey conducted by the World Bank in 2010, 66% of the participants noted that Russia was not rich enough to help other nations while also improving its domestic welfare policies, and 82% believed Russia should be more concerned with its domestic problems (Brezhneva and Ukhova, 2013). Criticism has even emerged from within the government. According to the director of the Federal AIDS Center, Vadim Pokrovsky, "the problem is that Russia helps the Global Fund but does not increase funds for the fight against HIV/AIDS within the country" (quoted in Quinn, 2014, 1). Others comment that "international prestige and the wish to be accepted among the group of G8 countries thus apparently had a higher priority for the Russian government than the development of an effective domestic response to HIV/AIDS" (Pape, 2014, 218). What is even more ironic is that the government felt compelled to fund methadone treatment and harm reduction strategies through the Global Fund for other countries while vehemently resisting the funding of such policies in Russia (Quinn, 2014). When an activist from the ESVERO (Russian Harm Reduction Network) NGO approached an anonymous international donor to help finance its harm reduction activities, the funder was baffled, allegedly stating: "Wait, you yourselves [Russia's government] are giving us money for this" (quoted in Quinn, 2014, 1).

Despite the government's seemingly renewed commitment to domestic and global HIV/AIDS policy, several policy shortcomings remain, especially with respect to the efficacy of federal funding and improved prevention and treatment programs. In contrast to Brazil, India, and China, even as Russia's leadership began to pay more attention to HIV/AIDS, this attention did not lead to a strong, effective, and ongoing policy response.

For example, by 2008, in response to the government's concern about its financial situation, the Putin administration decided to reduce the national budget for HIV/AIDS (Gutterman, 2008), thus failing to provide sufficient funds for medical treatment and the MOH's various Regional AIDS Centers (Brown, 2006). Furthermore, researchers subsequently discovered that the increase in federal funding for prevention programs between 2006 and 2007 did not lead to any substantive improvements and/or the creation of new prevention and treatment programs (Kucheryavenko and Gómez, 2016). Yet, HIV/AIDS officials emphasized that more funding for specific policy efforts was needed: specifically, funding for programs targeting Russia's largest at-risk groups such as IDUs, the gay community, and sex workers. In fact, according to Pokrovsky, despite an increase in federal spending, the programs at that time almost completely neglected those groups most intensely affected and in need (Schwirtz, 2011). At the same time, others claimed that of the 400 million rubles (US$6.1 million) provided for the national AIDS program in 2009, much went missing (*ITAR-TASS*, 2009a). Worse still, this occurred even after Putin reemphasized the threat posed by HIV/AIDS to national security in the publication *National Security Strategy of the Russian Federation until 2010* (Kucheryavenko and Gómez, 2016). Figure 5.2 shows the change in funding of programs in Russia from 2004 to 2015.

Only recently has federal spending for the Federal AIDS Center been increased. In 2014, 18 billion rubles (US$274 million) were allocated (Agence France-Presse, 2015), increasing to 20.42 billion rubles (US$306 million) in 2015 (fig. 5.2). However, this level of funding is deemed wholly insufficient, considering that most of the funds are used for the purchase of ARV medications rather than prevention programs for at-risk groups (Agence France-Presse, 2015; Reuters, 2015b).

Pokrovsky has also continued to express his ongoing frustration at the lack of political support for his efforts to obtain funding for prevention programs. In addition to repeatedly criticizing the government for its lack of focus and the absence of a coherent national strategy, Pokrovsky has complained

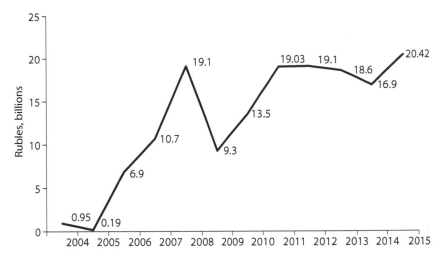

Figure 5.2. Federal budget for domestic HIV/AIDS programs in Russia (billions of rubles), 2004–15. Source: Kucheryavenko and Gómez, 2016.

constantly about the absence of concrete political and financial support. He even presented the MOH and Duma with ongoing problems such as the shortage of ARV medications (Kucheryavenko and Gómez, 2016). Pokrovsky's opposition to the state's conservative views and his support for western-based, proven scientific approaches to HIV/AIDS prevention, treatment, and policy recommendations have contributed to this lack of political support within government. It also contributes to ongoing tensions between the Kremlin, the MOH, and the Federal AIDS Center. In this context, and in sharp contrast to what we saw in Brazil and India, Pokrovsky has had very little autonomy and essentially no financial and political support for the prevention programs that he and the international scientific and policy community believe are essential to stem Russia's burgeoning tide of HIV/AIDS cases.

The inability to secure ongoing financial support for prevention programs has been one of the main reasons that the epidemic persists (Arkhangelskaya, 2015; Schwirtz, 2011). As the disheartened HIV/AIDS activist Anya Sarang, president of the Andrey Rylkov Foundation for Health and Social Justice, once commented: "there [was] zero money in the federal budget to fund focused HIV prevention and education" programs (quoted in Gorst, 2010, 1). To this day, there is not a single piece of national legislation requiring sex education in schools, general state-sponsored propaganda messages about safe sex that provide simple information such as how to obtain and use condoms, the distribution of condoms to sex workers, or the distribution of clean needles (Mirovalev, 2016). Worse still, recently, when Pokrovsky lobbied the Moscow City Council for the introduction of sex education in schools, the head of the city council's health committee, Lyudmila Stebenkova, responded by stating that Pokrovsky was a "typical agent working against the national interests of Russia" (quoted in Fitzgerald and Kucheryavenko, 2015), claiming that his suggestion would only increase children's interest in sex and lead to a further increase in HIV infections. To this day, Pokrovsky claims that there is not a single MOH expert in charge of HIV prevention (Fitzgerald and Kucheryavenko, 2015).

Federal funding for Regional AIDS Centers also failed to increase after Putin's 2006 national security declaration. Burns (2007) claims that this mainly stemmed from the federal government's ongoing belief that regional AIDS authorities should respond to the epidemic on their own. Indeed, in 2006, even after Putin's proclamation, the federal government required that local governments start increasing their share of healthcare and other social welfare responsibilities through a new federal law on "local self-government" (Burns, 2007, 30). This led to the MOH's decision in 2013 to decentralize the responsibility of purchasing all ARV medications to the *oblast* governments (Quinn, 2014), thus imposing an addition financial burden. Even before this decision was made, when the MOH controlled all AIDS funding, the states still received inadequate financial support (Thatchenko-Schmidt et al., 2010). Indeed, Kiselev (2010) claims that government-run AIDS clinics received only about 20% to 40% of the funding to which the Federal AIDS Center said they were entitled.

The government also continued to fall short of ensuring an adequate supply of ARV medications (Vangelder, 2011). According to Pokrovsky, at least one in three HIV-positive persons in Russia were unable to receive treatment due to shortages of medical supplies in the Regional AIDS Centers (Stolyarova, 2010). In 2008, he further commented that despite the expectation that the government would provide free ARV medications, only 35,000 individuals had received treatment (*Moscow Times*, 2008). This situation worsened over time, as there has been a repeated shortage of ARVs due to federal financial shortfalls (instigated by an ongoing economic recession) and high costs, which means provision of ARVs cannot keep pace with the burgeoning rate of HIV infection. But these medication shortfalls also reflect a reduced supply due to the government's efforts to create its own domestic market of generic medications to replace expensive imported—and arguably better quality—ARV medications, which have comprised 80% of all medications purchased by *oblast* governments (Rozhdestvensky, 2015). Currently, most doctors can treat only about one in five patients due to the shortage of several new and complex ARV medications, which are mainly found abroad (Goble, 2015a). Other estimates suggest that of all the AIDS cases in Russia, only 200,000 people are being treated with ARVs, with preference given to individuals with malfunctioning immune systems (Arkhangelskaya, 2015). As of 2015, the MOH reported that approximately 30% of the population in need of ARV treatment did not have access to it (*Chicago Tribune*, 2015).

Yet another challenge is the government's ongoing reluctance to provide methadone treatment for IDUs—a scientifically proven, WHO-prescribed treatment—or to provide social workers who can distribute clean needles and teach drug users how to avoid infection (Clark, 2016; Reuters, 2015b). Worse still, any individual or institution suspected of selling methadone for treatment can face up to 20 years in prison (Bennetts, 2016).

But geopolitics has also mattered. Moscow's ongoing reluctance to adopt the WHO's recommendation for methadone treatment, which is on the WHO's list of "essential medicines," and the free distribution of needles provides yet another example of the pernicious effects of the government's negative geopolitical positioning. That is, politicians ignore international advice and seek policy design and implementation on their own, at their own pace, based on their own beliefs and cultural values, reinforced through their position as a sovereign power, and indifferent to world opinion. Journalists at the Pulitzer Center, Nora Fitzgerald and Oleg Kucheryavenko (2015, 1), summarized this situation nicely: "It's clear that the government of President Vladimir Putin has decided to significantly reduce any outside influence over the country's AIDS policies, which prevents foreign financial and technical assistance or cooperation with the international AIDS community. The Putin administration's unrelenting efforts to reestablish Russia as a world power has encouraged the medical community and officials to ignore all international AIDS policy recommendations and technical assistance, while banning the presence of foreign NGOS."

At a special UN meeting on June 8, 2016, the secretariat called on all member states to put an end to the epidemic by 2030. The Russian delegation revealed its continuing unwillingness to adopt the UN's policy recommendations. The resolution voted on at this meeting was to establish three targets to be reached by 2030: (1) reducing new HIV infections, (2) reducing mortality rates, and (3) eliminating HIV discrimination in AIDS prevention and treatment policies (Loyce, 2016). A political declaration was adopted by the 193-nation General Assembly that stressed the importance of HIV prevention programs for IDUs, sex workers, gay men, transgender people, and prisoners. Russia immediately rejected the declaration, calling for an amendment that did not require assistance for the gay community, drug addicts, prisoners, diplomats, or civil societal groups (Loyce, 2016). By requesting this amendment, Moscow was essentially rejecting the UN's resolution to decriminalize homosexuality and drug use for the purposes of prevention and treatment policies. When defending Russia's position, the government's health minister, Veronica Skvortsova, stated that Russia and other governments should have a "sovereign right" to decide their own public health strategies (Radio Free Europe, 2016).

The government's ongoing lack of commitment to adopting the international community's suggested prevention and treatment programs is also fueled by the government's high regard for the Russian Orthodox Church. Since the epidemic emerged, the Church has had a track record of influencing the AIDS policy views of presidents and Duma leaders, especially under Putin's conservative, dominant Pro Unity political party (Gómez, 2006). The Church's ongoing influence has motivated the government to heed the Church's repeated condemnation of drug substitution therapies—notwithstanding the escalation of HIV cases attributable to intravenous drug use (Schwirtz, 2011). Putin has made an effort to appeal to more conservative segments in society— primarily middle-aged Russians and blue-collar workers, many of whom are members of the Russian Orthodox Church—by promoting a return to family and moral values. This has created few incentives for Putin and his party to support treatment and prevention programs deemed by this conservative community as immoral, such as methadone treatment, sex education in schools, and funding for the gay community (Agence France-Presse, 2015; Bennetts, 2016). As if this were not enough, in 2015 influential bishops lobbied the government to accept the Church's proven approach to HIV prevention (confirmed through its application to an estimated 10,000 children and college-age students): the promotion of chastity, faith, and patriotism (Reuters, 2015a). The Church vehemently opposed the free distribution of condoms, sex education, and methadone treatment, perceiving these approaches as both ineffective and immoral.

Nevertheless, noticing the ongoing need to strengthen the government's policy response, in the spring of 2015 the MOH announced the creation of the Five-Year Strategy for Fighting HIV. This strategy seeks to increase spending, provide new initiatives such as HIV/AIDS education, promote and facilitate international collaboration, increase the effectiveness of HIV testing and treatment, and encourage the production of domestic generic ARV medications (Rozhdestvensky, 2015). To date, however, the strategy is still in development and no credible information has been released as to how it will be funded and implemented.

In summary, in 2006, after realizing the threat posed by HIV/AIDS to national security, the government heightened its attention and response to the epidemic (Gorst, 2010; Pape, 2014). But to what end? The threat to national security did not guarantee that the government would enact a sustainable, stronger policy response. Some new policy initiatives were established, but the response appears to have weakened within the past five years: insufficient federal funding for HIV/AIDS prevention policies, *oblast* health departments, and ARV medications persists. This situation has recently forced Director Vadim Pokrovsky of the Federal AIDS Center to comment that the government "has in effect stopped fighting the spread of HIV/AIDS" (quoted in Goble, 2015b, 1). Anything close to creating a strong centrist policy response, as seen in Brazil, does not appear anywhere on the horizon.

Needless to say, the government has not created a centrist policy response. As I explained in chapter 1, a centrist policy response requires three components: the creation and ongoing financial and administrative expansion of federal agencies, the development of effective prevention and treatment programs (particularly, universal access to medicines), and formal and informal strategies to increase the central government's policy influence in a context of healthcare decentralization. In Russia, however, the government has not maintained its commitment to increased administrative spending for the NAP, has not introduced an effective universal ARV policy, and has never engaged in efforts to formally increase the MOH's influence over state AIDS policies through the provision of conditional grant assistance for HIV/AIDS programs. In addition, and as I explain in more detail shortly, because of the MOH's weak partnership with NGOs, it has not informally worked with them to monitor policy implementation at the oblast level.

Because of this situation, and in sharp contrast to its BRICS counterparts, Russia saw the number of HIV cases increase to 900,000 (the highest in Europe) in 2015 (Arkhangelskaya, 2015), up from an estimated 50,000 in 2010 (Luhn, 2015). Moreover, approximately 10,000 new HIV cases are reported annually, which is likely to increase by 250% over the next five years (Goble, 2015a). The government's own health minister, Veronika Skvortsova, recently admitted that Russia's AIDS situation is "out of control" (quoted in Goble, 2015a, 1).

In 2014, this worsening situation motivated Prime Minister Dmitry Medvedev to approve an eight-year, 212 billion ruble (US$6.4 billion) plan to help the MOH identify drug addicts and fund programs that promote healthy lifestyles and sports (Bennett and Kravchenko, 2014). And in October 2015, Medvedev announced that the MOH would increase funding for HIV/AIDS prevention to US$600 million (Bennetts, 2016). Many remain skeptical, however, especially when considering the innumerable failed promises made in the past. In fact, just two months after this announcement, when the federal budget was announced in December 2015, funding for HIV/AIDS care and prevention *decreased* by US$600,000 (Bennetts, 2016). Activists also recall that in 2011, less than 150 million (US$2.2 million) of the 500 million rubles (US$7.6 million) allocated for prevention was spent, with the rest returned to the treasury for no apparent reason. Much of the federal funding allocated for the purchase of ARV medications has gone to the Russian company Rostec—which is, incidentally, led by a close friend of Putin, Sergei Chemezov, like Putin a former KGB officer (O'Hanlon, 2012).

But why has the government been repeatedly incapable of strengthening its policy response to HIV/AIDS? Yet another contributing factor has been the absence of a strong partnership between the bureaucracy and NGOs, providing few allies that bureaucrats could use to potentially obtain more political support for their programs.

The Absence of Strong Bureaucratic-Civil Societal Partnerships

Historically, social movements and organizations in Russia have developed separately from the government. Before the 1917 Bolshevik Revolution, during Russia's tsarist period, the activist community flourished and was committed to solving its own problems (Conroy, 2006; Hosking, 2001). Social clubs that were focused on poetry, music, and art thrived, and volunteer groups—often organized by the youth—arose to lend a hand where needed. Teenagers in Moscow created the Timur Teams, formed to help the elderly (Topolev and Topoleva, 2001). Business philanthropy thrived, donating generously (Conroy, 2006).

The government helped to foster this volunteerism. Primarily, this encouragement stemmed from the government's difficulty in providing social services to remote areas. The tsars often encouraged the formation of volunteer civic organizations to provide social services for the poor in such areas. Under Catherine II and Alexander I, local participatory governments, called *Zemstvo*—composed of voting peasants, nobles, and the business class—thrived (Conroy, 2006; Hosking, 2001). *Zemstvo* eventually replaced state boards in their responsibility for providing social welfare services, particularly medical attention, to the poor (Conroy, 2006). By the late nineteenth and early twentieth centuries, a rich tradition of participatory self-governance and volunteerism had emerged (Conroy, 2006; Topolev and Topoleva, 2001).

When it came to public health, local doctors and healthcare practitioners, known as *feldshers*, did not pressure the central government for immediate policy intervention whenever new diseases emerged. In fact, the opposite situation occurred: *feldshers*, steeped in their beliefs in participatory self-governance and encouraged and invited by friends within the *Zemstvo*, preferred to work on their own, without the help of central government officials. In fact, the *feldshers* viewed the central government as an impediment to their work at the grassroots level. Up through the early twentieth century, then, local governments and physicians were primarily responsible for responding to epidemics on their own (Hosking, 2001).

Social movements and organizations were certainly present during this period, sharing concern and interest in containing the spread of disease. But in contrast to what we saw in Brazil, they were either ineffective in or apathetic toward establishing close partnerships with public health officials and asking for their assistance. Though a Social Hygiene movement emerged during the late 1700s—seeking to transform the MOH's focus to preventive (rather than curative) healthcare, universal healthcare, and an understanding of the social determinants of health—the movement's leaders repeatedly failed to gain traction and influence at the national level. The movement eventually received the endorsement of the national Commissariat of Public Health, N. A. Semashko, but he did not have much influence and even faced political resistance for his policy ideas (Solomon, 1990).

Civic organizations that were focused on public health also flourished, though they did not seek central government intervention. In major cities, pharmacy societies began to emerge, working with local government officials and engineers for cleaner water and food. In addition, the Society for the Preservation of Public Health first emerged in St. Petersburg in 1880, with approximately 300 volunteers. Within a few years, however, this organization had spread to several cities, where it focused on sponsoring research and increasing public awareness (Conroy, 2006). The MOH endorsed much of the society's work—which supports historians' views that the MOH needed the organization's help in reaching out to distant communities.

Despite the emergence of proactive physicians, *feldshers*, and social movements and civic organizations focused on public health, these individuals and groups never proffered ideas for immediate central government intervention in response to disease epidemics. They flourished in their ability to work alone, under *Zemstvo* auspices, to eradicate disease (Hosking, 2001). There was an ongoing belief that local physicians and community members were, in fact, more capable than the central government in containing the spread of disease.

After the 1917 revolution, and especially under the Soviet Union, these social movements and civic organizations gradually disappeared. There was a brief increase in civic activity shortly after the revolution, but by the 1930s, the government had supplanted civic organizations and social movements with new ones organized by the Communist Party (Evans, 2006a). Soviet Communism and its self-proclaimed infallibility and totalitarianism took over all of Russian society, leaving little room for questioning or doubt (Mead, 1955). By 1935, Evans (2006a) explains, essentially all of the civic organizations and social movements that stemmed from years of civic freedom under the tsars, including those committed to public health, had come to an abrupt end. This left an enduring negative imprint: the Russian people's unfamiliarity with the importance and effectiveness of civic mobilization and a fear to mobilize.

Societal activism's second chance came with the downfall of the Soviet empire and the transition to democracy. This opportunity was short lived, however. Under the head of the Communist Party, Mikhail Gorbachev (1985–91), subsequently elected as Russia's first president in March 1990, the government encouraged the development of social movements and NGOs, mainly in an effort to monitor national and state governments and therefore increase political accountability (Evans, 2006a). NGOs nevertheless lacked sufficient funding, while concerned individuals in society had little knowledge about or trust in social movements that for years had done nothing to help people (Evans, 2006a; Nemyria, 2002). Furthermore, under the Boris Yeltsin (1991–99) administration, the extreme concentration of power under the president and the lack of government attention to NGOs further undermined development of the NGO community (Evans, 2006b). By the 1990s, at the height of the HIV/AIDS epidemic, NGOs were financially insecure, socially and politically marginalized, and incapable of influencing policy (Evans, 20016b; Nemyria, 2002; Topolev and Topoleva, 2001).

The arrival of the Vladimir Putin administration did not help. Perhaps more so than any other president since Stalin, Putin, from the beginning of his administration, made it clear that he did not trust any independent movement in society (Evans, 2006b). Putin lambasted any NGO working closely with international organizations, especially those in the West, as well as charitable groups (Evans, 2006b; Topolev and Topoleva, 2001). While he encouraged the presence of NGOs in public, Putin's version of an NGO was one that was wholly subservient to his needs (Evans, 2006b). This naturally led to the endorsement of only those NGOs that were working in support of Putin's interests.

These historical and political preconditions contributed to the absence of an immediate and effective NGO response to HIV/AIDS (Gómez and Harris, 2015; Wallander, 2005). The NGOs that first emerged, AIDS Infoshare in 1993 and Siberia AIDS-Aid (in the state of Tomsk) in 1995, received little recognition and support from the government (Gómez, 2006; Gómez and Harris, 2015; Wallander, 2005). Heavily influenced by conservative communist tenets and the Russian Orthodox Church, politicians and MOH officials viewed any civic organization working with the gay and drug-using community as immoral and unworthy of government support. As occurred under the Soviet Union, only those NGOs viewed as nationalistic and morally upright and those staffed and guided by the state were supported; these views deepened under Putin (Evans, 2006b; Pape, 2014).

Despite this challenging environment, by the late 1990s several AIDS NGOs had emerged throughout Russia (Pape, 2014; Wallander, 2005). The first type to arise were well-organized, internationally funded NGOs in major urban centers, such as Focus Media, AIDS Infoshare, ESVERO, and Siberia AIDS-Aid. As described by Pape (2014), these organizations focused on increasing public awareness, pressuring the government to adopt prevention and treatment programs, information gathering, and the exchange of policy ideas and experiences in various public venues. Several national-level NGOs emerged that were focused on establishing networks of service providers throughout Russia, with a focus on access to medical and harm reduction services. These included ESVERO, the All-Russian Association of PLWH, and the National Forum of AIDS-Service NGOs. A plethora of smaller regional and community-based NGOs also emerged to increase awareness, provide prevention and treatment services, and encourage self-help initiatives and groups. Finally, several federal and regional NGOs were established with the support of the government's Federal and Regional AIDS Centers, such as the Federal Russia Healthcare Foundation (RHF). The RHF was primary responsible for creating large public awareness campaigns such as the "AIDS Stop" motor rallies in 2007 and 2008, for implementing prevention and ARV treatment programs, and for palliative care. The RHF was criticized by the domestic and international NGO community for being a bureaucratic arm of the state, working in close partnership with MOH bureaucrats rather than with NGOs.

As Pape (2014) notes, there was a considerable amount of inequality in the financing and organizational capacity of these NGOs by the turn of the twenty-first century. While the large NGOs working in major urban centers had ample volunteers and support from international donors, smaller regional and community-based NGOs often lacked adequate funding, technical expertise, and human resources (Pape, 2014; Wallander, 2005). This situation led to a high level of competition and an unwillingness to share resources and experiences at the regional level (McCullough, 2005). At the same time, because of its close association with the Federal AIDS Center, the RHF was able to secure a steady stream of funding, though this was mainly used to sustain careers within RHF rather than introduce innovative, western-based prevention and treatment programs (Pape, 2014).

In the mid-2000s, the larger NGOs working mainly in Moscow and St. Petersburg received an injection of support, and thus of potential policy influence, from the international donor community. In 2004, Focus Media and AIDS Infoshare partnered with foreign-based NGOs in these cities—namely, the Open Health Institute, AIDS Foundation East-West, and Population Services International. Together, they successfully bid for a grant from the Global Fund in the amount of US$109 million for prevention and treatment programs (Pape, 2014). What emerged from this project was the GLOBUS consortium, the largest externally funded project focused on providing funds for a variety of NGOs working on prevention and treatment services. ESVERO, an NGO that united 33 regional harm reduction NGOs, also received a grant from the Global Fund in 2006 in the amount of US$14 million. The RHF received a grant of US$136 million (Brown, 2006; Pape, 2014).

In 2006, shortly after Putin's HIV/AIDS and national security speech, Putin and MOH bureaucrats began to voice their support for the work that these NGOs were doing, emphasizing the government's commitment to working with them (Brown, 2006). The political momentum in favor of supporting NGOs' response to HIV/AIDS seemed to have finally emerged. Those NGOs that benefited the most from this were the well-funded ones located in Moscow and St. Petersburg, which had not only funding but also access to key government officials (Pape, 2014).

But this political attention and support did not last long. In July 2009, Putin and the MOH decided to no longer fund the GLOBUS consortium through the Global Fund (Cohen, 2010). This move reaffirmed suspicions that Putin and the MOH were not fully committed to working with the HIV/AIDS community. This had serious implications. Some NGOs receiving grants through the GLOBUS consortium, such as LaSky, an NGO dedicated to prevention services for the gay community, had to let go several employees due to insufficient funding; other NGOs faced the specter of being shut down (Cohen, 2010). Several NGOs saw a decline in federal funding not only for their organizations but also for the MOH's HIV/AIDS prevention efforts, leaving the NGOs to fill in the gaps for services previously provided by Regional AIDS Centers. NGOs that were focused on harm reduction strategies, such as ESVERO, quickly discovered that no AIDS bureaucrats had any experience or interest in harm reduction (Toor, 2015). Worse still, those NGOs that were providing harm reduction services, methadone treatment, and the distribution of condoms were told to stop providing these services and to decrease their staff (O'Hanlon, 2012).

The ability of HIV/AIDS NGOs to continue providing such services is waning. Their major sources of funding, international donors, are starting to leave Russia. For example, existing Global Fund grants are due to expire in 2017. This is the result of the Global Fund's decision to withdraw from Russia because of the government's substantial reduction in funding support in 2009 and the fund's decision to do the same, as well as its reclassification of Russia as an aid donor rather than recipient in 2010. Furthermore, in 2012, international bilateral donors such as USAID and philanthropic organizations such as the

Open Society Foundation, which previously provided funding to approximately 200 NGOS for harm reduction programs, were asked to leave the country. They were viewed by the Kremlin as conspiring to influence domestic politics through the provision of grants (*Chicago Tribune*, 2015; Quinn, 2014). This unmasked the Putin administration's interests in curtailing the West's influence in domestic politics and HIV/AIDS policy (Bennett and Kravchenko, 2014).

These interests were solidified through the passage of a federal law in 2012 that required all foreign organizations providing funding to Russian NGOs to register themselves as "foreign agents." In so doing, NGOs became subject to random government investigations, and in some instances this led to the detention, arrest, and interrogation of staff (Mirovalev, 2016; Toor, 2015). Other domestic NGOs have simply been denied registration based on their work. For instance, the Silver Rose, an NGO based in St. Petersburg, has been denied registration three times because of its work with sex workers and its acceptance of western funding (Mirovalev, 2016). Through these efforts, the ability of external donors to support NGO prevention and treatment efforts has declined considerably. As if that were not enough, the government has denied funding to NGOs once they have been perceived as allies to western institutions and their policy ideas. In fact, Ilya Lapin, an activist working for ESVERO, recently stated that after requesting funding from the MOH, ESVERO was told "that we are foreign agents, that we promote pedophilia, homosexuality and drug addiction. It all comes back to that" (quoted in Quinn, 2014, 1).

The NGO community has also been the victim of information censorship and violation of civil liberties. Organizations that have posted information on their websites about the advantages of methadone treatment, for example, have seen their websites shut down by the government, in accordance with state law on "drug propaganda." Other NGOs have been forced to remove any statements supporting methadone treatment. These efforts suggest that the government has lost trust and confidence in NGOs and that it does not agree with them on how to treat the HIV/AIDS epidemic (Toor, 2015).

As a result, NGOs have essentially had to work on their own, striving to make a difference where they can. The Andrei Rylkov Foundation for Health and Social Justice is a good example of an NGO that is reaching out to the at-risk community in Moscow, providing condoms and being the only organization in the city to provide clean needles to IDUs (Bennetts, 2016). Meanwhile, activists continue to complain of the government's ongoing lack of attention to their needs. Ilya Lapin recently commented in a newspaper that "organizations like ours inform him [Putin], we send him reports, we do independent reports, we study international recommendations . . . we talk about this, but he doesn't hear us" (quoted in Luhn, 2015, 1).

In this context, HIV/AIDS NGOs have had little impact on the design of national policies (Gómez and Harris, 2015; Pape, 2014). And it is easy to understand why national AIDS bureaucrats have never viewed AIDS NGOs as strategic, influential partners that they could work with to increase bureaucrats' legitimacy, influence, and ability to secure ongoing program support from the government. In the eyes of key politicians and senior health officials, HIV/AIDS NGOs, especially those pursuing prevention and treatment efforts encouraged by external donors, are not trustworthy and lack credibility (Pape, 2014). As Pape (2014, 228) notes, today the government has essentially "turned a deaf ear to the proposals of NGOs." The ideas and visions that NGOs provide stem not from historical pride in central government intervention (which never existed) but rather from ideals, interests, and beliefs deriving from international policy recommendations such as the importance of methadone treatment, harm reduction, condom distribution, and prevention programs for the gay community; these policies have not been supported by the Putin administration (Pape, 2014). Even if the MOH and Pokrovsky's Federal AIDS Center strove to establish a partnership with NGOs, Putin's administration and his conservative dominant party in the Duma would more than likely not provide support. However, this has not stopped Pokrovsky from doing what he can to meet with and educate society about HIV prevention. He has been relentless in protecting society, especially Russia's youth; he has proactively met with local schools and attended conferences to share knowledge, lend support, and provide encouragement (Panina, 2016).

In sum, although Russia's negative geopolitical positioning eventually motivated the government to respond to HIV/AIDS because of its perceived national security threat, such a threat proved insufficient for amassing a stronger policy response; worse still, in the absence of strong bureaucratic–civil societal partnerships, Russia's AIDS bureaucrats joined their Indian and Chinese counterparts in being hampered in their ability to achieve a centrist policy response.

Responding to Tuberculosis

By the 1980s, in tandem with the growth of HIV/AIDS cases, Russia was experiencing a resurgence of TB. Several factors contributed to this reemergence of TB, including the introduction of a free market system and an increase in unemployment and poverty (Kazionny et al., 2001; Shilova and Dye, 2001); increased incarceration rates in congested prison centers (Shilova and Dye, 2001); drug use and the AIDS virus (Dimitrova et al., 2006); and a steady decline in federal funding for TB prevention and treatment, due mainly to the collapse of the Soviet system and the financial inability to sustain a federally funded vertical program (Dimitrova et al., 2006; *ITAR-TASS*, 1998; Perelman, 2000; Shilova and Dye, 2001). Major socioeconomic transformations, new health threats, and a weakening public health system all contributed to the resurgence of a disease that had been controlled for several decades through the Soviet government's historically well-funded public health system (Perelman, 2000; Shilova and Dye, 2001).

The epidemiological profile of TB varies from one state to another. In some states, imprisonment and poor sanitary conditions have been the main contributors to the resurgence, while in major cities, HIV is the principal cause of infection. Initially, most TB cases emerged among prisoners and the poor, but they have now spread to the general population (Dimitrova et al., 2006).

As figure 5.3 illustrates, beginning in the 1990s, the number of registered TB cases began to surge, increasing from 34.1 per 100,000 in 1991 to 85.1 per 100,000 in 2008 (Russia, Ministry of Health [MOH], 2009). Furthermore, due to a steady decline in the number of TB-positive individuals who adhered

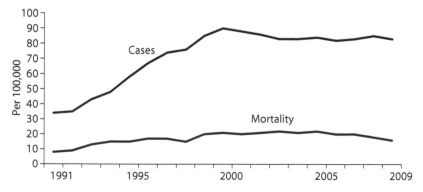

Figure 5.3. Tuberculosis cases and mortality in Russia (per 100,000 population), 1991–2009. Source: Demikhova and Karamov, 2011.

to the prescribed medical treatment (mainly through DOTS), cases of multidrug-resistant TB (MDR-TB) have burgeoned. MDR-TB arises when individuals with TB fail to adhere to a specific drug regimen, thus strengthening the bacterium's ability to adapt to and resist the antibiotic medication. People's inability to be in areas where DOTS treatment is provided, such as prisons or sanitariums, or a simple inability to travel for treatment can lead to MDR-TB. In 1999, 6.7% of all newly reported TB cases in Russia were confirmed to be MDR-TB; this increased to 10.7% by 2008 (Russia, MOH, 2009).

The government's initial response to this resurgence of TB is best characterized as apathetic and delayed. In contrast to the government's response to HIV/AIDS, it was not conservative moral tenets and discriminatory views toward those with TB that affected the government's perceptions of and response to the TB epidemic. Instead, it seems that TB was viewed as a disease that had already been controlled for several decades through an aggressive Soviet system of case notification, detection, and treatment (Perelman, 2000). Consequently, despite the increase in new notification rates in the 1980s, the government and most MOH officials did not see the resurgence as posing a serious national health threat—TB, it was thought, was already under control. During the 1980s and 1990s, moreover, the presence of multiple health threats and increasingly scarce financial resources further contributed to the government's and MOH's lack of attention to TB. The disease also did not pose a serious threat to the military, thus eliciting few fears of an impending national security threat (Feshbach, 2008).

This lack of attention and political apathy, when combined with a waning federal budget for infectious diseases, eventually led to the dismantling of Russia's national TB programs. The well-funded Soviet system of case detection, notification, and treatment came to an abrupt end with the fall of the Soviet Union in 1991 (Perelman, 2000; Shilova and Dye, 2001). Consequently, the MOH and related federal centers working on TB control, such as the Federal Research Institute—which is responsible for developing regulations, training staff, monitoring cases, and supervising TB policy—did not receive adequate funding throughout the 1990s (Associated Press, 1997; Russia, MOH, 2009).

The government briefly contemplated reinstating the national TB program in 2000, but this did not occur. The closest the government came was the creation of a federal law in 1998, decree no. 582, Immediate Measures to Control TB in 1998–2004 (Perelman, 2000). Falling under the auspices of the MOH and widely touted in the media (*Rossiyskaya Gazeta*, 1998a), decree no. 582 was focused on reducing TB mortality rates through several key measures: establishing the modern treatment for patients with TB; training healthcare personnel and educating the public about TB; implementing preventive medicine for incarcerated individuals; adopting prophylactic policies to curb disease among animals; and establishing the domestic production of drugs and vaccines such as BCG and BCG-M. The estimated cost of this program, which was to be implemented in several stages, was 17.5 billion rubles (US$267 million). This included funds from several sources, including approximately 7.7 billion rubles from the federal budget and 9.5 billion rubles (US$145 million) from the states (*Rossiyskaya Gazeta*, 1998b). Nevertheless, as Atun et al. (2005) found, the Duma failed to provide adequate and consistent financial support for the program's implementation.

By 2001, the MOH budget for TB programs in regional *oblast* governments had also decreased (Atun et al., 2005). Consequently, "the money available per patient with TB declined from 1542 Russian roubles [US$23] in 2000 to 1291 Russian roubles [US$19.7] in 2001" (Atun et al., 2005, 219). During this period, federal spending on acquiring TB medications also decreased, leading to a massive shortage of medications at the height of the epidemic. Scholars note that there was essentially no federal funding going toward eradication of TB at that time (Farmer, 2001).

The decline in federal assistance for regional governments was also emerging at a time when municipal health agencies were lacking sufficient beds and infrastructure to treat patients with TB. By the late 1990s, a report published by the MOH indicated that the number of TB beds for adults was reduced by 28%. Similarly, there was a dearth of healthcare workers and practitioners for implementing DOTS treatment (Russia, MOH, 2009). Along with these challenges, the government seemed indifferent to the resurgence of an epidemic that would soon place Russia on the WHO's list of the top 20 nations with the highest prevalence of TB.

International Criticism and Pressure

Russia's lackluster response to the resurgence of TB prompted a surge of international criticism and pressure, at approximately the same time as international reactions to Russia's poor response to the HIV/AIDS epidemic. At a three-day meeting in London in 1998—just five years after the WHO declared TB a pandemic threat—the WHO and health officials from several nations convened to examine how the 22 most-affected nations (with 80% of all

TB cases) were faring in achieving the WHO's goal of reaching a 70% TB detection rate and 85% cure rate by the year 2000. Russia was selected as one of several countries having the highest global TB burden (Agermose, 1998). Later that year, a WHO report was released stating that Russia was a "hot zone" area for TB and was "spiraling out of control" (*KyivPost*, 1998, 1). The media also chimed in with criticism. In 1998, the *Guardian* (London) newspaper stated that TB was now "pouring into the streets of Russia, blamed poor regulation and medical treatment in heavily congested prisons as the main culprit (Meek, 1998, 1).

For an emerging nation, international criticism and pressure typically prompt reform—as we saw in Brazil, India, and China. Russia's MOH could have suddenly reversed its course and engaged in a new federal campaign to eradicate TB. But this did not happen. As in its response to HIV/AIDS, the government was not influenced by this international criticism and pressure (Garrett, 2005; Gómez, 2013b). Once again, the government's negative geopolitical positioning generated few incentives for Russia's political leaders to increase the nation's international reputation in health through a stronger policy response. Instead, the government decided to work on its own and at its own pace. A policy response to TB eventually emerged, but it was due mainly to the government's becoming concerned about the resurgence of TB cases by the mid-2000s rather than pressure from the international community (*ITAR-TASS*, 2000b).

The Absence of National Security Threat and Instituting Reforms

Further compelling the government not to strengthen its policy response to the TB epidemic was that, unlike HIV/AIDS, TB did not pose a serious threat to Russia's national security. Indeed, researchers note that military officials were never concerned about its effects on military recruitment and preparedness, notwithstanding reports that TB infections were increasing by 10 percentage points a year. This failure of response was perhaps attributable to the significantly fewer enlistees being discharged for TB than for HIV/AIDS and other diseases (Feshbach, 2008). When combined with the serious effort by the military to monitor and treat TB (Akimkin, 2009), this seems to have generated little concern within the government about TB's national security threat.

Despite these government perceptions, with the number of cases burgeoning and the MOH's growing concern, the government did begin to take the

TB issue more seriously. This interest came mainly in the form of federal laws and mandates, without the creation of a new federal agency and/or subdivision for TB. In 2001, in response to a surge in case notification rates due to both the enhanced reporting of TB and the growth of the epidemic (*ITAR-TASS*, 2000b), the Duma, in collaboration with the MOH, implemented the Federal Law and Ordinance on the Prevention of Tuberculosis Spread in the Russian Federation, no. 77-03 of 18.06.01. Several other ordinances required heightened attention to regulating, monitoring, and preventing the spread of the disease (Russia, MOH, 2009). In addition, federal orders no. 109 (2003) and no. 50 (2004) established the guidelines for therapy, detection, and reporting of TB (World Bank, 2011). These orders were also designed to adhere to international DOTS treatment recommendations.

In 2006, the MOH also created the National Priority Project in Public Health and the Federal Target Program, Prevention and Control of Socially Significant Disease (2007–11). These programs called for additional spending for TB prevention and treatment, totaling 38.5% of the program's overall budget (Russia, MOH, 2009). Moreover, they sought to increase funding for TB control activities from federal and subnational governments—9.8 million rubles (US$148,000) and 16.5 million rubles (US$244,000), respectively—for improving treatment, early diagnosis, and prevention of complications associated with TB, and more funding for healthcare facilities (Russia, MOH, 2009). With this support, by 2009 the MOH claimed to be engaged in a multisectoral response to TB, recognizing the epidemic's complex, multidimensional socioeconomic characteristics.

Federal spending for TB programs continued. In 2012, on World TB Day, it was announced that within five years the MOH would increase spending for TB diagnosis and treatment fourfold. Twelve Russian regions received an additional 6 billion rubles (US$91,000) from the MOH, with the expectation that this would increase by another 1 billion rubles (US$15.2 million) in 2013 (Bruk, 2013). Federal spending for TB programs in federal prisons was also expected to increase (Yablonski et al., 2015).

As we saw with HIV/AIDS, the government also sought to increase the federal budget for foreign aid to help other nations combat TB. Beginning in 2010, the government agreed to provide the Global Fund with US$20 million for the period 2011–13 to fund TB and other disease programs (Rakhamgulov, 2010). For 2010–18, the MOH also committed US$80 million to the Advance Market Commitment, which pools funding from G8 nations to provide funds to manufacturing companies for research and development of new vaccines for TB and other infectious diseases. This also helps to ensure a steady supply of medications to lesser-developed nations (Russian Federation, n.d.). In 2016, the MOH also organized a conference with the WHO on enhancing international collaboration on national TB research strategies, with Russia emphasizing its commitment to sharing its research strategies and findings with other nations (WHO, 2016). Beginning in 2006, Russia provided bilateral assistance to several nations in Eastern Europe to help fund TB prevention programs and strengthen laboratory capacity, training for specialists, and organizational and methodological support for health systems (Russia, Federal Service for Surveillance, 2015).

The MOH also assumed a global leadership role. In 2015, at a BRICS health meeting in Brazil, Russia's health minister, Veronika Skvortsova, proposed the creation of an international forum for the BRICS to address how they could coordinate their resources to help other nations eradicate TB (*Moscow Times*, 2015). Russia also invited WHO representatives to attend the meeting. In addition to helping fund this TB initiative, Skvortsova stated, Russia would allocate more than US$600 million for HIV programs in 2016 (Russian Presidency, 2015). Much like what we saw with HIV/AIDS, these efforts revealed the government's intention to use foreign aid for TB to enhance its international leadership and superpower status. Putin believed that it was "demeaning" and "unfitting" for a country that claimed to be a global leader and donor to receive external assistance in health (Bohm, 2016).

The Putin administration's decision to provide foreign aid rather than receive it has had its costs, however. Russia was once a recipient of Global Fund and USAID funding for TB, but since 2012, any new funding from these sources has been eliminated (Anders, 2014). Consistent with the Putin administration's negative geopolitical positioning, in 2011 the MOH refused an offer from the Global Fund in the amount of US$127 million to finance TB projects, deciding instead to pursue the financing and implementation of projects on its own, at its own pace (MacDonald, 2013). And in 2012, Putin ordered USAID to stop providing assistance for TB and other health sectors, which some critics believed was done to show that Russia "no longer needs U.S. help because President Vladimir Putin has turned the country into a self-sufficient global power" (Bohm, 2016, 1). Again, as with HIV/AIDS, this decision has upset many, as the government still has not done a sufficient job of ensuring the provision of medical supplies, facilities, healthcare personnel, or infrastructure for its own population, especially in rural areas (Smith, 2015).

Despite the government's increased commitment to improving its domestic and foreign aid policies for TB, several ongoing challenges remain. Although federal spending for TB has increased, this endeavor alone has not ensured that health systems have been adequately strengthened (Smith, 2015). Furthermore, no effort has been made to ensure that the money provided to regional governments is being used appropriately—no conditionalities or working with regional health officials and NGOs to monitor how the money is being allocated, which are a key aspect of building an effective centrist policy response. This situation worries international health policy experts and advocates. In 2015, Lucica Ditiu, executive secretary for the international Stop TB Campaign, stated that "we don't know where the money is being invested . . . I think a lot of the money going into hospital care and other intervention are [*sic*] not the most cost-efficient" (quoted in Smith, 2015, 1).

In this context, regional governments have had to take the initiative in introducing policies and resources to ensure a steady decline in the number of TB cases. This, in turn, has led to considerable variation in the capacity of regional governments to implement reliable TB and MDR-TB diagnosis, DOTS treatment, and effective infection control practices (Yablonski et al., 2015). One successful instance is the state government of Voronezh, where the health ministry has introduced an innovative inclusionary approach to TB and MDR-TB management by strengthening awareness and coordination among all hospital staff and ensuring harmonious commitment to effective DOTS treatment (*LillyPad*, 2016). This has also helped to build staff discipline and commitment to treatment and, with this, a reduction of TB and MDR-TB cases by more than a half.

Shortcomings have also emerged regarding the federal government's provision of medications for TB treatment. By 2009, MOH officials complained that they were not receiving adequate funding for medications through the national health insurance system (*Washington Post*, 2009). To make matters worse, in an effort to stabilize its budget, in 2011 the MOH announced that it would no longer provide free medications for more complex TB strains through the national health insurance system (Goble, 2011). This decision forced many people to pay out of pocket for complex, expensive medications—disproportionately affecting the lower income classes where TB is most prevalent. There continues to be a shortage of these specialized TB medications now removed from most insurance-covered preferred drug lists in several regional health departments (*Z-News*, 2016). Medication shortages are most apparent in remote rural areas, where hospitals are not supplied with sufficient quantities and the MOH has failed to provide support (Smith, 2015).

Healthcare infrastructure has also been a problem. MOH and regional health officials described a shortage of hospital beds, and approximately 40% of all hospitals lacked adequate medical equipment (Russia, MOH, 2009). In 2009, the number of TB sanitarium beds "decreased by 14.5% (22.6% for adult TB patients and 9.8% for children)" (Russia, MOH, 2009, 136). The number of rural TB clinics where individuals can get tested and treated decreased from 2,050 in 2005 to 1,840 in 2007, and few sanitariums exist for individuals in hard-to-reach rural areas.

To this day, most hospitals continue to employ outdated approaches to TB treatment, such as large waiting rooms for patients, which were adopted under the Soviet system but subsequently found by western researchers to contribute to the spread of the disease (Smith, 2015; Stracansky, 2014a, 2014b). And with respect to human resources, the situation is so grave that even the MOH has admitted that the "number of TB staff decreases year after year." From 2000 to 2008, the number of persons employed in TB services in the MOH system decreased by 8.3%, including physicians—by 14.2% (from 9,181 to 8,517). The physician-to-population ratio in 2008 was 0.6 per 10,000 population (Russia, MOH, 2009). Among TB physicians, 63.6% have received certification for specialization, and 33.3% have received the highest category of certification (Russia, MOH, 2009). These shortages persist, which poses a particular challenge for ensuring a sufficient number of healthcare personnel to provide effective treatment (Smith, 2015).

Nor has any effort been made to address the growing TB epidemic within prisons, which many consider to be one of the main epicenters of the epidemic (Goble, 2015c; Stracansky, 2014a, 2014b; C. Thompson, 2014). Overcrowding issues, poor hygiene and nutrition, and discrimination toward those with TB continue (Stracansky, 2014). It has been estimated that approximately 50% of MDR-TB infections in Russia come from the spread of infection among inmates and to visiting family members (Goble, 2015c). To curtail the spread of MDR-TB and to protect the broader population, more effort needs to be placed on greater consistency in drug treatment and improved living conditions within prisons. Yet, to this day, the MOH has not made an earnest effort to work with the *oblast* penal systems to achieve this (C. Thompson, 2014).

In sum, the government does not seem firmly committed to taking the TB situation seriously (Stracansky, 2014). The MOH has not been able to achieve a strong policy response and, needless to say, a centrist policy response. While government spending for the MOH's TB programs has increased, funding has not been used effectively, no successful universal TB medication programs have been implemented, and the MOH has not tried to formally increase its policy influence over the oblasts through conditional grant assistance while informally partnering with NGOs to monitor policy implementation.

Indeed, while the government has boasted about its joining the UN resolution to eradicate all forms of TB by 2034, analysts note that "the Russian authorities have done little to reach that goal and almost nothing at all in the penal system where tuberculosis remains rife" (Goble, 2015c, 1). Although the number of TB cases has gradually decreased, with new cases now at a rate of approximately 80 per 100,000, the scientific community is mainly concerned with the ongoing growth of MDR- and XDR-TB (extensively drug-resistant TB) (Tyurin, 2016), especially among children and prisoners (MacDonald, 2013). Currently, Russia is home to one of the highest incidences of these arguably more deadly forms of TB infection (WHO, 2015).

Why has the government been incapable of pursuing a stronger policy response to TB? Critically examining NGOs' response to the epidemic and the MOH's partnership with NGOs provides additional insight into this matter.

The Absence of Strong Bureaucratic-Civil Societal Partnerships

Similar to the situation described above for HIV/AIDS, MOH bureaucrats did not have access to social health movements and NGOs that they could partner with to help expand their federal TB programs. First, there were no civic organizations working on TB when it reemerged in the 1980s. Not only did a repressive Soviet state generate few incentives for civic mobilization (Evans, 2006a; Nemyria, 2002), but social stigma associated with TB and the general belief that the disease had already been controlled created little interest among activists and scientists in creating TB NGOs. Second, even if TB NGOs had emerged in the 1980s, there were no civic organization or social health movement predecessors advocating policy ideas that bureaucrats could have used when working with NGOs to increase their legitimacy and influence in seeking funding from the Duma.

Nevertheless, over time, international NGOs began to emerge in response to the dearth of domestic NGOs working on TB and the need to address its resurgence. For example, in 2001, the Russian chapter of the International Federation of the Red Cross received a grant in the amount of US$3.4 million from USAID to begin a three-year awareness and treatment program to prevent the spread of TB (Interfax, 2001). The Red Cross continues to provide financial support and to work with local volunteers and doctors through these endeavors (International Federation of the Red Cross, 2015). The Red Cross also began to train medical staff and community leaders to increase awareness about TB, going as far as to host conferences in Geneva with officials from the Global Fund, to share knowledge and strategies in activism and treatment (Advocacy Partnership, 2010). In 2012, the LHL Tuberculosis Foundation, another international NGO, emerged to provide treatment services and awareness campaigns in western Russia (Arkhangelskaya, 2015). The Lilly Foundation has helped the Red Cross in funding large TB information campaigns targeted to migrant communities, such as the 2015 Programme to Strengthen Advocacy and TB Prevention Measures in Economic Migrant Communities (International Federation of the Red Cross, 2015).

While the Global Fund's presence in Russia has helped to increase civic mobilization for diseases such as HIV/AIDS, it did not have such a direct impact for TB. Most of the Global Fund grants for TB—specifically, rounds 3 and 4—were provided for organizations that were not exclusively focused on TB (Global Fund, 2011). No recent grants have gone to civic organizations and/or other groups that concentrate on TB. This is partly because, as mentioned earlier, in 2010 the Global Fund reclassified Russia as a donor nation, and the Putin administration has not allowed local TB NGOs to apply for new grant funding. To temporarily get around this dilemma, the Global Fund has contributed additional money to preexisting Global Fund HIV and TB programs with the intent that this extra funding help AIDS NGOs provide additional TB services (Zaardiashvili, 2016).

As we saw with HIV/AIDS, many of the domestic and foreign-based NGOs working on TB in Russia will be challenged by their inability to receive donor support in the future, hampering their development and the possibility of partnering with the bureaucracy. Since 2012, major donors such as USAID and the Open Society Institute have been forced to leave Russia. Consequently, NGOs such as Partners in Health, which was funded by USAID, and several other smaller community-based NGOs have had to close down their projects and dismiss their staff (MacDonald, 2013). The Russian Red Cross had to return USAID funding for 11 projects across the worst-hit areas in Russia, leading to the closing of 5 projects. The government's reason for denying the presence of these external donors was once again political, as we saw with HIV/AIDS: the Putin administration suspected these western donors of trying to influence Russia's TB programs, interfering with internal political matters, and undermining state sovereignty (MacDonald, 2013; Smith, 2015).

There is no evidence to suggest that national TB bureaucrats are even trying to work closely with NGOs. These bureaucrats have a long track record of not only refraining from partnering with NGOs but also ignoring their specific policy requests (Golichenko, 2016). This has forced NGOs such as the Andrey Rylkov Foundation, Chance Plus, and Ural-Positive to appeal to the UN and file a formal complaint. Moreover, most NGOs working on TB are foreign organizations that have been delegitimized by the Putin administration, thus providing few incentives for MOH bureaucrats to work closely with them. Those community-based NGOs that are present are simply too small to offer national TB bureaucrats much legitimacy and influence. And many of these organizations, such as the Andrey Rylkov Foundation, Chance Plus, and Ural-Positive, have worked closely with western donors and are thus considered suspect, making a potential bureaucratic partnership with them less appealing.

Thus, in the absence of TB's national security threat, a stronger policy response was never pursued due to Russia's international isolation and apathy toward international pressure and reputation building, products of the government's negative geopolitical positioning. Moreover, MOH bureaucrats once again proved unwilling to establish a strong partnership with NGOs, thus hampering their ability to pursue a centrist policy response.

Conclusion

In contrast to what we saw in Brazil, India, and China, political leaders in Russia essentially ignored international criticism and pressure and were never interested in using a stronger policy response to HIV/AIDS or TB to increase the government's international reputation in health. Furthermore, no effort was made to pursue international financial and technical assistance. While the government would eventually begin to provide foreign aid to other nations struggling with these diseases, these efforts were pursued to augment the government's reputation for being a global leader in health. In essence, Russia's response reflected the government's negative geopolitical positioning, which was influenced by a foreign policy tradition of Russia as a superpower, a world leader, a nation shaping international diplomacy while working independently of external interference. In this context, Russia's leaders would respond to HIV/AIDS only when it was perceived as posing a credible threat to national security—although this never occurred for TB. For both health sectors, however, the government did not strengthen its policy response, and the absence of a strong partnership between health bureaucrats and NGOs further hampered any efforts in this regard. With growing political hostilities toward independent activist groups supported by international donors, the bureaucracy's ability to develop a stronger partnership with NGOs does not seem likely. The Putin administration continues to display little interest in strengthening its policy response to HIV/AIDS, TB, or other diseases.

NOTE

1. According to Hardley (1999), approximately 30% of Russian government personnel in high-level posts held these conservative beliefs.

6

Responding to HIV/AIDS and Tuberculosis in South Africa

Along with South Africa's transition to democracy in 1994 and its unwavering commitments to political stability and economic growth, in the 1990s it joined the other BRICS nations in confronting the threat of health epidemics. As in Russia, HIV/AIDS and TB posed such a threat. When its poor response to the epidemics aroused international criticism and pressure, South Africa's leaders did not use this situation to pursue a stronger policy response with an eye to bolstering the government's international reputation in health. Instead, building on a long foreign policy tradition of state sovereignty, independence, and international and regional leadership, the government's reaction to the international community reflected its negative geopolitical positioning. That is, political leaders ignored the international pressure, resisted international financial and technical assistance, and decided to respond to these epidemics at their own pace and in their own way. South Africa joined Russia in responding to HIV/AIDS, though not to TB, only when the epidemic threatened national security—including the economy, government, and military performance. Though the South African government also briefly joined its BRICS counterparts in providing foreign aid assistance for HIV/AIDS and TB programs, as in Russia, its intent was not to increase its international reputation but rather to solidify its regional leadership. Over time, however, South Africa's bureaucratic and policy reforms proved to be ineffective, revealing the inability of the Department of Health (DOH) to obtain a sufficient amount of parliamentary funding for prevention and treatment programs, much needed investments in human resources and infrastructure for policy implementation, and financial and technical assistance for provincial health departments.

These ongoing challenges were also shaped by the absence of strong bureaucratic–civil societal partnerships. For both HIV/AIDS and TB, bureaucrats never sought to partner with NGOs to improve their ability to obtain ongoing political and financial support for their programs. This challenge reflected the historically weak relationship between the bureaucracy, activists, and those afflicted by disease in the area of public health, the resulting lack of expectations and motivation for working with each other, NGOs' subsequent inability to effectively mobilize and respond and receive the political attention needed to influence policy, and thus a lack of interest and incentive for bureaucrats to partner with them. Without a strong bureaucratic–civil societal partnership, the government has not been able to achieve a centrist policy response.

Responding to HIV/AIDS

AIDS first emerged in South Africa in the city of Johannesburg in 1982 (Ras et al., 1983). Of the 215 South Africans who died of AIDS during the mid- to late 1980s, 26 were flight attendants for South African Airways. The virus was mainly contained within the white gay community during this early period, but by 1986 had transitioned to the black heterosexual and IDU community (Wren, 1990). Figure 6.1 traces the increase in AIDS cases in the 1980s and 1990s.

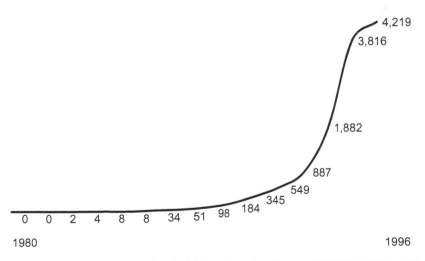

Figure 6.1. HIV/AIDS cases in South Africa, 1980–96. Source: UNAIDS, 2004. *2004 Update. South Africa. Epidemiological Fact Sheets.*

Motivated by fear and misunderstanding, National Party members and health officials exercised a great deal of discrimination toward the gay and black communities (A. Butler, 2005; Marias, 2000; Wren, 1990). Homophobia hampered policy attention to the gay community's needs, creating an excuse for the government not to respond (A. Butler, 2005; S. Karim et al., 2009; Marias, 2000; Wren, 1990). Meanwhile, racism toward the black community comported with the National Party's policy of racial segregation, resulting in little healthcare assistance (A. Butler, 2005; S. Karim et al. 2009; Lieberman, 2009; Marias, 2000; Wren, 1990). Feeling increasingly threatened by the rising and prosperous black population, and fearing that whites would one day be outnumbered, some Nationalist politicians celebrated the possibility that AIDS might finally eradicate the black population (A. Butler, 2005; Maxmen, 2009). These sentiments dovetailed with a general disbelief and denial within the Nationalists that HIV/AIDS had, in fact, emerged in their country.

As we saw in China and Russia, a deep conservative moral impulse ran through the veins of South Africa's National Party government. Conservative politicians, doctors, and medical workers believed that HIV/AIDS was the result of immoral activity among gays and the drug-using community—viewed as the "other," as sinners, those partaking of naughty western vices and immoral lifestyles (Marias, 2005).

But other factors contributed to the government's unresponsiveness. First, there was little epidemiological evidence suggesting that HIV/AIDS posed a serious national threat. Rates of HIV prevalence did not escalate until the late 1980s, with the first official case of AIDS being reported to the government in 1982 (Van der Vliet, 2004). Moreover, AIDS prevalence was low throughout the early 1990s. Consequently, in the absence of strong international pressure to respond, the government was not particularly concerned about the epidemic, focusing instead on what it considered to be more pressing health and political matters (A. Butler, 2005; Marias, 2000; Schneider and Stein, 2001). Because the National Party bureaucracy exhibited little interest in and commitment to healthcare, especially AIDS (Chirambo, 2004), the government decided to focus exclusively on the worsening political situation (Chirambo, 2004; Strand et al., 2007).

These factors created few incentives for the apartheid government to strengthen its policy response. No effort was made to construct a national AIDS program within the DOH (Gauri and Lieberman, 2006; Lieberman, 2009; Marias, 2000; Schneider, 2002). Although the DOH created a National AIDS

Advisory Group in 1985, which mainly provided biomedical advice to the government, followed by an AIDS Unit and a National AIDS Council in 1989 (Lieberman, 2009), these agencies were not well supported and were ineffective (Van der Vliet, 2004). In fact, the National AIDS Council was dismantled in 1992 (Lieberman, 2009). The bureaucrats staffing these agencies also had little autonomy and policy influence; this persisted even after the transition to democracy in 1994 (A. Butler, 2005; Chirambo, 2004; Johnson, 2005).

During this period the government did not provide any assistance to provincial or municipal governments. For example, by 1991, only R 2.1 million (rand; US$147,787) had been provided by the DOH for municipal governments to fund HIV/AIDS educational awareness and prevention efforts. Of this money, most went to the white urban centers, while rural black communities received essentially nothing. The largest predominantly black community, Sweto, for example, saw no funding for its innovative Township AIDS Program. Consequently, the central government by the early 1990s had lost all credibility in its efforts to assist marginalized AIDS communities (Wren, 1990).

Essentially operating on their own, provincial health departments created their own AIDS organizations, the AIDS Training, Information, and Counseling Centers (ATICCs), which opened house in eight provinces prior to the 1994 democratic transition As described by Marias (2000), the ATICCS (located mainly in urban centers), though poorly staffed and funded, provided training and counseling services. Despite the emergence of 18 ATICCs by the late 1990s, the African National Congress government saw them as "part of the old order," which motivated national and local health officials appointed by the ANC to have little trust in the ATICCS staff. With little support and funding and a loss of legitimacy, by the late 1990s most ATICCs were forced to close down. And this occurred despite UNAIDS's declaration in 1988 that ATICCs served as a good example of the important work being done at the community level.

These weak institution-building efforts notwithstanding, in the late 1980s some exiled ANC politicians, academic researchers, and NGOs were mobilizing and pressuring the government to respond more effectively to HIV/AIDS (Zhu, 2007). These efforts benefited from the presence of a highly vocal, well-organized pro-democratic movement pressuring for democratization, human rights, and participatory governance (Schneider, 2002; Zhu, 2007). Members of the exiled ANC and its medical community, NGOs, medical researchers, and healthcare workers banded together to join the growing pro-democratic coalition fighting not only for human rights but also for equal and equitable access to healthcare. Scholars note that by the early 1990s, NGOs, which were essentially nonexistent in the response to AIDS during the 1980s (Chirambo, 2004; Parkhurst and Lush, 2004), worked closely with the exiled ANC to raise awareness about AIDS while pressuring the government for a more effective policy response (Johnson, 2005; Zhu, 2007).

By 1992, activists and people living with HIV/AIDS had joined aspiring ANC leaders to voice their concerns through the organization of a conference, the National AIDS Convention of South Africa. At this conference, a national nongovernmental umbrella organization named after the conference, NACOSA, was created and served as the primary inspiration and backbone for a potential shift in the government's response to AIDS. NACOSA's primary focus was to define and establish the principles and strategies for a coherent and comprehensive national policy response (A. Butler, 2005). It was grounded in the spirit of civic participation and involvement in policymaking, thus pushing for strong state–civil societal "synergy" (Schneider and Stein, 2001). NACOSA therefore embodied and brought together the prevailing social democratic movement and an unwavering dedication to civic representation, inclusiveness, and equality, with the need for a comprehensive national AIDS plan that built upon and deepened these principles.

In 1993, based on NACOSA's recommendation, the government's first National AIDS Plan emerged. The plan consisted of six key elements: education, counseling, healthcare, human rights and law reform, welfare, and research (Marias, 2000). For the first time, it seemed that South Africa had a plan that proposed a holistic and multisectoral response to HIV/AIDS (Johnson, 2005). Moreover, it assigned a central role to the government in leading, financing, and implementing a coordinated national response to AIDS, while proposing that the plan be managed in the office of the presidency (Johnson, 2005; NACOSA, 1994).

Against this backdrop, and with the election of Nelson Mandela in 1994 as the democratic ANC president (serving from 1994 to 1999), new efforts were made to increase the government's response to HIV/AIDS. Mandela fully embraced the National AIDS Plan (Marias, 2000; Schneider and Stein, 2001; Wouters, van Rensburg, and Meulemans, 2010). There was now an expectation within and outside government and civil society that a coherent and effective national AIDS program would be implemented (Johnson, 2005; Schneider and

Stein, 2001). As a sign of his commitment, Mandela appointed the first director of the National AIDS Plan, Quarraisha Karim, and retitled the plan the HIV/AIDS and STD Program (referred to hereafter as the national AIDS program, NAP) (Wouters, van Rensburg, and Meulemans, 2010). AIDS policy was assigned presidential "Special Status," thus locking in more presidential commitment and potential resources (Marias, 2000; Schneider and Stein, 2001). A new Inter-Departmental Committee on AIDS was also established, along with an AIDS Advisory Group; the former sought to increase interagency collaboration in policymaking, while the latter sought to institutionalize civil societal participation in this process (Marias, 2000). During this period the NAP freely distributed condoms, a process that had begun in 1988 (Lieberman, 2009), and prevention and awareness campaigns were gradually implemented.

In 1994, the DOH also introduced policies to assist the provincial governments in implementing AIDS policy. The new "quasi-federal" constitution required that all nine provincial governments be responsible for social welfare policy; HIV/AIDS fell into this category (Johnson, 2005). In an effort to assist provincial governments, in 1994 the NAP authorized the creation of Provincial AIDS Commissions (PACs), which served as delegated arms of the NAP, staffed by health officials from the MOH. The goal was to work with the provincial health departments in implementing NAP policies and providing technical assistance and guidance (Marias, 2000).

By the end of the 1990s, multiple problems had begun to emerge. Several scholars characterize the 1994–98 period as one of bureaucratic and AIDS policy failure at all levels of government (A. Butler, 2005; Johnson, 2005; Parkhurst and Lush, 2004; Schneider, 2002; Schneider and Stein, 2001). At the national level, Mandela and the ANC gradually began to give less political attention and support to the NAP (Bisseker, 1997; Marias, 2000; Wouters van Rensburg, and Meulemans, 2010). The program's director, Quarraisha Karim, also had little autonomy and was essentially subservient to the DOH and the president's interests. Funding was provided for the program, but between 1994 and 1996, due to a lack of bureaucratic resolve and commitment and to inefficiency (Johnson, 2005), the program *underspent* the money allocated to it by the parliament. And funding for NGOs fell by a half, to R 12 million (US$845,100), in 1998 (Marias, 2000; Schneider and Stein, 2001). While the number of AIDS program staff increased (Marias, 2000), this was deemed insufficient given the needs at the time (A. Butler, 2005; Whiteside and Sunter,

2000). Karim complained that she never received sufficient guidance on how to manage the NAP (Johnson, 2005).

By the late 1990s, the NAP's support for the provincial PACs had also decreased. First, there was a two-year delay in most of the appointments of national staff to PAC field offices (Marias, 2000). Second, insufficient financial resources were flowing from the DOH to the PACs and local health clinics, which were bereft of medical staff and supplies (Bisseker, 1997; Marias, 2000). Finally, the PACs were essentially powerless, working as what Marias (2000, 19) referred to as "submissive comrades" to provincial health department authorities. By the late 1990s, PACs were essentially meaningless groups of federal bureaucrats with no influence over local AIDS policy.

Though the NAP had done a commendable job in funding the distribution of condoms and ensuring a safe blood supply (Lieberman, 2009), there still was no universal policy for use of medications. Brazil had already enacted national legislation mandating the universal provision of ARV medications such as AZT by 1996. South Africa's NAP was far from achieving that benchmark. Under the subsequent Thabo Mbeki administration (1999–2008), the DOH started questioning the efficacy of such medications, suggesting that they were potentially more toxic than helpful in combating the virus.

Indeed, despite the claims of scientists in Europe and international health agencies that AZT was effective, the DOH did not immediately disburse the drug (T. Jones, 2001). The resistance mainly stemmed from Mbeki's denial that HIV contributed to AIDS deaths; he instead blamed other illnesses as well as increased poverty (Lodge, 2015). Mbeki's denialist beliefs ultimately led to the DOH's refusal to provide public hospitals with AZT from 1998 to 2001 (T. Jones, 2001). Activists subsequently claimed that the delay in providing this treatment contributed to the deaths of approximately 300,000 individuals (ACTSA, 2016).

HIV/AIDS prevention policies that were focused on educational awareness began to emerge during this period, but they seemed to favor white rather than black school districts. Moreover, the NAP failed to target its prevention messages to the most at-risk groups, such as labor migrants, miners, and commercial sex workers (Lieberman, 2009).

International Criticism and Pressure

Similar to the situation for the other BRICS nations, the international community soon began to express criticism, pressure, and expectations for a stronger policy response. This occurred rather late for South Africa: in the late 1990s, compared with the late 1980s for Brazil, the early 1990s for India, and the mid-1990s for China (Dernberger, 2014; Easterly, 2006). Scholars have argued that this delay was mainly due to the international community's apathy about the rising number of HIV/AIDS cases in South Africa: they decided to respond, Easterly points out, "only after a truly massive number of people were infected" (quoted in Dernberger, 2014, 3). The international community was also sidetracked by the government's transition to democracy in 1994 (Easterly, 2006). As we will see, however, and as we saw for Russia, this criticism and pressure did not have any impact on the government's subsequent policy response.

In 1998, UNAIDS and the UNDP released a report blaming the apartheid legacy of poverty, inequality, and political and economic alienation for the rise in HIV/AIDS cases. The report further stated: "It is clear, for example, that the formal health system will not be able to cope with the increased demands of those infected with HIV and Aids" (SAPA, 1998c, 2). Such claims underscored the UN's belief that even the pro-democratic ANC regime, proud of proffering its commitment to combating AIDS even before entering office, did not have the health system capacity needed to eradicate the disease.

The World Bank followed up with critical comments of its own. In 1998, bank analysts projected that by 2005–10, infant mortality in South Africa would "be 60 percent higher than it would have been without HIV/AIDS (61 deaths per 1,000 infants born rather than 38 per 1,000 in the absence of AIDS)." Bank officials went on to claim that "in 1998, South Africa accounted for over half of all new infections in Southern Africa and for one in seven new infections in SSA [Sub-Saharan Africa]" (World Bank, 1998, 13, 14).

In 2000, the director of UNAIDS, Peter Piot, concluded that South Africa had joined Botswana in having the worst AIDS situation in all of Africa, remarking that the situation in South Africa was "tragic today, in spite of this 'period of grace' and in spite of the increasing amount of knowledge about the virus and the means of combating it" (*Afrol News*, 2000, 5). Piot even chastised Mbeki for his denialist claims.

How did the ANC respond to this criticism and pressure? One might assume that because of South Africa's recent reintegration into the international community with its transition to democracy, as well as its interest in bolstering its international credibility as an emerging economy, the government would respond positively through a stronger policy response, striving to build its international reputation in health—as seen in Brazil, India, and China. One might further assume that South Africa would join these nations in proactively seeking financial and technical assistance from the international community and thus helping to mold its domestic policy in accordance with international scientific views and prescriptions.

Unfortunately, this did not occur. In a move that revealed the government's negative geopolitical positioning, the president and senior health officials essentially ignored the international criticism and pressure—thus emphasizing its sovereign status and the ANC's belief in its ability to respond to AIDS on its own (Lieberman, 2009). In contrast to what we saw in Brazil, India, and China, at no point was the ANC interested in positively responding to international pressure through stronger policy reforms to bolster its international reputation in health. Worse still, and further consistent with the government's negative geopolitical positioning, the ANC vehemently resisted any kind of international financial and technical assistance (Lieberman, 2009). Lieberman (2009, 137) claims that "after 1994, the South African government steadfastly rebuffed offers of [international donor] aid and assistance, particularly from the World Bank." Even at the height of the HIV/AIDS epidemic, Mbeki and the government vehemently resisted financial and technical assistance from other nations, such as the US President's Emergency Plan for AIDS Relief (PEPFAR) (Downie, Jackson, and Angelo, 2016). In 2003, the Mbeki administration even attempted to block a grant from the Global Fund to Fight AIDS, Tuberculosis, and Malaria to the province of KwaZulu-Natal for the distribution of ARV medications (McGreal, 2002; Nunn et al., 2012). Moreover, Mbeki and the DOH continued to ignore the scientific evidence and international pressure to adopt AZT and other medications (A. Butler, 2005).

In fact, the only time Mbeki positively responded to international criticism and pressure was when international leaders threatened to exclude him from important G8 meetings because of his repeated reluctance to address the biomedical aspects of AIDS (A. Butler, 2005). Anthony Butler (2005, 606) writes: "Ultimately, however, international opinion—notably Canadian Premier Jean Chretien's reported threat to exclude discussion of Mbeki's New Partnership for Africa's Development from the G8 agenda unless government policy on HIV/AIDS was turned round—was to prove significant in forcing the government to engage publicly with the biomedical paradigm," a paradigm that South Africa's government had ignored for years. In other words, international criticism and pressure about the AIDS situation and the deteriorating health and deaths of thousands of South Africans were not enough for Mbeki to listen to science and consider a policy change. The only issue that appeared to matter for Mbeki was the threat of being excluded from important G8 discussions, which could have tarnished South Africa's status as a world leader.

This is telling. This response suggests that Mbeki at the time believed that South Africa was a regional power, a leader, not a follower of international advice or recipient of technical assistance. It provides insight into why presidents Mandela and Mbeki ignored international criticism and pressure and why they were indifferent to increasing their international reputation in health. Like his counterparts in Russia, by the turn of the twenty-first century Mbeki seemed to believe that South Africa was a leader within the region and that he knew more than the international community about how the AIDS virus was transmitted and how his government should respond. But why did Mbeki behave in this manner? Analyzing South Africa's historical record in foreign policy and international diplomacy may provide some insight into the government's negative geopolitical positioning.

Geopolitics and the Rise of a Regional Leader

Like Russia, South Africa had a long history of pursuing foreign policies that could display the government's geopolitical importance as a leader in foreign diplomacy. For instance, during the First World War, prominent South African diplomats played important roles in helping to form an international consensus for the peace. Trained in classical philosophy at Cambridge University, Jan Smuts was a South African diplomat who took the lead in these endeavors and was admired for his unwavering passion for peace and equality (Hancock, 1962). Smuts played a critical role not only in working with the British to fend off German occupation during the First World War (Vandenbosch, 1970) but also in helping to build a peaceful resolution after the war. Smuts took the initiative to author and propose the "Terms of Peace," which among other resolutions outlined the need for the creation of an international organization of peace—that is, the League of Nations (Vandenbosch, 1970).

Smuts proceeded to help position South Africa as a small but independent nation eager to make a difference (Hancock, 1962). As Klotz recounts (2004), during the early twentieth century, South Africa was a nation striving to gain political independence from Great Britain; it was trapped within the confines of British command of South African foreign policy. South Africa soon joined other British dominions in demanding independence; this led to the signing of the Balfour Declaration in 1926, which granted its request—especially in the area of foreign policy making. South Africa quickly solidified this process by establishing its own Department of Foreign Affairs in the following year.

But even before this, because of Smuts's efforts, South Africa slowly began to be recognized as an independent nation with an important role in establishing world peace and diplomacy through the League of Nations (Hancock, 1962; Vandenbosch, 1970). It was a time when Smuts promoted among his political leaders the view that South Africa should be seen as an equal with Britain, as an independent, free-thinking state capable of shaping international relations, signing treaties, establishing global peace and order, and formulating its own foreign policy. Smuts's efforts eventually led to South Africa's placement as a permanent member of the League of Nations. In contrast, Brazil's delegates never strove to lead and contribute to the league's mission, and Brazil did not ultimately become a permanent member—nor did China, Russia, or India (Leuchars, 2007). Though small in size and influence compared to the predominant US and European states involved in the league, South Africa was becoming recognized as an important nation helping to shape international agreements through this institution (Vandenbosch, 1970). And on becoming prime minister in 1917, Smuts further amplified his nation's recognition and influence at the international level (Hancock, 1962).

In the next attempt to establish an international organization committed to international peace and development, South Africa again took a leadership role. When delegates from the United States, Britain, France, Italy, China, and Brazil were called to San Francisco in the summer of 1945 to draft the UN charter, Smuts appeared at the meeting as a delegate for Britain and South Africa (Vandenbosch, 1970). He took an active part in forming the UN charter, going as far as to chair one of the four working group committees while serving as president of the Commission on the General Assembly (Carter, 1959; Vandenbosch, 1970). Through these institutions, Smuts also strove to limit the role of veto powers in the UN Security Council (Hancock, 1968). And even before delegates met in San Francisco, Smuts took the lead in drafting a preamble to the UN charter to ensure that there would be sufficient international support behind its implementation (Mazower, 2008). In contrast, other nations such as Brazil decided to engage in less creative leadership, playing a more cooperative role in the discussions and votes contributing to the formation of UN institutions such as the Security Council, due in part to disagreements over the lack of adequate representation of Latin American nations in the UN (Garcia, 2012). Therefore, South Africa's efforts were once again different from those of Brazil and China: South Africa strove to lead discussions and establish consensus on the creation of the UN's governing structures, whereas Brazil's and even China's delegates were only agreeable voting participants on these matters.

South African diplomacy and international influence changed with the election of the National Party in 1948. With its stern, morally inspired belief in apartheid, the National Party's segregationist laws and discrimination toward the native population and immigrants led to global condemnation (Carter, 1959; Garcia, 2012; L. Thompson and Prior, 1982). South Africa quickly slipped into a dark period of geopolitical isolation and was viewed by the international community as a pariah state (Flemes, 2007). During this period, the UN took a particularly critical, hostile stance toward South Africa, accusing the government of racial segregation and violating human rights (Spence, 1975). In the 1960s and 1970s, a phalanx of UN resolutions were passed calling not only for the imposition of economic sanctions on South Africa but also for its removal from the UN (McClellan, 1962; Spence, 1975; L. Thompson and Prior, 1982). South Africa resisted, blaming the UN for violating its agreement not to intervene in the domestic politics and policies of its member states (Carter, 1959).

What is important to emphasize here is not South Africa's resistance to the UN's decision but the government's ongoing belief in its nation being an independent, sovereign state, unshakable in the government's views, capable of solving its own problems. By this point, South Africa had become a proud, arrogant, successful nation, believing in international cooperation but from a tolerable distance, while rejecting any international influence—especially from the UN (Siko, 2014).

Scholars indeed note that, despite the UN's repeated condemnation and pressure for reform, the National Party found its strength in its independent resolve. Burgeoning international pressure and threats from the UN eventually backfired. As Carter (1959, 382) explained, "this collective [international] pressure has hardened the determination of the ruling National Party to pursue its own line of policy." During this period, South African prime ministers and National Party members were proud to be fending off international pressure, standing alone, ensnarled in the romanticism of "a small, proud nation embattled for survival against a greedy hostile world" (Legum and Legum, 1964, 86). This sense of geopolitical independence persisted, shaping not only the government's foreign policy objectives but also, as we will see, its relationship with the international community during the HIV/AIDS epidemic.

With a growing economy and strong military and political institutions, apartheid leaders believed South Africa to be the strongest nation on the continent. Leaders believed that they had the capacity and responsibility to lead and develop Africa (Vandenbosch, 1970). In a speech to his constituents, Prime Minister Balthazar Vorster (1978–79) commented: "We are of Africa . . . we understand Africa . . . and nothing is going to prevent us from becoming the leaders of Africa in every field" (quoted in Vandenbosch, 1970, 273–74). These views persisted and deepened under future, democratic administrations.

One area in which the government expanded its regional leadership and influence was in the provision of healthcare assistance to neighboring states. From the 1940s through the 1980s, Pretoria's health ministry sent scores of medical doctors and veterinarians to Botswana, Lesotho, Malawi, Swaziland, and Zimbabwe to provide medical training (S. Chan, 1990; Geldenhuys, 1984). Pretoria also shipped vaccines for diseases such as yellow fever, polio, cholera, TB, tetanus, gangrene, and typhus (S. Chan, 1990). South Africa's foreign policy ambition was to use this medical assistance to strengthen its regional influence, gradually building a coalition of supportive African states that South Africa could trade with, thus expanding the economy while helping protect Pretoria from potential European—mainly communist—influence (S. Chan, 1990; Siko, 2014).

Since South Africa's independence from Great Britain in 1910 and through to the transition to democracy in 1994, unlike other BRICS nations, Pretoria did not try to expand its leadership presence in the area of global health. As described by Siko (2014), this mainly stemmed from the delayed formation of South Africa's foreign policy autonomy,[1] as well as the government's increased isolation from the UN during the apartheid era. With the exception of Prime Minister Smuts's early diplomatic leadership endeavors, prime ministers had shown very little interest in strengthening South Africa's foreign policy influence. More emphasis was instead placed on domestic racial, economic, and political issues, with periodic efforts to improve the government's relationship with neighboring states in order to restore confidence and to advance economic trade and Pretoria's regional influence. As I discuss later, South Africa's commitment to helping other nations combat disease would resurface after the government rejoined the international community and after the economy was growing—and, with that, the government's albeit brief attempt at providing foreign aid in health.

In the 1970s, new efforts were made under Prime Minister Vorster (1966) to improve South Africa's image through several means, mainly opening up competitive sports to multiracial foreign teams, as well as engaging in diplomatic and economic relations with neighboring African states (South African History Online, 2011). In contrast to what happened in other authoritarian regimes in Latin America and Asia during this period (McGuire, 2010), reformation of health policy to enhance the government's international reputation was never of interest. Public health policies were strictly run by the federal government and biased in favor of serving the white community, while remaining autonomous from international influence. By the 1980s, however, these efforts were still failing to acknowledge the wave of international opposition and, by that point, outright boycotting of South Africa (Pfister, 2000; South African History Online, 2011).

With the election of the ANC in 1994, the government's foreign policy objectives changed. Breaking from years of isolationism, the government pursued a closer relationship with the international community and rejoined the UN and other international organizations. For the first time, South Africa joined the Organization of African Unity and the Non-Alignment Movement (Flemes, 2007; Pfister, 2000). Mandela's primary foreign policy objectives nevertheless fell mainly into two camps: first, becoming the regional leader on the African continent; and second, transforming global institutions and power relations in order to increase the representation of previously marginalized third world nations (Flemes, 2007).

Mandela essentially viewed South Africa as the leader of the African continent (Flemes, 2007). He and the administrations after him believed that because of the nation's unique position in the region, its resource wealth, and its history as an oppressive hegemonic power in the region (Pfister, 2000), they must lead by example to help other African nations promote human rights, better race relations, peace, and economic prosperity through economic and political modernization. During Mandela's administration, it became clear that leading and developing the African continent was the government's primary foreign policy objective (Habib, 2009, 2011; Kornegay, 2007; Pfister, 2000). The government's commitment to leading and developing Africa also stemmed from its deep nationalist impulse (Habib, 2009, 2011) and was focused on several issues: maintaining regional stability and peace through strategic diplomatic and military intervention; developing regional organizations and institutions; popularizing the African agenda in the international community; making development in the region a priority for the G8 and international organizations such as the World Bank and IMF; and investing heavily in industrial development throughout the region (Flemes, 2007; Habib, 2009). These goals and initiatives persisted under the Jacob Zuma administration (Habib, 2011).

As a regional leader, South Africa nevertheless continued to maintain its historical foreign policy commitment to state sovereignty and independence from international—especially western—influence. As if to return to Smuts's original call for a globally integrated yet independent nation, both Mandela and his minister of foreign relations, Mbeki, pursued the same strategy and made it clear that neither the West nor any international institution would influence their domestic policies (Habib, 2009; Kornegay, 2007; Salifu, 2010). Both leaders believed that South Africa and other developing nations should have complete autonomy and sovereignty in their foreign and domestic policymaking and should not continue to fall prey to international influence (Kornegay, 2007; Salifu, 2010).

Why was there continuity in the foreign policy approaches of the Apartheid Nationalist Party (NP) government and the ANC to sovereignty and independence from international influence? It is important to emphasize that ANC leaders did not intentionally adopt the NP's position on this foreign policy issue, giving the impression that there was some sort of policy legitimacy associated with the NP's foreign policies. Instead, it was the personal interests, experiences, and ambitions of Presidents Mandela and particularly Mbeki (1999–2008) that shaped the ANC's interest in state sovereignty and independence from external interference, views that were reinforced by constitutional amendments empowering the office of the president in the area of foreign affairs (Siko, 2014).

During the Mandela and, especially, Mbeki administrations, no previous NP leader or interest group influenced the president's foreign policy interests and decisions. In fact, Mbeki was well known for distancing himself from others' opinions, taking a strong personal interest in foreign affairs. His strong views on foreign affairs mainly emanated from his experience as leader of the ANC's Department of International Affairs during the ANC's exile from politics (Siko, 2014). It was during this time that Mbeki developed a suspicion of international—notably western—influence over South Africa and other African nations, for he had developed deep anticolonial and anti-imperial sentiments, moving him to believe in the continent's liberation from western colonial rule. These views shaped Mbeki's stance on state sovereignty and independence, while inspiring his belief in an African renaissance; he thus recommended continental policies that would revive Africa's economic independence and cultural richness (Ajulu, 2001). His views were also reflected in "The Foreign Policy of the Future South Africa," a position paper that "elucidated a strongly anti-imperialist foreign policy" for the transitioning ANC government (Siko, 2014, 625). When Mandela entered office in 1994 and ANC diplomats assumed positions within the outgoing apartheid regime's Department of Foreign Affairs, they brought with them their preexisting beliefs in regional solidarity, contested interstate power relations, established alliances with western nations only if initiated by and benefiting South Africa, and ensured sovereignty and independence from external—mainly western—interference (Siko, 2014; Thakur, 2015).

The government's sense of independence, arrogance, and pride in its decision-making abilities therefore persisted after the ANC's rise to power. As in the past, the new ANC government believed that it had the experience, knowledge, and commitment needed to create and implement effective policies on its own, and that it knew more about its political, economic, and social context than did any other nation or international institution (Habib, 2009). This helps to explain why Mbeki and the DOH were so reluctant to obtain donor aid assistance for HIV/AIDS and other programs (Lieberman, 2009). Indeed, Zhu (2007, 11) writes that Mbeki's belief, as a leader of Africa, involved "moving away from Western dependency, including in areas of financial, logistical, and practical support for the AIDS issue."

The Zuma administration, from 2009 to the present, maintained Mandela's and Mbeki's foreign strategies. But Zuma also made it clear that he wished to formally join the ranks of BRIC nations, going beyond his leadership role in the Africa region. In 2009, Zuma was upset that the Putin administration in Russia failed to invite him to a BRIC emerging economies summit in Yekaterinburg, Russia (Kornegay, 2009). After complaining, in 2010 Zuma was extended an invitation to join the BRIC coalition—now BRICS.

National Security Concerns and Instituting Reforms

As we saw in Russia, it seems that the government did not improve its response to HIV/AIDS until the epidemic posed a serious threat to national security. The year 1998 stands out in this regard, the year that the opposition Democratic Party claimed that the ANC government finally "woke up" to the HIV/AIDS situation (SAPA, 1998a). In that year, according to the *Johannesburg Saturday Star,* Deputy President Mbeki stated that he finally perceived the HIV/AIDS situation as one that went beyond its health implications, having grave economic and social implications (Baleta, 1998). The *Saturday Star* went on to comment that "the reality of the devastating HIV/AIDS statistics seems to have finally convinced the Government to summon 200 leaders of South African society to Pretoria to finally begin to tackle the AIDS epidemic on all fronts, . . . the key message was that AIDS was no longer just a health problem, but had the potential to devastate economic and social reform and had to be tackled from all fronts" (Baleta, 1998, 1).

At an urgent meeting organized by Mbeki in 1998, government officials learned that approximately 150,000, or one in seven, public servants had been infected with the virus (Baleta, 1998), thus potentially destabilizing government performance. Economists at the meeting emphasized the disastrous implications of AIDS for the economy. Reports were trickling in that AIDS was going to adversely affect South Africa's global economic competitiveness, due mainly to a loss of productivity and workdays (Bisseker, 1997). In 1999, it was estimated that the percentage of the South African workforce infected with HIV would rise from 11% in 1999 to 18% by 2005, thus making AIDS the biggest crisis facing the business community (Vass, 2005).

By the late fall of 1997, the government had also become increasingly concerned about rising HIV/AIDS infections in the military. As reported in *Business Day* (1997), some claimed that AIDS cases in the military had now reached an all-time high. The director of South Africa's International Civil-Military Alliance compared South Africa's AIDS situation to the high prevalence rates in Angola and Zimbabwe, while stating that soldiers were two-and-a-half times more likely than civilians to contract the virus. Fearful of a continued scale-up in infection rates, a new South African Civil-Military Alliance was formed in 1997 to prevent AIDS among "the military, paramilitary, police personnel, military families and communities where these groups are located" (*Business Day*, 1997, 1). The new alliance also provided AIDS prevention courses and published a quarterly newsletter. Director Miller of the alliance maintained that the government now believed that AIDS was contributing to an increase in overall medical costs, while compromising military security and foreign military deployments—mainly due to concerns about blood safety, field first aid, and contact with local populations (*Business Day*, 1997). Mbeki could no longer avoid the security threat. Immediate action was needed. The government acted.

At a rally organized in the fall of 1998, Mbeki announced that the time had come to respond more aggressively to HIV/AIDS. During his address, he launched the Nationwide Partnership against AIDS. For the first time, Mbeki's discussion of AIDS transitioned from a purely health issue to a broader socioeconomic problem, while noting that it was *all* of South Africa's problem. Mbeki called on a new collective effort to combat the epidemic, arguing that discrimination and fear needed to be stopped and that a more proactive effort was needed to scale up prevention and awareness (SAPA, 1998b).

But was the threat to national security the primary reason that the government began to take HIV/AIDS more seriously? Perhaps the government was responding to the rapid growth of AIDS cases and deaths. This cannot be the case, however, as the DOH had recognized the AIDS epidemic several years earlier (Dernberger, 2014). Alternatively, perhaps Mandela and Mbeki were striving to use AIDS policy as an electoral issue to keep the ANC in power and increase its legitimacy and support. This thesis also does not hold: at no point did Mandela or Mbeki campaign on the AIDS issue, nor did Mbeki's AIDS-denialist claims in the past hamper his electoral prospects. In fact, Lodge (2015) claims that by 2006, Mbeki's job approval rating had reached 77% (before dipping to 55% in 2008). Many attribute this to society's unwillingness to take the HIV/AIDS situation seriously, which reflected not only a lack of general knowledge about AIDS but also the prevailing conservative views in society that put blame on the immoral individual rather than the government.

Seeking to strengthen the government's response, one of the first initiatives the Mbeki administration undertook was creation of the South African National AIDS Council (SANAC) in January 2000. Under the auspices of the DOH, SANAC was and continues to be the primary plenary institution responsible for creating and coordinating, with other government agencies, the drafting and implementation of HIV/AIDS policies. The PACs are accountable to SANAC, which consists of representatives from government, activists, people living with HIV/AIDS, and the private sector—16 state and 17 nonstate actors, to be exact. In 2000, SANAC released the 2000–2005 HIV/AIDS Strategic Plan for South Africa, which proposed new managerial, policy, and epidemiological goals to be achieved by 2005 (Chirambo, 2004). Amid escalating demands for a more multisectoral, coordinated response (Bothma, 1998), SANAC wholeheartedly committed itself to meeting this need (Chirambo, 2004). SANAC symbolized the government's commitment to creating a stronger policy response to HIV/AIDS (Sidley, 2000).

To further ensure SANAC's effectiveness, in May 2000 Mbeki created a special 30-member Presidential AIDS Advisory Panel. Striving to overcome ongoing criticism of his unorthodox denialist views, Mbeki invited into the panel several prominent scientists, including virologist and Nobel Prize recipient Luc Montagnier, who subscribed to the orthodox view and could provide keen insight into treatment policy. At the same time, however, Mbeki appointed several scientists and policymakers supporting his denialist views. The end result was a panel that could not agree to anything, thus contributing to years of policy deadlock and delay (Lamberti and Sidley, 2000).

In 2000, SANAC also introduced policies to increase its distribution of resources to the provinces. For example, the National Integration Plan on AIDS was introduced to provide fiscal transfers to the provincial health departments. These transfers were conditional, such that their continuation depended on state health departments' appropriate and effective use of the money. In 2002, the DOH established the Joint Financing and Health Department Resources initiative. This program increased the federal government's commitment to providing ARV medications to the states. It was established to ensure joint responsibility for managing ARV financing, thus tying into the DOH's new emphasis on interagency harmonization and collaboration (Schneider, Hlophe, and van Rensburg, 2008).

The Joint Financing initiative was a prelude to the government's perhaps most successful and important policy initiative during Mbeki's tenure: the Plan for Comprehensive Treatment and Care for HIV and AIDS (the Plan). Established in 2003, the Plan called for the purchase and universal distribution of all ARV medications for those in need (Marshall, 2004). After several years of Mbeki's reluctance to consider the provision of ARV medications— mainly due to the high costs, the lack of proven scientific evidence of their efficacy, and Mbeki's denialist beliefs (Overy, 2011)—the president acquiesced to heightened domestic demands for the increased distribution of ARVs. These demands stemmed mainly from aggressive civil societal protests and law suits from influential NGOs such as the Treatment Action Campaign (TAC) (Baleta, 2003)—a lobbying process discussed in more detail below.

Through the Plan, the DOH agreed to distribute ARV medications through service points in every health district within a year and in every municipal health department within five years. The goal was to treat 1.2 million people by 2008 (Marshall, 2004). This landmark legislation seemed to be a turning point in the government's proven commitment to fighting the epidemic.

During this period, the NAP also maintained its commitment to increasing HIV/AIDS prevention and awareness. Condoms were being distributed to local clinics, free of charge. Approximately 340–540 million condoms had been provided by 2004 (Lieberman, 2009). Several HIV/AIDS public media campaigns were aired by the DOH, such as LoveLife, which targeted 12- to 19-year-olds and sponsored social activities for youth to receive sexual health information. Soul City and Soul Buddyz were government-sponsored multimedia campaigns targeting children and adults, mainly through television advertisements and radio messages, to increase awareness about HIV and provide sex education. The government also provided funding for schools for sex education, while financing NGO initiatives on these endeavors (Avert, 2015). In 1999, the Department of Basic Education, in collaboration with the DOH, created the program titled National Policy on HIV and AIDS, for Learners and Educators in Public Schools, and Students and Educators in Further Education and Training Institutions (Republic of South Africa [RSA], 2012a). Through this program, the government sought to increase teaching about HIV/AIDS in school curricula and to reduce discrimination in schools. In 2000, the Department of Basic Education followed up with creation of the HIV and AIDS Life Skills Education Program, implemented in all public primary and secondary schools, which integrated HIV education into the school curriculum and provided social support for HIV-positive students (Avert, 2015). And finally, the government maintained its long-held commitment to ensure a safe blood supply (Lieberman, 2009).

By 2006, President Mbeki, the DOH, and SANAC endorsed creation of the HIV/AIDS and STI Strategic Plan for South Africa, 2007–2011 (in brief, NSP 2007–11). This initiative established new policy goals, such as the heightened provision of ARV treatment, increased HIV testing, and improved diagnosis, to be achieved by 2011. NSP 2007–11 also aspired to reduce infection rates by half and to make ARV medications accessible to 80% of people in need by 2011 (*Nature*, 2007).

By the mid-2000s, however, several problems began to emerge, suggesting that the government was still not fully committed to ensuring a stronger policy response. First, with respect to ARV treatment, Mbeki and the DOH were still reluctant to adopt HAART (highly active antiretroviral therapy), and ARV medications were allegedly distributed too slowly (Lieberman, 2009). What is puzzling is that this occurred even after the government worked closely with TAC and the Congress of South African Trade Unions to successfully lobby international pharmaceutical companies for a reduction in ARV prices in 2001. Even more puzzling was the DOH's efforts to promote the use of natural herbal medicines such as beets, spinach, garlic, and olive oil as a remedy for HIV, suggesting that Mbeki's unorthodox denialist views were still present in government (Lethbridge, 2009). Second, a lack of coordination and respect existed between federal AIDS institutions and the presidency. While SANAC was experiencing a host of intraorganizational challenges and inefficiencies, its recommendations to Mbeki were often ignored, and the DOH provided SANAC with little autonomy in agenda setting and policymaking. Some believe that the DOH was creating and managing all AIDS policies on its own, without coordinating with SANAC members (Chirambo, 2004).

Finally, SANAC also failed to provide assistance to the provincial governments. There continued to be a shortage of medical personnel in urban and especially rural health clinics (Lethbridge, 2009). The ongoing dearth of full-time doctors and nurses complicated the NAP's ability to achieve its policy goals (*Nature*, 2007).

In response to these ongoing problems, as described by Simelela and Venter (2014), the newly elected 2009 Zuma administration decided to address the issues head on. Zuma's impetus stemmed from overwhelming data revealing the ongoing adverse effects of AIDS not only on mortality rates but also on the economy and societal relations. Zuma acknowledged that the government had spent the past "10 years pedaling backwards" in AIDS prevention and treatment and that the time had come for a stronger response. His ambitions were not influenced by international pressure or reputation building but arose more from the realization that the government had failed to adequately address the HIV/AIDS epidemic for several years.

Zuma's initial step in strengthening the government's response was to fortify SANAC. In addition to providing more political and financial support, he reorganized SANAC to ensure increased coordination between health agencies, activists, and people living with HIV/AIDS (Simelela and Venter

2014). Zuma's approach also marked a radical turn from Mbeki's unorthodox denialist views by emphasizing not just the orthodox idea that HIV does in fact lead to AIDS deaths but also that testing is important to find and treat individuals while reducing stigma (RSA, 2010). Shortly after entering office, Zuma implemented a program for providing free test centers in rural health clinics and training nurses on how to properly administer the tests. And in an effort to incentivize people to get tested, he publicly underwent the HIV test and disclosed his results in 2010 (Dugger, 2010). Zuma also supported massive efforts to increase domestic and international funding for the NAP (Bearak, 2010).

New efforts were also made in the areas of prevention. In 2011, the DOH authorized creation of the 2012–2016 National Strategic Plan for HIV, STIs, and TB (NSP 2012–16). This plan was more progressive than its predecessor, NSP 2007–11, because of its emphasis on addressing critical areas of HIV prevention such as male circumcision and funding of harm reduction programs for IDUs, sex workers, the gay community, truckers, and adolescents, while ensuring ongoing ARV rollout (RSA, 2013; Simelela and Venter, 2014). In April 2010, in an effort to prevent the transmission of HIV from female to male, the DOH created the Voluntary Medical Male Circumcision campaign, with the goal of reaching 80% of HIV-negative men by 2016 (Avert, 2015). Later that same year, the DOH launched the National HIV Counseling and Testing Campaign, which led to an increase in voluntary testing, from an estimated 19.9% in 2008 to 37.5% in 2012 for men, and from 28.7% to 52.6% for women (Avert, 2015). In 2013, the National Department of Education and the DOH implemented the Integrated School Health Program, which ensures HIV/AIDS awareness education in schools, comprehensive sex education, and sexual and reproductive health services This school health program has been deemed critical for addressing the nation's most at-risk group: girls and young women between the ages of 15 and 24 (RSA, 2013).

The Zuma administration also ensured greater access to ARV medications and treatment. As reported in the government's *Global AIDS Response Progress Report* (RSA, 2013), in April 2013 the DOH expanded its commitment to providing ARV treatment for all women who are HIV-positive during pregnancy and breastfeeding, all infants born to these mothers, and all HIV-positive individuals with TB. In 2010, the prevention of mother-to-child transmission (PMTCT) program guidelines had been amended to include AZT treatment from the early stages of gestation, HAART for all pregnant women with CD4 cell counts less than or equal to 350, and nevirapine prophylaxis for all infants for the first six weeks or until one week after ending breastfeeding. These efforts contributed to a significant reduction in mother-to-child transmission, from 3.5% in 2010 to 2.7% in 2011. The number of infants in need of AZT also decreased from approximately 26,000 in 2009 to 17,000 in 2012. To sustain this success rate, in 2011 SANAC established two programs: the South African Framework No Child Born with HIV by 2015 in South Africa; and Improving the Health and Well-being of Mothers, Partners, and Babies. Implemented at the federal and state levels, these action frameworks were linked to NSP 2012–16 and focused on improving policy strategy, financing, management, and monitoring of programs and their outcomes. Finally, the DOH has worked with provincial governments to increase the number of public health clinics providing treatment; it increased from 362 in 2008 to approximately 3,000 facilities by 2013 (Bekker et al., 2014).

By 2016, an estimated 3.4 million people were receiving ARV medications in South Africa, making SANAC's treatment program the largest in the world (Downie, Jackson, and Angelo 2016). South Africa had also far surpassed the other BRICS nations in the number of individuals taking ARV medications (fig. 6.2)

South Africa did not surpass the BRICS when it came to providing foreign aid for HIV/AIDS policies. Although the Mbeki administration did use the provision of foreign aid assistance in HIV/AIDS to help bolster South Africa's

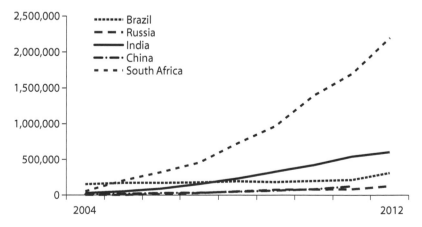

Figure 6.2. Number of individuals receiving ARV therapy in the BRICS, 2004–12. Source: UNAIDS, 2014. *Antiretroviral therapy coverage.* The World Bank Group Databank. Washington, DC. http://data.worldbank.org/indicator/SH.HIV.ARTC.ZS.

reputation as a regional leader (Cooke, 2010; Osih and Masire, 2012), these efforts were short-lived and did not become an ongoing foreign policy priority (Cooke, 2010). Under Mbeki, providing foreign aid in health—and in other social welfare sectors—was primarily used to help improve the government's relationship with other African nations and the international community, following years of geopolitical isolation and conflict over apartheid (Besharati, 2013). In achieving these objectives, Mbeki provided US$10 million to the Global Fund and pledged another US$20 million over 20 years to Gavi, the Vaccine Alliance (formerly, Global Alliance for Vaccines and Immunization); any further commitments were hampered by Mbeki's denialist views (Cooke, 2010). When Zuma entered office, his focus was more on strengthening the government's response to HIV/AIDS in South Africa than on helping other nations (Cooke, 2010; Osih and Masire, 2012). As one of Zuma's health officials put it, the administration's focus was to "put its own house in order" first before going global (quoted in Cooke, 2010, 43). Moreover, Zuma never shared Mbeki's ambition of displaying South Africa's global and regional leadership through increased foreign aid for HIV/AIDS. This mainly reflected Zuma's foreign policy beliefs in noninterventionism, state sovereignty, and independence—a tenet that, as we saw earlier, had a long foreign policy precedent in South Africa (Cooke, 2010; Osih and Masire, 2012).

The foreign assistance that Zuma has authorized for helping other nations respond to HIV/AIDS has been limited in scale, shaped more by the government's commitment to building solidarity and unity in South-South relations than by seeking international fame and influence. The government has mainly focused on providing technical research assistance through the India–Brazil–South Africa Dialogue Forum (IBSA), a coordinating forum that brings India, Brazil, and South Africa together for the purpose of strengthening their partnerships, establishing a common policy view, and engaging in development cooperation with other developing nations (Cooke, 2010; Osih and Masire, 2012). For instance, through this forum South Africa has worked with India to provide vaccine research and policy recommendations in the areas of HIV/AIDS, TB, and malaria. The government has also provided a limited amount of direct bilateral technical assistance to several nations in the southern African region to help control the spread of malaria (Osih and Masire, 2012). Finally, although the Mandela administration authorized domestic pharmaceutical companies to produce generic ARV medications—despite vehement protests and court actions from pharmaceutical companies accusing South

Africa of violating the WTO's TRIPS rulings (Bekker et al., 2014)—neither the Mbeki nor the Zuma administration sought to make use of the successful resistance to these industries to bolster the government's international reputation in health (as we saw in Brazil).

South Africa has joined its BRICS counterparts—save for Russia—in being receptive to international donor aid assistance. Beginning in 2004, the DOH received funding from PEPFAR (totaling US$3.7 billion) and from the Global Fund for the nation's PMTCT and ARV programs (Bekker et al., 2014). However, this funding was requested mainly by select South African provinces and NGOs, circumventing Mbeki's resistance to external donor support, particularly in the area of funding for ARV drug distribution. It also dovetailed with an increase in the targeting of foreign donor aid to local governments and NGOs rather than to the central government (Bekker et al., 2014; Nunn et al., 2012). To the government's credit, Mbeki did not seek to prohibit the donor community's work with NGOs (McGreal, 2002)—as Putin had done in Russia. The majority of domestic AIDS program funding has nevertheless consistently come from the government, not from the international donor community, which comports with the government's long history of policy independence, sovereignty, and negative geopolitical positioning—going it alone when it came to HIV/AIDS (Avert, 2016; McGreal, 2002). About 25% of the costs for the government's HIV/AIDS programs, which includes funding for NGO activities, is from donors; multilateral and bilateral donor aid is expected to decrease in the near future (Lodge, 2015). As I discuss shortly, this reduction in donor support will hamper the NGO community's ability to respond to the epidemic.

Despite South Africa's limited presence at the global level, it has remained committed to increasing domestic spending for HIV/AIDS. As figure 6.3 illustrates, government spending for HIV/AIDS increased from an estimated R 966 million (US$68 million) in 2003 to R 11.2 billion (US$789 million) in 2013 (LaCock, 2015). However, this spending was soon deemed to be insufficient. In 2013, the government itself acknowledged that this funding needed to be better targeted at prevention programs for higher-risk groups, especially young women and girls. More funding has also been needed for scaling up evidence-based HIV prevention efforts (RSA, 2013). These shortcomings have led scholars to conclude that, despite an increase in federal spending, prevention programs are not expanding to meet the needs of the groups at highest risk (Bekker et al., 2014).

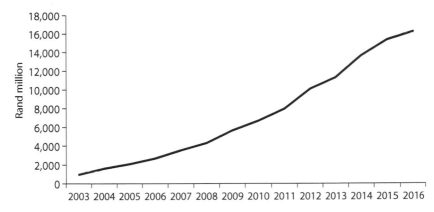

Figure 6.3. Consolidated HIV/AIDS spending in South Africa (million rand), 2013–16. Source: LaCock, 2015.

Despite the increase in federal spending for SANAC, this, too, has not been enough. For example, for the 2013–14 period, SANAC's total operational costs were R 25 billion (US$1.7 billion), but parliament authorized only R 19.9 billion (US$1.4 billion). Since 2013, SANAC has requested from parliament an additional R 1.6 billion (US$112 million) each year, which has not been provided (Bekker et al., 2014). This additional funding is needed to keep up with the burgeoning demand for ARV treatment, which has expanded due to increased patient longevity and further government commitments to ARV distribution. The funding gap is expected to grow, while future predicted expenses, especially hospitalization costs, are expected to well exceed the current funding sources available (Avert, 2016; Lodge, 2015).

Several health system challenges also persist, which are mainly associated with the DOH's decision to decentralize ARV treatment services (Bekker et al., 2014). Ensuring an adequate supply of medical doctors and nurses at the provincial level is a constant problem, reflecting limited provincial government spending and inadequate financial support from the central government (Downie, Jackson, and Angelo, 2016). Shortages in this area have challenged SANAC's and the provinces' ability to carry out prevention programs and especially ARV treatment and HIV testing (Downie, Jackson, and Angelo, 2016; RSA, 2013), both encouraging early testing and tracking and retaining patients in their ARV treatment (Bekker et al., 2014). Although the number of nurses trained and responsible for delivering ARV treatment increased from 250 certified in 2010 to 10,000 by 2012, the supply of nurses is still limited, especially in rural areas. This situation has contributed to a decline in the overall quality of care, an inability to effectively manage and maintain patients on ARV treatment, and longer wait times in hospitals. Furthermore, there is an ongoing limitation of primary health care facilities, which since 2004 have had primary responsibility for administering ARVs; those that exist are inundated with new and returning patients. Limited infrastructure, such as clean working spaces and access to equipment, especially in rural areas, has further complicated these endeavors (Bekker et al., 2014; J. Cohen, 2016).

In the area of HIV/AIDS prevention, improving educational awareness and behavioral change has also been an ongoing challenge. While the government has increased the budget for the DOH's and the Department of Basic Education's HIV/AIDS programs, both the federal and provincial governments have not done a good job of guaranteeing the quality of sex education: ensuring high teaching standards and addressing the reluctance in some schools to provide condoms (Heywood, 2016; Van der Merwe, 2015). According to a Human Sciences Research Council's survey of South African households published in March 2014, there has been an overall decline in condom use, while the number of sex partners has increased and knowledge about HIV transmission has decreased (Van der Merwe, 2015).

Despite the sizable increase in the number of individuals receiving ARV treatment, a shortage of ARV medications continues in some areas (Lodge, 2015; Van der Merwe, 2015). As Lodge (2015) reports, a national survey conducted in 2013 of 2,139 public health facilities found that more than one-fifth, 459, had experienced shortages of ARV and TB medications in the previous three months. Poor logistical planning and management and a lack of sufficient federal financial support and adequate patient reporting systems were blamed. In 2013, this prompted the DOH and the Treasury Department to carefully monitor and control the drug procurement systems in several provinces, such as Limpopo, Gauteng, and the Eastern Cape.

Although recent government efforts have led to a steady decline in HIV cases, the number is still high. In 2016, the DOH reported that HIV incidence for adults dropped from a high of 1.67% in 2005 to 1.22% in 2015 (J. Cohen, 2016). Yet this still equates to approximately 330,000 new infections each year. When combined with the fact that only 2.7 million of 6.2 million HIV-positive individuals are receiving ARV medications, this situation has convinced pundits that HIV/AIDS in South Africa is still a "public health crisis" (S. Allison, 2015).

The government has improved its policy response to HIV/AIDS, but why has SANAC not been capable of achieving a stronger or, better yet, centrist policy response? As I explained in chapter 1, a centrist policy response entails the creation and ongoing financial and administrative expansion of federal agencies, the development of effective prevention and treatment policies (especially, universal access to medicine), and formal and informal strategies to increase the central government's policy influence in a context of healthcare decentralization. In South Africa, however, the government has not engaged in an ongoing financial commitment to SANAC, and prevention and ARV treatment programs have fallen short of achieving their goals. At the same time, the DOH has not formally tried to increase its central policy influence through the use of conditional fiscal transfers to the provinces, nor has it informally worked with NGOs to monitor provincial health departments and hold them accountable for policy implementation. As the next section explains, the latter failure has emerged because of the consistently weak partnership between the DOH and NGOs. Indeed, as seen in Russia, India, and China, South Africa's inability to achieve a centrist policy response seems to stem in part from the bureaucracy's inability to establish a strong partnership with NGOs.

Absence of Strong Bureaucratic-Civil Societal Partnerships

South Africa's public health system does not have a long history of serving the entire population, with health bureaucrats working closely with all segments of society. Instead, the deep racial divide that grew out of European colonialism (Davenport and Saunders, 2000), mainly through Dutch and British settlers, led to the emergence of public healthcare systems that were segregated along racial lines. Since the nineteenth century, white European colonists had created and relied on their own western-style healthcare systems, while the black population mainly relied on traditional medical practices and tribal healers. These healers possessed a considerable amount of influence in local communities, whereas westernized medical services and basic care were unevenly distributed. There were ample numbers of tribal healers, providing each family with a healthcare practitioner (Kalipeni, 2000; Miti, 2013).

The presence of this influential tribal healing system generated few incentives for civil society to organize and create social health movements or public health associations. Indeed, during the nineteenth century, no civic movement arose that was dedicated specifically to combating disease (Miti, 2013). In large part this stemmed not just from the existence of a well-integrated traditional healing system but also from the absence of a unified public healthcare system that most of the general population could access (Kalipeni, 2000). Consequently, social health movements and/or civic organizations proffering a more central-ized, universal policy response to diseases never emerged. Nor were there public health officials willing to work with and serve the entire population, regardless of racial identity (Hausler, 2013; Miti, 2013).

Civic mobilization among the marginalized and suppressed black population began during the nineteenth and twentieth centuries, though its influence was isolated and focused mainly on political liberalization and antiapartheid senti-ment. As an outgrowth of historical social movements originating in the nine-teenth century over the right to vote, by the 1960s and 1970s voluntary civic organizations began to emerge throughout the nation (Bundy, 2000). Like movements in the past, this civic response emerged in opposition to central-ized and oppressive political rule, in a form of antinationalist sentiment (Adler and Steinberg, 2000; Bundy, 2000). Many of these movements and organizations had been forcefully suppressed in the 1950s (Bundy, 2000). Activists were forced into exile, and limited incentives remained to mobilize. Civic movements and organizations did emerge, but they operated in isolation at the local level and were peaceful and seemingly nonconfrontational toward the government (Adler and Steinberg, 2000; Miti, 2013).

In the late 1980s, proactive civic mobilization and protest heightened in support of the ANC's return to power. A flurry of pro-democratic and civil rights NGOs began to emerge (Chirambo, 2004; Johnson, 2005; Miti, 2013). However, these new pro-democratic movements did not immediately translate to the presence of well-organized AIDS NGOs with influence on policy (Schneider, Hlophe, and van Rensburg, 2008). The NGOs that did emerge included the AIDS Foundation of South Africa in 1988, which focused on pro-viding community-based prevention and treatment interventions in rural ar-eas (Oxfam, 2015); the Gay Association of South Africa in 1982; and the AIDS Consortium Project in 1992. These organizations pressured the government for prevention programs and especially drug treatment, grounded in the princi-ples of nondiscrimination and individual rights. But these NGOs were small in size and influence and consequently could not get the government's atten-tion (Mbali, 2005). The Gay Association, for example, was not even invited to participate in the DOH's initial Aids Advisory Group—which provided expert advice on policy—even though it represented the largest community affected by HIV/AIDS at that time. Add to this the fear of mobilizing in a context where gay and lesbian sexual activity was illegal and the state had the legal right to suppress movements opposing the government (Gómez and Harris, 2015; Mbali, 2005). Moreover, the limited number of AIDS activists that emerged could not justify their need for government assistance on the grounds of a historically based, strong partnership with public health bureaucrats who were proffering similar policy ideas about state intervention in times of health crisis (Miti, 2013). Consequently, AIDS bureaucrats were not accustomed to having a strong partnership with activists and those affected by disease and so did not seek to work closely with the AIDS NGOs (Guari and Lieberman, 2006).

Even after the return to democracy in 1994, the ANC and the DOH still did not try to improve this situation. For example, the AIDS Advisory Council, which was explicitly designed to formally incorporate the views of scientific experts, NGOs, and people living with HIV/AIDS, was shut down in 1997 after its critiquing of the government's policy progress (Chirambo, 2004; Johnson, 2005; Zhu, 2007). Although NGO activists and people with HIV/AIDS were represented at the 1993 NACOSA conference, their representation seemed to be more ceremonial than effective in influencing policy. In fact, despite their representation in NACOSA, NGOs incessantly complained of being unable to access top-level AIDS policymakers (Johnson, 2005; Marias, 2000; Zhu, 2007) and of poor coordination with national and local AIDS bureaucrats (Bisseker, 1997). Even provincial PAC administrators failed to reach out to NGOs (Johnson, 2005). For almost 10 years, from 1999 to 2008, Mbeki ignored the opinions of NGO activists and scientific experts on AIDS advisory bodies. The NAP became increasingly reclusive, failing to establish strong partnerships with NGOs (Hausler, 2013; Lethbridge, 2009; Miti, 2013; Nunn et al., 2012; Zhu, 2007). DOH and AIDS bureaucrats simply did not consider NGOs to be valued partners in the policymaking process (Parkhurst and Lush, 2004; Zhu, 2007). This was reflected in the DOH's decision to reduce the subsidies going to AIDS NGOs from R 20 million (US$1.4 million) in 1996 to R 12.5 million (US$880,564) in 1997 (Bisseker, 1997).

This weak partnership between the DOH and NGOs emerged for several reasons. First, there was no history of the health bureaucracy's commitment to partnering with civil society to eradicate disease or seek policy suggestions (Johnson, 2005; Miti, 2013). Second, Mbeki's denialist beliefs prohibited a partnership with progressive activists (Gómez and Harris, 2015). Third, the government had decided in 1998 to refuse funding for pilot programs providing ARV treatment to pregnant women. Fourth, initiatives taken by the NAP were viewed as both corrupt and disrespectful toward the NGO community: specifically, the NAP's usage of R 14 million (US$985,815) for funding a musical play, *Sarafina II*. Funding for this play was taken from the NAP and PAC budgets without consulting SANAC or the NGOs (Gómez and Harris, 2015). When questioned about this allegedly scandalous activity, the DOH director, Nkosazana Dlamini-Zuma (1994–98), stated that "the department could not be expected to consult every NGO. AIDS doesn't consult, it infects people" (quoted in Johnson, 2005, 122). And finally, to add insult to injury, in 1997 the DOH decided to mandate the disclosure of every individual found to be HIV-positive. This flew in the face of AIDS activists' clamoring for the right to medical privacy (Schneider, 2002).

Nevertheless, the DOH's unwillingness to partner with NGOs did not in any way affect the latter's efforts to mobilize and directly pressure the government for much-needed legislation. In fact, if anything, Mbeki's denialist claims and unwillingness to work with NGOs further incentivized their mobilization efforts and pressure on the government (Lodge, 2015).

For instance, by the late 1990s, NGOs such as the Treatment Action Campaign and the AIDS Law Project emerged to pressure the government and to use newly established democratic institutions such as the Constitutional Court to persuade the Mbeki administration to provide treatment services. TAC was formed in Cape Town in 1998 as a network of groups such as unions, churches, and gay rights and healthcare workers' organizations, fused together by a human rights–based belief in access to HIV/AIDS prevention and treatment services. It arose to mobilize and to demand that the DOH provide ARV medications, such as nevirapine for HIV-positive pregnant women. In 2002, after lobbying and organizing mass demonstrations, TAC, with the assistance of the Congress of South African Trade Unions, sued the DOH in the Pretoria High Court on the grounds that the government was violating the 1996 Constitution by not providing this medication. The suit was based on the Constitution's health-related socioeconomic rights stipulations. In 2003, the high court decided in TAC's favor and forced the DOH to start providing nevirapine for pregnant women. In 2004, the government followed up with creation of the PMTCT program, though with considerable resistance and delay. That same year, TAC engaged in an aggressive civil disobedience campaign through mass protests and activist arrests, ultimately forcing the Mbeki administration to reverse its decision not to support the distribution of ARV medications (Bekker et al., 2014; Mbali, 2005; Nunn et al., 2012; Yawa, 2016).

In 1997, instead of working in opposition to the state, TAC had partnered with the DOH to win a court battle against the Pharmaceutical Manufacturers' Association to ensure that the government had a legal basis for producing and importing generic ARV medications (Overy, 2011). This earlier partnership suggests that, at times, the government was willing to work with NGOs to ensure access to medicine. But it also suggests that the government was inconsistent in its partnership with NGOs, seeking to work with them only when that suited its interests.

TAC's and other NGOs' eventual success in pressuring the government for policy reform, we should note, occurred only *after* the government had already decided to improve its policy response—albeit, to a limited extent. This had occurred at the end of the 1990s, after the Mbeki administration perceived AIDS to be a national security threat.

Much as we saw in Russia, in the past two to three years the departure of international donor support for TAC and other AIDS NGOs has challenged their ability not only to provide critical health and social services but also to hold the DOH accountable for ensuring an ongoing, adequate supply of ARV medications and a stronger public health system. Both of these are necessary for high-quality treatment interventions. In November 2014, for example, DFID permanently withdrew its funding for TAC, allegedly worth R 8 million (US$563,561), on the grounds that South Africa's government had already made excellent progress in the area of ARV treatment and now had sufficient resources to sustain this response. TAC has argued, however, that it still needs more funding to carry out its work and that, due to budgetary shortfalls, it has had to reduce its organizational staff (S. Allison, 2015). It is not clear whether the government will fill this gap with additional funding.

The Zuma administration, SANAC, and the DOH have also recognized the important role that AIDS NGOs are playing to increase awareness and provide social and medical services (Gómez and Harris, 2015). And yet, since Mbeki, there is no evidence to suggest that AIDS bureaucrats have tried to strengthen their partnership with NGOs to justify an increase in parliamentary funding for prevention programs for at-risk groups and ARV medications. At the same time, the parliament has become reluctant to work with NGOs and SANAC to increase public transparency and accountability for how AIDS funds are being used. In 2014, for example, the parliament ignored NGOs' request to reinstate parliament's Joint Committee on HIV and AIDS, which was created in 2012 to monitor and evaluate programs and funding allocations (Sonke Gender Justice, 2015). The parliament suggested that politically, even if SANAC and the DOH could establish a stronger partnership with NGOs, the government might still not take their requests seriously.

In sum, despite South Africa's apathy toward international pressures and reputation building and its resistance to international aid, when HIV/AIDS began to pose a national security threat, the government began to take the epidemic more seriously and pursued policy reforms. Before these national security interests emerged, while AIDS NGOs were forming and pressuring the government for a stronger policy response, the MOH did not effectively respond to their needs. Moreover, even after the government began to take HIV/AIDS more seriously, MOH bureaucrats did not try to establish a strong partnership with NGOs. This hampered the government's ability to pursue a centrist policy response.

Responding to Tuberculosis

The resurgence of TB in South Africa in the 1980s was attributable to a combination of historical conditions, economic transformation, government policy, and the emergence of HIV/AIDS. In the 1930s, poor urban and rural conditions, congested housing, and fragmented and inadequate healthcare services had contributed to the spread of TB. An estimated 60% of the black population had TB. The thriving goldmining industry and the lack of employers' interest in TB prevention contributed to its further spread, not only in the mines, but also in the communities where workers lived (Edington, 2000; Fourie, 2011; S. Karim et al., 2009). High-TB conditions in poor black communities persisted under apartheid, fueled some would claim by government-funded, congested squatter settlements, underdeveloped healthcare systems, and swelling ranks of migrant labor (S. Karim et al., 2009). Figure 6.4 shows the increase in TB cases from the mid-1990s to mid-2000s.

As in Russia, the TB epidemic resurfaced in the 1980s mainly because of HIV (Achmat and Roberts, 2005; Loveday and Zweigenthal, 2011). By the mid-1990s, it was estimated that approximately 40% of people with TB were HIV-positive (Bamford, 1999), with TB eventually becoming the leading cause of death for people with HIV. To this day, TB along with influenza and pneumonia are the leading causes of death for the entire population (Merten, 2014).

The government's initial reaction to the TB resurgence was marked by a high degree of political and bureaucratic contestation (Achmat and Roberts,

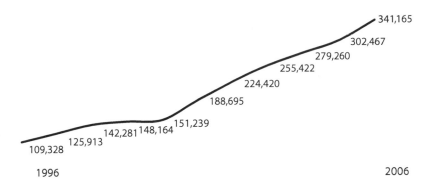

Figure 6.4. TB cases in South Africa, 1996–2006. Source: RSA, Department of Health, 2011.

2005; Karim et al., 2009). Politicians and most health officials could not agree that there was sufficient epidemiological evidence that TB posed a serious national health threat. Other politicians simply denied that TB had resurfaced as the main cause of death for people with HIV/AIDS (Achmat and Roberts, 2005). Yet others insisted that politicians were in denial, inept, and trying to undermine scientific evidence as a basis for policy reform (S. Karim et al., 2011). Under apartheid rule, most politicians were indifferent to the living and health conditions in poor black communities, where TB was mainly concentrated. And where TB was rapidly reemerging, such as in highly congested mining plants, business owners were reluctant to invest in TB awareness and prevention services, given the large pool of unemployed laborers available (Stuckler, Basu, and McKee, 2010).

The apartheid government's policy response also highlighted its lack of commitment to the issue. Despite the government's acknowledgment of the resurgence, scholars note, the DOH delayed creating an effective response (Q. Karim et al., 2011). While some analysts claim that some health policies were implemented as early as 1979 in response to TB, these responses were characterized as "patchy," inadequately funded, and poorly managed (Bamford, 1999). During this period, moreover, the DOH, which administered the TB programs, had a difficult time coordinating policy implementation with 18 different subnational governing districts (Edington, 2000).

The DOH's response in rural areas further emphasized the government's lack of commitment to responding adequately to the TB epidemic. In these areas, TB was often underdiagnosed because there were not enough health clinics to administer testing; this contributed to the spread of the disease (Edington, 2000). This revealed that the DOH was not providing provincial governments with the financial, technical, and human resources needed for an adequate response.

Finally, during this period, the DOH was not working closely with activists and those living with TB to devise a more effective strategy against the disease. At no point was there any organized attempt to involve local communities in the decision-making process. No effort was made to create new public awareness campaigns or to disseminate information about TB (Edington, 2000). With respect to TB, HIV/AIDS, and other diseases, apartheid's divided governance and discrimination toward poorer, black communities did not bode well and did not encourage the development of strong bureaucratic–civil societal partnerships (Kalipeni, 2000).

International Criticism and Pressure

Eventually, the government's inadequate response to TB not only kindled social unrest but also aroused international criticism and pressure. However, that international attention to TB did not occur until 1993, when the WHO officially declared the disease a pandemic threat. By the mid-1990s, the WHO, other international organizations, and the medical community began to criticize nations for their delayed response, as well as their biased attention to HIV/AIDS. Of course, South Africa was not exempt from these criticisms.

International criticism in response to South Africa's TB situation began to emerge in the mid-1990s. In 1996, for example, after being invited by the South African government to evaluate its TB policies, WHO officials wrote a report essentially condemning the government for its failure to respond effectively. More specifically, the report stated that the government needed to declare the seriousness of the TB epidemic; that it needed to strengthen its policy management; that it needed to effectively implement the DOTS strategy (officially adopted in 1996); and that it needed to invest adequate resources at the national and subnational levels (Bamford, 1999). The WHO report found that TB management systems (including financial commitments) were lacking at the national and provincial levels and that there was an inefficient use of financial and administrative resources. It also found that the new TB register was inadequately used, TB microscopy services were not being provided, and patients were not being treated effectively. In essence, the WHO report found that despite adequate financial resources within the DOH, national and subnational heath departments' failure to take the TB issue seriously was leading to inefficiency in resource management and inadequate policy outcomes (Edington, 2000). In 1998, at a three-day conference in London, the WHO once again criticized South Africa, among other nations, for its lackluster policy response to TB (Cookson, 1998).

But what consequences did this international criticism and pressure have? Did it motivate the South African government to strengthen its response to TB? Or was the government just as apathetic toward the international community's response as it had been for HIV/AIDS?

Once again, the international criticism and pressure had no impact on domestic bureaucratic and policy reform. In fact, shortly after the WHO had pointed its finger at South Africa, McNeil (1996) stated that the South African government's sense of urgency surrounding these criticisms had faded within several months. While the DOH was temporarily concerned about the epidemic, even prompting Health Minister Zuma to publicly state in 1996 that TB was "a national priority" (Bamford, 1999; Fourie, 2011), the government once again decided to ignore international pressure. It would do what it had always done: remain independent and resolved in its own ability to understand and respond to epidemics, at its own pace, regardless of international opinion.

Absence of National Security Threat and Instituting Reforms

If international criticism and pressure did not elicit a government response to TB, then perhaps the threat to South Africa's national security would. As I discussed in chapter 1, when governments engage in negative geopolitical positioning we should expect a threat to national security, such as military readiness and the economy, to prompt reforms. Did this occur in South Africa for TB? In contrast to what we saw with HIV/AIDS, the answer is no, for several reasons.

With regard to military readiness, research suggests that the number of TB cases within the military did not reach epidemic proportions. In large part this was due to the ongoing early-detection policies in place in the military, given the well-known coinfection problem with HIV/AIDS (RSA, 2007). As outlined in the Tuberculosis Strategic Plan for South Africa (2007–11), the military is responsible for engaging in early detection of TB, appropriate treatment and referral, increasing awareness about the disease, and reporting of all cases within the military (RSA, 2007). Through these initiatives the military seems to have been able to avoid major infection within its ranks. With respect to the economy, TB was not projected to impede economic growth. While the epidemic did adversely affect workers' capacity and employment in some mining industries (Stuckler, Basu, and McKee, 2010), and while family members lost a considerable amount of income due to days lost at work (Bond et al., 2008), TB never posed a serious threat to economic growth.

The absence of credible threats to national security notwithstanding, in 1998 the DOH introduced the National TB Program (NTBP). The timing of its implementation suggests that it may have emerged in response, not to any national security threats, but to an increase in international criticism and pressure, which emerged by the late 1990s. The NTBP called for a heightened commitment to DOTS treatment and appointed new provincial- and district-level TB coordinators to ensure effective DOTS therapy and other healthcare services (Bamford, 1999; Fourie, 2011). But a closer look at the NTBP and subsequent policy initiatives reveals that this program was not created in response to this pressure or to enhance the government's international reputation. Analysts note that the NTBP suffered from weak federal guidelines on how to administer policy and on monitoring and evaluation systems, inadequate administrative resources and capacity at the provincial and district levels, poor planning skills at these levels, and low levels of administrative accountability (Bamford, 1999; Fourie, 2011). Meanwhile, others claimed that the overall pace of policy implementation was too slow, as if to suggest a lack of government commitment to strengthening the NTBP (Fourie, 2011).

In 2004, in response to the burgeoning HIV/AIDS-TB coinfection problem, the DOH established the HIV/AIDS and TB Unit and the HAST (HIV/AIDS/STI/TB) Initiative to work at the provincial and district levels (Loveday and Zweigenthal, 2011). Analysts nevertheless note that the DOH and the HIV/AIDS and TB Unit were never clear on what HAST did or how HIV/AIDS and TB services were to be integrated (Eley, 2010; Loveday and Zweigenthal, 2011). Furthermore, there was no sharing of healthcare service providers and staff. For many observers, these challenges indicated the DOH's apathy toward ensuring effective integration and coordination between the HIV/AIDS and TB sectors.

The DOH also demonstrated an unwillingness to be transparent and accountable with the national TB budget. Whereas in other countries, TB budget details were often publicly disseminated (such as on websites), in South Africa this was never the case. NGOs working on TB issues, such as TAC, complained that because of this lack of transparency and accountability, they could not determine how federal funding was being allocated (Treatment Action Campaign, 2011).

In 2007, the DOH appeared to have strengthened its policy commitment to TB by creating the Tuberculosis Strategic Plan for South Africa 2007–2011 (TSPSA). The overall goal of this plan was to improve the government's response to TB and MDR-TB, to acknowledge and respond to the HIV/AIDS-TB coinfection problem, and to offer all TB patients voluntary HIV testing (Mseleku, 2007). The plan also provided new NTBP guidelines in the curriculum for basic training for doctors and nurses; appointed two full-time staff at the national NTBP office, who would be responsible for human resource development activities; mobilized new funding schemes; and created the National TB Crisis Management Plan, which was designed to further intensify efforts at TB control (Eley, 2010; WHO, 2007). The TSPSA also sought to strengthen the overall health systems response to TB, to work collaboratively with all care providers, to empower NGOs to get more involved in the response to TB, to coordinate and implement TB research, and to strengthen infection control (S. Karim et al., 2009).

Nevertheless, scholars note, the DOH was not successful in implementing the TSPSA. First, S. Karim et al. (2009) found that while the DOH had sufficient financial resources, it did not increase these resources to meet ongoing TSPSA needs, especially in several specific areas: prevention; treatment, care, and support for patients; legal and human rights; and research, monitoring, and evaluation. In addition, at the lowest tiers of government, there was an ongoing shortage of infrastructural resources such as beds and x ray machines as well as insufficient space to treat TB patients in hospitals and clinics (Atkins, 2011; Treatment Action Campaign, 2011). There was an ongoing shortage of healthcare providers, including doctors and nurses; this required lay workers to be trained as nurses to provide TB services. There was also an ongoing need for healthcare worker training to administer DOTS and other TB services (Atkins, 2011). Finally, even those who were trained to provide such services, and their service provider managers such as TB and communicable disease coordinators, did not spend enough time taking care of TB patients (Strachan, 2000).

Further DOH efforts were made in 2012 to address these and other needed reforms through the National Strategic Plan for HIV, STIs, and TB 2012–2016. This plan, NSP 2012–16, is NSP 2007–11 with the addition of TB—because it is the highest-prevalence disease associated with HIV/AIDS and shares similar levels of stigma and similar high-risk groups.[2] As described by the Soul City Research Unit (2015), NSP 2012–16 sets out to further ensure the integration of prevention and treatment services for HIV/AIDS and TB at the primary care level as well as improved guidance and monitoring of policy implementation. This program provides a general policy vision to address these diseases simultaneously while adhering to UNAIDS's suggested goals of achieving zero HIV/AIDS-TB coinfection, zero discrimination, and zero preventable deaths, with the ultimate objective of zero TB mortality by 2032. Through this program, NSP 2012–16 sought to reduce the number of TB infections and deaths by 50% and the number of self-reported cases of TB-related stigma by the same percentage.

In the area of TB prevention, new annual voluntary testing campaigns are included as part of NSP 2012–16, to be carried out at a variety of public venues, with a focus on the most at-risk groups—including HIV-positive patients, current and former prisoners, and children (Soul City Research Unit, 2015). In 2011, moreover, the NTBP also introduced a multifaceted TB screening program in high-burden districts, which included door-to-door inquiry, community mobilization, HIV counseling and testing services, and screening of high-risk populations (Churchyard et al., 2014). As further reported by the Soul City Research Unit (2015), to more effectively discover new TB cases, the NTBP also implemented the Xpert MTB/IRF test as a replacement for sputum smear microscopy, as well as a central data-monitoring system to monitor this process remotely. Detection has been facilitated by efforts to enhance the monitoring and reporting of TB through the introduction of electronic recording and reporting systems for MDR-TB strains (EDR.net) and drug-susceptible strains (ETR.net). This reporting system is used at the district levels. And finally, in 2015, on World TB Day, Deputy President Cyril Ramaphosa launched the Comprehensive TB Screening and Testing Campaign. The focus of this campaign is to mobilize all South Africans to ensure increased screening and testing, especially in isolated, high-risk places such as prisons, mines, and schools.

Beginning in 2011, the DOH also pursued a more decentralized approach to TB management and care to enhance patients' access to testing, diagnosis, treatment, and home care. To facilitate this process, the DOH published the *National Tuberculosis Management Guidelines 2014*, for distribution at health facilities and community centers (Soul City Research Unit, 2015). The guidelines provide advice for introducing prepaid diagnostic tests for MDR-TB, new medicines for treating MDR- and XDR-TB, and more primary care outreach teams with a focus on improved home care (Soul City Research Unit, 2015).

The government has not tried to provide foreign aid assistance for TB to enhance its international reputation in health and/or its status as a regional leader. While the Mbeki administration sought to briefly achieve the latter with respect to HIV/AIDS, Zuma's administration has instead focused more on eradicating TB, HIV/AIDS, and other diseases at home (Osih and Masire, 2012; Ravelo, 2014a). South Africa has been a recipient, along with other southern African nations, of a US$30 million grant from the Global Fund for its national TB programs, with a focus on at-risk groups such as workers in the mining sector (Nyaka, 2015). South Africa also received bilateral support from USAID for TB programs—approximately US$10 million by 2010 (Ravelo, 2014b). While the Global Fund has continued to provide grant support for South Africa's TB programs since 2011, most of its funding has been for HIV/AIDS, despite the growing need for more investment in the government's TB programs (Ravelo, 2014b). When compared with domestic government spending, this external donor support has been minimal, which reflects the government's ongoing interest in designing and funding its own TB programs (Ravelo, 2014b; RSA, 2016). Analysts maintain, however, that the government is not financially or politically ready to do this (Ravelo, 2014b). This response comports with the government's ongoing negative geopolitical positioning: it continues to believe in its ability to solve its own public health problems and to rely less on international support and policy advice. Considering the ongoing domestic budgetary shortfalls for the NTBP's and SANAC's program endeavors, as well as the Zuma administration's ongoing domestic focus, it is doubtful that the government will seek to provide financial and technical assistance to other nations.

Despite the government's recent TB policy reforms, several challenges remain. Studies suggest that the NTBP still receives insufficient funding for its policies. Despite NSP 2012–16 addressing both diseases and other STIs, HIV/AIDS still receives the bulk of parliamentary budgetary support. From 2011 to 2013, AIDS funding increased from R 12.7 billion (US$894 million) to R 17.9 billion (US$1.2 billion), whereas TB funding increased from R 3.3 billion (US$232 million) to R 3.7 billion (US$260 million) for the same period (RSA, 2016). Because of these problems, some have argued that TB should have its own separate, vertical program under the DOH so that it can obtain more funding (Ravelo, 2014b). Furthermore, and as mentioned earlier, SANAC, which is primarily responsible for coordinating with the PACs to implement NSP 2012–16, is not receiving sufficient funding for its program initiatives (RSA 2012b, 2016). A government report in 2012 suggests that the NSP needs an increase of 15% of its operational budget to achieve its objectives (RSA, 2012b).

Since the provision of TB medications was decentralized in 2011, the provinces have also experienced repeated problems in ensuring sufficient revenue for their treatment programs, as well as for human resources and infrastructure—especially in poorer provinces and townships (Bosworth, 2014; Churchyard et al., 2014; Khumalo, 2014). In contrast to the centrist policy response that we saw in Brazil, there have been no conditional federal grants incentivizing the provinces to adhere to the NTBP's goal of timely testing and treatment. In this context of little accountability to the national program, the provinces have varied in their capacity and willingness to meet these objectives (Bosworth, 2014). Studies also show that there is a shortage of provincial government primary care outreach teams and mobile clinics for detecting (e.g., through the 2011 house-to-house visit campaign) and managing new TB cases. And there is no clear policy or practice for TB screening among local healthcare workers (Churchyard et al., 2014; Soul City Research Unit, 2015). Given the projected high costs associated with hiring more TB healthcare workers, the government has shied away from this option (Low, 2016). A shortage of healthcare workers may account for the estimated 25% of TB-positive patients whom these workers do not follow up to initiate treatment. Studies also point to the ongoing dearth of hospital beds needed to treat TB patients, especially in rural areas (Churchyard et al., 2014).

With respect to the provision of TB medicines and treatment, the number of individuals defaulting on their standard TB treatment has increased; in most provinces this fails to reach the national target of a less than 5% default rate (Soul City Institute, 2015). In 2012, only 42% of patients diagnosed with MDR-TB started treatment, and the successful completion rate was estimated at only 40% (Bosworth, 2014). A high percentage of patients receiving MDR-TB treatment are not followed up for adequate treatment service, and approximately 40% have not received the appropriate initial treatment (Churchyard et al., 2014). Successful treatment rates among those with drug-resistant TB have remained low, at approximately 42% for MDR-TB and 18% for XDR-TB (Churchyard et al., 2014). In this context, while the number of standard pulmonary TB cases has declined, the number of MDR-TB and XDR-TB cases, infected with the deadliest strains, continues to increase (Bosworth, 2014; Churchyard et al., 2014). The emergence of drug-resistant cases is worrisome because of the difficulty of acquiring effective second-line drugs for these strains and the government's limited funding (Bosworth, 2014).

In contrast to what we saw with HIV/AIDS, then, in South Africa's isolated geopolitical context, it is the absence of a credible national security threat that explains the lack of incentives for the government to strengthen its policy response to TB. And at no point was the government close to achieving a centrist policy response—that is, it never provided ongoing funding for the national TB program, prevention and TB drug treatment programs were limited and ineffective, and the DOH never sought to increase its policy influence over provincial governments formally through the use of conditional fiscal transfers or informally by contracting NGOs to monitor and hold local governments accountable for their policy shortcomings. But why did this occur? As we saw with HIV/AIDS, part of the answer seems to lie in the absence of a strong partnership between NGOs and national TB bureaucrats.

Absence of Strong Bureaucratic-Civil Societal Partnerships

The TB epidemic in South Africa, much like HIV/AIDS, did not elicit a strong civil societal response. The lack of social awareness of and interest in a disease that had been around for decades, the association of TB with the poor, and the overwhelming attention to HIV/AIDS—all resulted in little interest in aggressive civic mobilization or formation of new NGOs dedicated to eradicating TB (Matholc et al., 2010). Just two NGOs had been formed in the past to address TB: the TB/HIV Care Association, founded in 1929 as the Nelspoort After Care Committee, and the South African National TB Association, established in 1945. While these organizations were important—and still are—for sustaining their tradition of providing prevention, treatment, counseling, employment, psychosocial support, and childcare services for people with TB during the Mandela and Mbeki administrations, they did not aggressively mobilize and lobby the government for a stronger policy response (Nicolson, 2015). In fact, by 2002, researchers found that only two new national-level NGOs were working on the TB crisis.

During this period, the DOH also demonstrated little commitment to partnering with these NGOs (WHO, 2007). Reports indicate that there were not only insufficient national and provincial government grants to support TB NGOs but also no political commitment to partnering with them (Kironde and Nasolo, 2002; WHO, 2007). Most of the government's and the international community's attention at the time was focused on the worsening HIV/AIDS situation (Kironde and Nasolo, 2002).

When the Zuma administration arrived in 2009, as well as a new health minister, Dr. Aaron Motsoaledi, who also chaired the South Africa STOP TB Campaign, NGOs sensed the government's renewed commitment to addressing HIV/AIDS and TB. The NGOs now emerged to pressure the government for a stronger policy response. Following a march to Cape Town's parliament on World TB Day, March 24, 2009, TAC and the TB/HIV Care Association publicized a memorandum insisting that the DOH commit to greater integration of TB and HIV/AIDS testing and treatment services at health clinics. Other NGOs that had initially focused on HIV/AIDS—including TAC, Médecins Sans Frontières, Sex Workers and Advocacy Taskforce, Sonke Gender Justice, the Desmond Tutu HIV Foundation, and the People's Health Movement—also joined to raise awareness about TB and to lobby the government for better detection and treatment (Mannak, 2009).

These organizations have also advocated for the continued decentralization of TB treatment and care services, so that diagnosis and treatment can be carried out quickly while sustaining strong adherence to drug regimens (Mannak, 2009). These groups have also pressured the DOH for reliable provision of second-line drugs for drug-resistant TB strains such as MDR- and XDR-TB, preapproval access to new MDR-TB medications such as delamanid, a decrease in prison crowding and more TB services in these facilities, the auditing of mines for safety, and the elimination of patent laws to allow the accelerated production and distribution of generic medications (Knoetze, 2015; Mannak, 2009). Moreover, TAC has been credited for the government's decision to make the new drug-resistant TB medication bedaquiline available before its approval by the government's Medicines Control Council. Through these efforts, by 2014 bedaquiline had reached approximately 150 patients (Knoetze, 2015). Recent efforts have seen international NGOs, including the Global Coalition of TB Activists, Médecins Sans Frontières, and the Global TB Community Advisor Board, join TAC, TB Proof, and the People's Health Movement to lobby the government for more international and domestic funding for TB programs and elevation of the TB epidemic to the level of "public health emergency" (Melorose, Perroy, and Careas, 2015). However, we should note that the DOH's policy initiatives began prior to the emergence of this civil societal pressure, and its success has been limited mainly to raising government awareness and access to medications.

Indeed, perhaps the most important policy issue that these NGOs have not managed to influence is increasing federal funding and commitment to strengthening the public health system. Realizing that the decentralization of TB detection and sustainable treatment services depends on a sufficient supply of community healthcare works, hospital staff, beds, and equipment (S. Karim et al., 2009), NGOs have pressured DOH minister Motsoaledi to address these shortages. Activists claim that Motsoaledi has not responded, mainly due to internal ANC political pressure not to intervene in provincial politics and not to hold ANC-supported politicians accountable for their reluctance to work with the DOH in addressing this issue. Moreover, a realization of the excessive costs involved in increasing human resources and infrastructure for TB creates few incentives for the parliament to address the shortages (Low, 2016). Consequently, activists claim, Motsoaledi has essentially ignored civil societal pressure in this area (Tobergate, 2013).

While the government has acknowledged the importance of NGOs in addressing the TB epidemic, in practice there has been little support for the concrete development of NGOs and their influence within government. The DOH has repeatedly failed to provide sufficient funding and technical support for NGOs (Kironde and Neil, 2004). TB NGOs therefore face the specter of closedowns because of their inability to secure additional funding from the government or from the international community. In 2013, the United Kingdom's DFID, for example, decided to stop funding NGOs that work closely with the TB/HIV Care NGO. This decision will inevitably force the latter to engage in extra activities and in writing grant proposals to sustain its TB services. South Africa's perceived emergence as a robust developing economy and its status as an emerging donor contributed to the DFID's decision (Ravelo, 2014b). Nevertheless, the authorized grants from the Global Fund will help to sustain other NGOs' work.

Finally, no evidence exists suggesting that national TB bureaucrats have tried to establish a stronger partnership with NGOs and to strategically use them to obtain greater political and financial support. As mentioned earlier, the parliament has not prioritized additional funding to address health systems reform and is reluctant to highlight provincial governments' deficiencies in human resources, infrastructure, and budgetary accountability (Tobergate, 2013). This situation, when combined with the insufficient attention to

TB within the DOH (especially when compared with HIV/AIDS), seems to have created few incentives for national TB bureaucrats to work with NGOs in lobbying the parliament and Zuma for additional funding and support. This problem is compounded by the fact that, with the exception of periodic lobbying efforts, there is still no aggressive, consistent, well-organized, influential social movement for—or social consciousness of and interest in—addressing the worsening TB situation. This has led an influential TAC director, Mark Heywood, to state that the "revolution [for TB] isn't yet forthcoming" (quoted in Nicolson, 2015, 1).

There is a ray of hope, however. In addition to Health Minister Aaron Motsoaledi's commitment to improving the TB crisis, in July 2015 he organized the launch of the National Coalition Against TB. This coalition consists of the DOH, the South African National TB Association, the South African Red Cross, and the National Religious Association for Social Development. The coalition is focused on working together to increase TB awareness, thus signifying the government's multisectoral commitment to addressing the epidemic (*Times Live*, 2016). As the TB epidemic worsens, Motsoaledi may use this new coalitional venue to strengthen his cause and seek greater political support.

In sum, in contrast to the government's response to HIV/AIDS, in a context in which South Africa's negative geopolitical positioning created no incentives to strengthen the government's policy response to TB in order to increase its international reputation while seeking assistance from the international community, the absence of a national security threat represented by TB likewise generated few incentives for the government to improve its policy response. Worse still, and similar to what we saw in Russia, MOH bureaucrats never strove to establish a strong partnership with TB NGOs, thus hampering the government's ability to pursue a stronger, or even centrist, policy response.

Conclusion

With the arrival of the HIV/AIDS and TB epidemics in South Africa, the government did not join Brazil, India, and China in striving to use a stronger policy response to increase its international reputation in health. Instead, with its long foreign policy history of state sovereignty, independence, and regional leadership, the government sought to ignore international criticism and policy pressure, refrained from immediately seeking international financial and technical assistance, and instead strove to determine when and how the government should respond on its own. These decisions reflected political leaders' negative geopolitical positioning. In this context, an epidemic's threat to the national security, though only for HIV/AIDS, would instigate an improved policy response. But even then, bureaucratic and policy reforms were for the most part unsuccessful, unmasking the bureaucracy's ongoing inability to secure adequate funding for prevention, treatment, and health systems reform— all critical for effective policy implementation. In the absence of government efforts to establish strong bureaucratic–civil societal partnerships for both health sectors, South Africa would never achieve a centrist policy response and, with this, the possibility of successfully controlling and eradicating these diseases.

NOTES

1. South Africa's foreign policy decisions were mainly made in London until the Balfour Declaration of 1926, which granted South Africa equal and autonomous status under the new commonwealth (Siko, 2014).

2. According to recent data, an estimated 70% of people living with HIV/AIDS in South Africa are also infected with TB (Avert, 2016).

7

Conclusion

Despite their similar ambitions to become more economically integrated and involved in the international community, the BRICS nations have differed considerably in their aspirations to develop effective public health systems. This became clear when the HIV/AIDS epidemic emerged in the 1980s, followed in the 1990s by the resurgence of tuberculosis and more recently by the obesity epidemic. Political leaders in all of the BRICS did not immediately respond to these epidemics, for a variety of political and cultural reasons unique to each nation, and when they did respond, they differed in the timing and depth of their policy response to these public health threats.

What factors accounted for the differences in policy outcomes? As I discussed in chapter 1, the existing literature has emphasized the importance of domestic electoral incentives, strong state capacity, and civil societal pressures as explanations for the timing and depth of policy responses to disease epidemics. But in the case of the BRICS, none of these factors were important. Instead, as I have argued in this book, the domestic policy response was shaped, first, by the criticism, pressure, and policy expectations emanating from the international community and how political leaders responded to this, and then by the strength of bureaucratic–civil societal partnerships and how this, in turn, affected the bureaucracy's ability to secure ongoing political and financial support.

To better understand how and why the international community played such an important role, I introduced the concept of *geopolitical positioning*. I define this as explaining the interests and incentives of political leaders to respond to international criticism and pressure through a stronger policy response to epidemics, the different domestic and foreign policy strategies that this entails, and leaders' willingness to pursue international financial and technical assistance to achieve their policy objectives.

Geopolitical positioning has positive and negative elements. *Positive geopolitical positioning* emerges when governing elites positively respond to international criticism and pressure by immediately pursuing a stronger policy response to epidemics in order to increase their government's international reputation in health, while at the same time pursuing international financial and technical assistance to ensure that their policies work effectively. To further enhance a nation's international reputation, positive geopolitical positioning also emerges when leaders seek to engage in acts of global health diplomacy by providing foreign aid assistance to other nations striving to eradicate disease. As we saw in chapter 1, all of these endeavors are shaped by historical foreign policy precedents, such as (1) governments' attempts to increase their international reputation as effective developing states with sound public health systems; (2) governments' willingness to engage in bilateral and multilateral cooperation, rather than striving to lead the world and establish international agendas; and (3) governments' receptivity to international financial and technical assistance to develop effective economic and healthcare systems.

Negative geopolitical positioning emerges when political leaders ignore international criticism and pressure and have no interest in building their nations' international reputation in health, while at the same time refraining from pursuing international financial and technical assistance. Rather, political leaders strive to pursue reforms for their own reasons and at their own pace, regardless of international criticism and pressure. This kind of negative geopolitical positioning reflects a historical foreign policy commitment to assuming an international leadership role in diplomacy and, in some instances, reflects foreign policy commitments to solidifying governments as influential superpowers, while establishing their sovereignty and independence from international—especially western—influence. In this geopolitical context, governments improve their response to epidemics only when they are perceived as posing a threat to national security. And while governments in this position may provide foreign aid assistance in health, this will be used only to enhance a government's international and/or regional influence, rather than for improving its international reputation in health.

Political leaders in Brazil, India, and China provide examples of positive geopolitical positioning. When confronting international criticism and pressure from influential institutions such as the WHO and the World Bank, these leaders immediately pursued a stronger policy response to the HIV/AIDS and obesity epidemics to strengthen their international reputation in health. At the same time, they requested financial and technical assistance from these international institutions, revealing their foreign policy tradition of engaging in multilateral cooperation while seeking foreign aid assistance. And to further enhance their international reputation in health, all three governments provided foreign aid assistance to other developing nations. In contrast, governments of Russia and South Africa provide instances of negative geopolitical positioning. Regardless of international criticism and pressure, leaders in these nations were never interested in pursuing a stronger policy response in order to improve the government's international reputation in health. It was only when HIV/AIDS, though not TB, was perceived as posing a threat to national security, such as military readiness and the economy, that leaders began to prioritize a response. At the same time, the Russian and South African governments opposed the idea of receiving international financial assistance and policy recommendations, deciding instead to pursue reforms on their own— while nevertheless providing foreign aid assistance and advice to other nations to reaffirm their position as international leaders. Eventually, however, Russia and South Africa proved incapable of achieving a strong policy response to HIV/AIDS and TB.

Among the BRICS, Brazil was the only nation to succeed, eventually, in creating a strong centrist policy response. Indeed, Brazil was the only government that remained committed to providing ongoing political and financial support, not only for public health administration and infrastructure, but more importantly, for innovative prevention programs for high-risk groups and the universal distribution of medications. At the same time, Brazil overcame the challenges of healthcare decentralization by augmenting its centralized policy influence through formal and informal processes. Formally, the Ministry of Health incentivized state governments into compliance with national policy guidelines by providing conditional financial grant assistance to municipal governments in need. Informally, the MOH maintained its centralized influence by working with NGOs and public health bureaucrats to closely monitor municipal governments' compliance with national policy goals, thus increasing local governments' accountability to the central government while incentivizing the former to ensure policy implementation.

Why did this occur in Brazil? Brazil was able to achieve a centrist policy response because of the presence of strong bureaucratic–civil societal partnerships. Indeed, Brazil's success underscores the importance of combining positive geopolitical positioning with strong bureaucratic–civil societal partnerships in public health.

When the HIV/AIDS and obesity epidemics emerged in Brazil, public health bureaucrats proactively sought to work closely with NGOs that were well-organized, influential, and committed to working with bureaucrats in building a centrist policy response. The bureaucracy's and civil society's centrist policy ideas were tightly fused, reflecting a long historical partnership in developing such ideas together since the early twentieth century. By partnering with NGOs that sustained these ideas and continued to work closely with the government, when the HIV/AIDS and obesity epidemics emerged, the bureaucrats had the legitimacy and influence necessary to obtain ongoing political and financial support for their centrist policy response.

For their own unique historical reasons, this kind of strong bureaucratic–civil societal partnership never emerged in the other BRICS nations. During India's and China's response to HIV/AIDS and obesity, health bureaucrats did not try to work closely with NGOs to increase the bureaucrats' legitimacy and ability to obtain ongoing political and financial support. The central government's suspicion of and general lack of trust in NGOs certainly complicated this process. But the absence of a strong bureaucratic–civil societal partnership mainly reflected a long history of the state's unwillingness to work closely with civil society in the area of public health, as well as civil society's unwillingness to create social health movements and/or NGOs focused on pressuring the government to intervene in response to disease outbreaks. This history led to a dearth of NGOs with which public health bureaucrats might have worked.

Similarly in Russia, in response to HIV/AIDS and TB, bureaucratic officials did not try to establish a strong partnership with NGOs. In Russia, historically, there has been no strong partnership between the state and civil society in the area of public health. Those social health movements that did exist were essentially eradicated during the socialist/communist era, leaving little interest or incentive to create NGOs in response to the HIV/AIDS and TB epidemics. When combined with a central government that remained hostile toward the NGO community and its western supporters, these conditions created few incentives for heath bureaucrats to establish a strong working partnership with NGOs. In South Africa, it was the historical division of public health services based on race, as well as forced political suppression under apartheid rule, that contributed to the absence of a unified collective movement and of NGOs pressuring and working closely with the state in the area of public health. When the HIV/AIDS and TB epidemics emerged during apartheid, most NGOs and social movements were focused on the transition back to democracy; few were focusing on eradication of HIV/AIDS and TB. And the government once again proved unwilling to work closely with civil society. NGOs such as the Treatment Action Campaign did eventually emerge to successfully pressure the democratic ANC government into improving access to ARV medications. However, in large part because of the historical absence of a strong partnership between the bureaucracy and civil society in public health, as well as President Mbeki's denialist claims and consequent lack of commitment to HIV/AIDS policy, health bureaucrats did not prioritize establishing a strong partnership with NGOs. While the Zuma administration has acknowledged the importance of NGOs in fighting HIV/AIDS and TB, health bureaucrats remain reluctant to partner closely with these organizations to obtain more financial and political support for their programs.

Although Brazil has demonstrated the best response to disease epidemics, one must keep in mind that this is not reflective of Brazil's entire healthcare system. Recent research shows that in other areas—such as strengthening the healthcare system through greater investments in hospital infrastructure and human resources, and ensuring access to medicine for various types of health conditions—Brazil joins the other BRICS nations in underperforming (K. Rao et al., 2014). The burgeoning need for public healthcare services among the poor, when combined with economic stagnation (to varying degrees) and limited healthcare spending, has adversely affected all of the BRICS nations. In recent years, the BRICS' healthcare systems, in general, have received insufficient political attention (Dréze and Sen, 2013; Y. Huang, 2013; K. Rao et al., 2014). While my focus on the HIV/AIDS, obesity, and TB epidemics has helped to better understand the conditions under which governments respond to public health crises—which is critical for understanding the factors that motivate political leaders to overcome their initial fears and prejudices and to meet medical needs—future research will need to compare the effectiveness of the BRICS' healthcare systems in their entirety. Moreover, researchers will need to examine why international pressure seems to have a greater impact on government responses to specific diseases than on the needs of the healthcare system in general.

Theoretical Advances and Policy Lessons

Several theoretical and policy lessons emerged from my comparative analysis of the BRICS nations. First, in contrast to what most scholarly work has argued about the politics of government response to disease epidemics, my findings suggest that the incentives for responding often reside at the *international* rather than domestic level, and that this is even more so for emerging nations that are eager to display their developmental potential and to integrate into the global economy. Indeed, because most of the BRICS were seeking to build their international reputation in health, criticism and pressure from powerful international institutions such as the UN and the World Bank provided more incentive to pursue reforms than did any domestic political, institutional, or civil societal considerations. These "high-level" politics and incentives, if you will, may also help to explain why lesser-developed nations with fewer geopolitical ambitions are not as influenced by the opinions of international institutions.

Second, the international relations literature has overlooked the advantages of combining different schools of thought. The linkages between international pressure and reputation building described in this book reveal the importance of combining the literature that emphasizes the role of such pressure in domestic health policy reform (Lieberman, 2009; Okuonzi and Macrae, 1995) with the constructivist literature that emphasizes the role of "soft power" through policy reputation building, at both the domestic and the foreign policy level (Feldbaum, Lee, and Michaud, 2010; Feldbaum and Michaud, 2010; Labonte and Gagnon, 2010; McGuire, 2010). When it comes to emerging economies such as the BRICS, for the reasons given above, peer pressure from international organizations and donor aid conditionalites can have a far greater effect on domestic political interests and incentives for policy reform. My effort to combine the literature on international pressure with this constructivist literature revealed that international pressure can motivate nations to improve their reputation in health through a stronger domestic policy response while providing foreign aid in health. This finding should encourage scholars to further explore the benefits of combining different schools of thought in international relations and global health diplomacy to better understand the broader effects that international institutions can have on nations that are rising in global prominence.

Some caveats nevertheless should be mentioned regarding the importance of international reputation building in health. That is, it is import to emphasize that not all healthcare issues generate these reputation-building interests. As I mentioned in chapter 1, these interests only emerge when influential international agencies, such as the WHO and the World Bank, prioritize responding to a particular disease or health issue and when they single out and pressure nations into improving their policy response; however, not all healthcare issues meet these two conditions. The need to improve health systems, governance— that is, institutional and political aspects driving health systems reform—and the response to other chronic diseases that are perceived as less immediately life threatening and do not draw sufficient media attention (for example, chronic pain, type 2 diabetes, and mental health diseases such as dementia and Alzheimer's) may not be prioritized by these international agencies and motivate them to criticize and pressure governments to improve their policy response.

In addition, what happens if the WHO loses its interest in particular diseases and eases up on pressuring governments to pursue a stronger policy response? Does this mean that governments will lose their interest in increasing their reputation for a particular health issue, leading to a decline in government support for these programs? This may indeed be the case. For example, while the WHO, PAHO, and international philanthropic organizations such as the Rockefeller Foundation worked with and pressured several developing nations to respond to diseases such as small pox, malaria, yellow fever, and polio during the early twentieth century, these institutions' reluctance over the years to prioritize responding to these diseases, pressuring governments to do so, and addressing general health systems challenges such as inadequate financing, human resources, and infrastructure appears to have decreased government incentives to invest continuously in prevention and treatment programs for these diseases (Miller, Barrett, and Henderson, 2006). Alternatively, perhaps these kinds of programs will be firmly entrenched in political and bureaucratic policy feedback processes (Pierson, 2003), ensuring that they continue to receive adequate government attention and support. Answering these questions will require researchers to examine how long the WHO and other international agencies prioritize disease, under what conditions they lose their focus on them, and whether this generates fewer incentives for governments to prioritize responding to these health issues.

Third, we need to better understand the different political motivations driving global health diplomacy. When it comes to providing foreign aid in health, as we saw in Brazil, India, and to a certain extent China, some nations provide this assistance to sustain and deepen their reputation for having effective public health systems, by providing aid and helping other nations through policy lessons learned from their own countries. Alternatively, leaders provide foreign aid to increase their international reputation in health while securing new markets and advancing their economic interests, as we saw in China. And finally, nations may provide foreign aid to solidify their international leadership roles and power, as we saw in Russia and, albeit briefly, in South Africa.

These findings comport with the constructivist literature highlighting the different issue frames that governments use when establishing their foreign aid objectives. As Van der Veen explains (2011), governments often use issue frames such as *reputation/self-affirmation, power/influence, security, enlightened self-interest, humanitarianism, obligation/duty,* and *wealth/economic self-interest* when establishing national discourses and discussions within legislative institutions to devise foreign aid policy. Similar to what we saw in Brazil in this book, Van der Veen claims that legislatures often employ reputation/self-affirmation frames to justify foreign aid in order to create a particular international image about a nation while improving the nation's international reputation. Similar to what we saw in China, Van der Veen claims that governments also employ wealth/economic self-interest frames when providing aid in order to enhance their economic position, such as gaining access to export markets. And, similar to what we saw in Russia, Van der Veen asserts that legislatures may use power/influence frames in order to increase a nation's international influence by bolstering a country's leverage over others through bilateral aid while acquiring supportive allies and prestige along the way. Other studies have joined Van der Veen and this book in underscoring the importance of foreign aid for building a nation's international reputation as a benevolent state (Hveem and McNeill, 1994), a government's economic trade intentions through foreign aid (Younas, 2008), and a government's interest in using foreign aid to augment its geopolitical power and influence (Milner and Tingley, 2013).

As we saw in this book, however, and what this literature to date has overlooked, is that history also matters. These differences in foreign aid motivations are often attributable to differences in nations' historical foreign policy goals and legacies. Nations that have historically sought to build their international reputations in economic development and public health, while at the same time working closely with international institutions—as seen in Brazil, India, and China—are more likely to provide future foreign aid in health for reputation-building purposes. Conversely, those nations that have foreign policy traditions of international diplomatic leadership and the pursuit of superpower status will provide future foreign aid to further solidify their power and leadership status in the world, as seen in Russia and to a certain extent in South Africa. Future research therefore needs to seek to better understand not only the different underlying political motivations guiding foreign aid in health but also how foreign policy legacies and expectations shape this process.

At the domestic level, findings from the BRICS also provide new insights into the role of civil society in periods of health crisis. A consensus has emerged suggesting that NGOs and social health movements are important for pressuring governments to respond more rapidly to disease epidemics through the provision of prevention and drug treatment programs (Barnett and Whiteside, 2006; Boone and Batsell, 2001; Lucker, 2004; Parker, 2003; Rau, 2006; Whiteside, 1999). Nevertheless, the BRICS case studies suggest that civil societal pressure was not the main reason that political leaders initially strengthened their policy response to epidemics and that, moreover, civil society's advisory role and influence within government often decreased during the first few years of an epidemic. An in-depth analysis of the BRICS revealed that, instead, civil society played a more important role *after* politicians had already strengthened their policy response.

Indeed, the findings presented in this book suggest that civil society's role became more important when bureaucrats sought to establish strong partnerships with civil society, partnerships that would provide mutual advantages for both parties. As seen in Brazil, after several years of failing to engage civil society and incorporate its views into the policymaking process, and after the emergence of international pressure and improvements to policy reform, AIDS bureaucrats began to seek the assistance of well-organized, influential NGOs to enhance their legitimacy and influence within government. This process helped bureaucrats secure the ongoing funding and political support needed to pursue a centrist policy response. At the same time, NGOs benefited by receiving support for additional prevention and treatment programs, while holding local governments more accountable for their policy actions.

This by no means suggests that civil society did not play an important earlier role in drawing attention to the emergence of new public health threats and to the need for a more aggressive policy response—especially in the area of drug treatment, as seen in Brazil and South Africa—while providing critical community services. Nevertheless, the bureaucratic behavior does suggest that future research needs to pay more attention to the historical trajectory of bureaucratic–civil societal partnerships—before and after policy reforms—and the additional motivations and incentives for bureaucrats to strategically use NGOs to advance their policy agendas.

My comparison of the BRICS nations' response to different types of public health threats also revealed several policy lessons. First, in a context of increased healthcare decentralization, where state and especially municipal governments have greater responsibilities in implementing public health programs, the central government still needs to play a proactive role in helping to fund and implement policy. This necessity is due to the ongoing inequality in financial, administrative, and infrastructural resources among local governments and thus the wide variation in policy performance. In this context, pursuing a centrist policy response through formal and informal channels, as we saw in Brazil, is critical for ensuring that policies are effectively implemented. More specifically, providing conditional fiscal grants to municipal governments in need, as well as working closely with NGOs and bureaucrats to monitor and report how the federal funds are being used, can hold local governments accountable to the central government, while sustaining the latter's influence even in a context of federalism and decentralization. As I mentioned in chapter 1, this centrist policy response by no means undermines the democratic principles of decentralization; rather, it can supplement and reinforce the benefits of decentralization by ensuring that policies work effectively.

Second, the BRICS case studies reveal that merely increasing government spending for public health programs does not always guarantee a stronger policy response. Instead, what matters more is how the money is spent. As we saw in Russia, inadequate spending for prevention programs targeting the groups at highest risk, despite increased spending on medication, will not help to ensure the eradication of HIV/AIDS and TB. Likewise in South Africa, the unwillingness of government to ensure sufficient funding for ongoing expansion of drug treatment services can lead to a shortage of drug supplies, inconsistency in patients' use of medication (which in the case of TB can lead to drug-resistant strains and worsening health conditions), and a lack of trust between the state and civil society. At the same time, if funding is not used to provide more healthcare infrastructure and healthcare workers, then prevention and treatment programs will be even more difficult to implement. Thus, strategically using an increase in federal funding to simultaneously invest in the strengthening of health systems, especially in rural areas, is vital for ensuring the effective implementation of policy.

Are the BRICS Really Emerging?

For many years, scholars' analysis of the BRICS nations was focused on economic performance and impact on global markets. Little attention was paid to analyzing how committed and successful they were in strengthening their social welfare policies. Consequently, most scholarly works overlooked the BRICS' domestic healthcare challenges, especially in the area of public health. This book is the first to address this lacuna in the literature. Its findings reveal that in the area of public health, for several decades, most of the BRICS were underperforming. Regardless of transitions to democracy and vociferous civil societal demands, the BRICS' delayed responses to different kinds of public health threats reveal that most of these nations did not prioritize meeting the healthcare needs of their citizens. For some of these nations, it would take strong international criticism and pressure to incentivize political leaders to improve their response to disease epidemics, in turn unmasking their lack of commitment to safeguarding their citizens and meeting healthcare needs.

Given these healthcare challenges, perhaps we were mistaken in labeling the BRICS as successfully emerging economies. For had we initially included public health, as well as other social welfare sectors such as education, infrastructure, and human rights, then perhaps our initial evaluation of this group would have been different. Indeed, perhaps Jim O'Neil, the financial analyst at Goldman Sachs who originally coined the term *BRICS*, would not have included some of these nations in this group. Going forward, and as I have argued elsewhere with respect to other recent acronyms used by financial analysts, such as the CIVETS (China, India, Vietnam, Egypt, Turkey, and South Africa) and the MINTS (Mexico, Indonesia, Nigeria, Turkey, and South Africa), perhaps it would be wiser to refrain from establishing these group acronyms in the first place, to avoid false hope and expectations, while describing these nations simply as they are: developing economies showing progress but with significant hurdles to overcome (Gómez, 2014).

Does this limitation suggest that we should lose hope in the BRICS' abilities to develop and prosper? In the light of the recent political scandals and economic problems in Brazil, Russia, and South Africa, analysts certainly appear to be losing confidence in the group's economic prowess, geopolitical influence, and developmental capacity (Nossel, 2016). Nevertheless, several factors should give us hope that the BRICS can overcome these problems and, in the process, develop more effective public health systems.

First, each of these nations has a vast pool of talented medical doctors, dedicated public health professionals, researchers, and civil societal organizations committed to improving the health, individual rights, and prosperity of their citizens. The BRICS therefore possess the "human capacity," if you will, needed to strengthen their public health systems. Second, collectively, the BRICS can provide important lessons: together they comprise the largest population in the world that is experiencing poverty and disease. Because of this, they are importantly positioned to have a significant impact on policy discussions within major international health agencies such as the WHO. And finally, through their recently created National Development Bank, the BRICS have the potential to help share their policy lessons and fund public health initiatives in other developing nations.

Researchers, analysts, and the activist community should strive to be less critical and pessimistic about the BRICS. Instead, they should endeavor to help the BRICS' governments develop the interest, incentive, and motivation needed to invest more in their public health systems and to ensure that these investments become a critical aspect of their future economic and development plans. While increasing international criticism and pressure could be an effective option, let us hope that in the future, such pressure will not be necessary and that political leaders in the BRICS will come to realize that investing effectively in public health will facilitate their path to economic prosperity and, more importantly, equitable and effective social welfare programs.

References

Abkowitz, Alyssa, and Hu Xin. 2015. "HIV/AIDS Prevention Classes, Now Coming to a Chinese School Near You." *Wall Street Journal*, August 14.

Abong, Portal dos Fundos Públicos, National AIDS Program, 2012. www.abong.org.br.

Achmat, Zakie, and Reid Austin Roberts. 2005. *Steering the Storm: TB and HIV in South Africa*. Policy report. Johannesburg: Treatment Action Campaign.

ACT+. 2014. *Civil Society Report on the Situation of Chronic Non-Communicable Diseases in Brazil*. São Paulo: ACT+ Press.

ACTSA. 2016. "South Africa: Thabo Mbeki on HIV/AIDS and TAC's Response." March 8. www.actsa.org/newsroom/2016/03/south-africa-thabo-mbeki-on-hivaids -and-tacs-response/.

Adler, Glenn, and Jonny Steinberg, eds. 2000. *From Comrades to Citizens: The South African Civics Movement and the Transition to Democracy*. New York: St. Martin's Press.

Advocacy Partnership. 2010. *Building Citizen Advocacy in Russia, Eastern Europe and Central Asia*. Source no longer available online.

Afrol News. 2000. "Politicising AIDS: Interview with Peter Piot." November 30.

Agence France-Presse. 2006. "WHO Urges China to Fight Nation's Top Killer— Chronic Diseases." May 9.

———. 2015. "Russia HIV-Aids Epidemic Worsening under Kremlin Policies." May 15.

Agermose, Stig. 1998. "WHO Warns of Massive Worldwide Tuberculosis Epidemic." March 18.

Ajulu, Rok. 2001. "Thabo Mbeki's African Renaissance in a Globalising World Economy: The Struggle for the Soul of the Continent." *Review of African Political Economy* 87:27–42.

Akimkin, V. G. 2009. "Epidemiology of TB in Armed Forces, TB Prevention Strategies." *Voyenno-Meditsinskiy Zhurnal*, August 18.

Alden, Chris, and Marco Antonio Vieira. 2005. "The New Diplomacy of the South: South Africa, Brazil, India, and Trilateralism." *Third World Quarterly* 26 (7): 1077–95.

All India Association for Advancing Research on Obesity. 2008. "AIAARO—Advancing Research in Obesity." December 1.

Allison, Roy. 2008. "Russia Resurgent?" *International Affairs* 84 (6): 1145–71.

Allison, Simon. 2015. "South Africa's Aids Programme under Threat as International Funds Dry Up." *Guardian* (London), December 1.

Altherton, Matt. 2016. "China: Childhood Obesity Rates 'Explode' as Western Lifestyles Take Over." *International Business Times*, April 27.

Altman, Dennis. 1986. *AIDS in the Mind of America*. New York: Doubleday Press.
Altman, Lawrence. 1996. "India Suddenly Leads in H.I.V." *New York Times*, July 8.
Alves, Ana Cristina. 2013. "Brazil in Africa: Achievements and Challenges." Unpublished manuscript, London School of Economics and Political Science.
Amon, Joe. 2010. "The Truth of China's Response to HIV/AIDS." *Los Angeles Times*, July 11.
Anders, Molly. 2014. "Can the BRICS Bank Rally Global Outcasts around TB Treatment?" *Inside Development*, November 6.
Andharia, Janki. 2009. "Reconceptualizing Community Organization in India." In *Interdisciplinary Community Development*, ed. Alice K. Johnson Butterfield and Yossi Korazim-Korosy, 91–120. Philadelphia, PA: Haworth Press.
Anugu, Akshay. 2015. "Is Obesity an Undermined Public Health Issue in India?" *News18*, November 23.
Aranha, Adriana, Alessandra da Costa Lunas, Carlos Américo Basco, Celso Marcatto, Crispim Moreira, Elisabetta Recine, and Francesco Pierri. 2009. *Building up the National Policy and System for Food and Nutrition Security*. Brasília: CONSEA, Office of the President.
Araujo, O. 1939. "As Tendencias Modernas no Luta Contra as Doencas Venerais." *Jornal de Sífilis e Urologia* 111.
Arbex, Alberto, Denise Rocha, Marisa Aizenberg, and Maria Ciruzzi. 2014. "Obesity Epidemic in Brazil and Argentina: A Public Health Concern." *Journal of Health, Population and Nutrition* 32 (3): 327–34.
Arkhangelskaya, Svetlana. 2015. "AIDS: Is There an Epidemic in Russia?" *Russia Beyond the Headlines*, July 3.
Arnquist, S., A. Ellner, and R. Weintraub. 2011. *HIV/AIDS in Brazil*. Cambridge, MA: Harvard Business School, Harvard University.
Arretche, M., and E. Marques. 2002. "Municipalização da saúde no Brasil." *Ciencia and Saúde Coletiva* 7 (3): 455–79.
Associated Press. 1997. "Highly Contagious Tuberculosis Spreading Rapidly in Russia." *Akron Beacon Journal*, October 19.
Atkins, Salla. 2011. *Improving Adherence: An Evaluation of the Enhanced Tuberculosis Adherence Model in Cape Town, South Africa*. Stockholm: Karolinska Institutet.
Atun, R., Y. A. Samyshkin, F. Drobniewski, N. M. Skuratova, G. Gusarova, S. I. Kuznetsov, I. M. Feorin, and R. J. Coker. 2005. "Barriers to Sustainable Tuberculosis Control in the Russian Federation Health System." *Bulletin of the World Health Organization* 83 (3): 217–22.
Avert. 2015. "HIV and AIDS in South Africa." May 1.
———. 2016. "Funding for HIV and AIDS." August 8.
Bakalova, Evgeniya, and Hans-Joachim Spanger. 2013. *Development Cooperation or Competition*. PRIF report no. 123. Frankfurt, Germany: Peace Research Institute.
Baleta, Adele. 1998. "Mbeki: HIV/AIDS 'Most Serious Crisis Yet' Facing S. Africa." *Johannesburg Saturday Star*, September 12. Accessed at World News Connection Online.
———. 2003. "South Africa Boosts Funding for HIV/AIDS." *Lancet* 362:1728.
Balfour, Frederik. 2010. "China Discovers the XXL Way of Life." *Bloomberg Businessweek, June* 7.
Balinska, Marta. 1995. "Assistance and Not Mere Relief: The Epidemic Commission of the League of Nations." In *International Health Organisations and Movements, 1918–1939*, ed. Paul Weindling, 81–108. Oxford: Oxford University Press.

Bamford, Lesley. 1999. "Tuberculosis." In *South Africa Health Review*, ed. Nicholas Crisp and Antoinette Ntuli, 23. Durban, South Africa: Health Systems Trust.

Bandeira, Luisete Moraes. 2016. Interview with the author, February 26.

Barbosa, Eduardo. 2008. Interview with the author, August 10.

Barboza, Renato. 2006. "Gestão do Programa Estadual DST/Aids de São Paulo: Uma Análise do Processo de Descentralizacão das Acões no Período de 1994 a 2003." Master's thesis, University of São Paulo.

Bardsley, Daniel. 2011. "Childhood Obesity on the Rise in China." *National World*, July 30.

Baria, Farah, Subhadra Menon, Subrata Nagchoudhury, Stephen David, and Vijay Menon. 1997. "AIDS—Striking Home." *India Today*, March 15.

Barnett, Tony, and Alan Whiteside. 2006. *AIDS in the Twenty-First Century*, 2nd ed. New York: Palgrave Macmillan.

Barreira, Draurio. 2012. Interview with the author, August 6.

Barris, Michael. 2014. "Yao Ming Puts His Weight behind Campaign against Obesity." *China Daily*, March 10.

Baruagh, Smita. 2008. "Never Mind the Numbers: India's HIV/AIDS Crisis Is Large Enough." *New York Times*, January 17.

Bava, Umma Salma. 2007. *New Powers for Global Change? India's Role in the Emerging World Order*. FES Briefing Paper 4. Friedrich Ebert Stiftung. March.

BBC News. 2001a. "India Obesity Fears." News article, October 5.

———. 2001b. "India Predicts Diabetes Explosion." News article, February 6.

———. 2003. "Brazil Close to a New Deal with IMF." News article, November 6.

———. 2004. "Chinese Concern at Obesity Surge." News article, October 12.

———. 2012. "Brazil Health Study Shows Growing Weight Problem." News article, April 11.

———. 2016. "Syria Conflict: US Suspends Talks with Russia." News article, October 5.

Bearak, Barry. 2010. "South Africa Fears Millions More H.I.V. Infections." *New York Times*, November 19.

Béja, Jean-Philippe. 2006. "The Changing Aspects of Civil Society in China." *Social Research* 73 (1): 53–72.

Bekedam, H. 2008. "The Challenge of Obesity and Related Disease Control in China." *Obesity Reviews* 9 (Suppl. 1): 4–5.

Bekker, Linda-Gail, Francois Venter, Karen Cohen, Eric Goemar, Gilles Van Custem, Andrew Boulle, and Robin Wood. 2014. "Provision of Antiretroviral Therapy in South Africa." *Antiviral Therapy* 19 (3): 105–16.

Bennett, Simeon, and Stepan Kravchenko. 2014. "Russian HIV Surge Shows Scourge Sochi Swagger Can't Mask." *Bloomberg Markets*, January 14.

Bennetts, Marc. 2016. "The Kremlin Shows the World How to Make AIDS Crisis Worse." *Newsweek*, January 26.

Berkman, Alan, J. Garcia, M. Muñoz-Laboy, V. Paiva, and R. Parker. 2005. "A Crucial Analysis of the Brazilian Response to HIV/AIDS." *American Journal of Public Health* 95:1162–72.

Besharati, Neissan. 2013. *South African Development Partnership*. Research report no. 12. Johannesburg: SAIIA.

Bijoy, C. R. 2010. *India: Transitioning to a Global Donor*. Reality of Aid Report. Quezon City, Philippines: Reality of Aid.

Bingqin, Li. 2012. "Social Welfare and Protection for Economic Growth and Stability—China's Experience." In *A Changing China: Emerging Governance, Economic and Social Trends*, 39–60. Singapore: Civil Service College.

Birch, Douglas. 2009. "AIDS Experts Say Russia Needs New HIV Strategy." Associated Press, October 28.

Bishwajit, Ghose. 2015. "Nutrition Transition in South Asia: The Emergence of Non-communicable Chronic Diseases." *F1000Research* 4 (8): 1–18.

Bisseker, Claire. 1997. "AIDS Costs Multiply: Study National AIDS Review." *Financial Mail* (Johannesburg), July 25. Accessed at Access World News, www.newsbank.com.

Blank, Stephen J. 1996. "Russia's Return to the Mideast Diplomacy." *Orbis* 96 (40): 517.

Bliss, Katherine, ed. 2012. *The Changing Landscape of Global Health Diplomacy.* Lanham, MD: Rowman and Littlefield.

Bloom, D. E., C. Fonseca, V. Candeias, E. Adashi, L. Bloom, L. Gurfien, E. Jané-Llopis, A. Lubet, E. Mitgang, C. O'Brien, and A. Saxena. 2014. *Economics of Non-communicable Diseases in India.* World Economic Forum. Boston, MA: Harvard School of Public Health.

BMJ. 2006. "China's One Child Policy." 333:361.

Bohm, Michael. 2016. "Putin's Pride Has No Price Tag." *Moscow Times*, August 3.

Bond, Virginia, Mutale Chileshe, Busi Magazi, and Clare Sullivan. 2008. *The Converging Impact of Tuberculosis, AIDS, and Food Insecurity in Zambia and South Africa.* Washington, DC: International Food Policy Research Institute.

Boone, Catherine, and Jake Batsell. 2001. "Politics and AIDS in Africa." *Africa Today* 48:3–33.

Bor, Jacob. 2007. "The Political Economy of AIDS Leadership in Developing Countries." *Social Science and Medicine* 64:1585–99.

Bortoletto, Ana Paula. 2016. Interview with the author, May 15.

Boseley, Sarah. 2003. "Richard Feachem, UN Global Fund Chief." *Guardian* (London), February 18.

Bosworth, Brendon. 2014. "South Africa Battles Drug-Resistant TB." Inter Press Service News Agency, August 16.

Bothma, Stephane. 1998. "Call for Comprehensive Plan." *Business Day* (Johannesburg), December 2. Accessed at Access World News, www.newsbank.com.

Bottelier, Pieter. 2006. *China and the World Bank.* Working paper no. 277. Stanford, CA: Stanford Center for International Development, Stanford University.

Bracken, Hillary. 2009. "Public Health or Rural Reconstruction? Developing Pratapgarh District, 1930–1940." Unpublished manuscript, Gynuity Health Projects, New York.

Branka, Francesco, Haik Nikogosian, and Tim Lobstein. 2007. *The Challenge of Obesity in the WHO European Region and the Strategies for Response.* Geneva: WHO.

Bräutigam, Deborah. 2011. "U.S. and Chinese Efforts in Africa in Global Health and Foreign Aid." In *China's Emerging Global Health and Foreign Aid Engagement in Africa*, ed. Xiaoqing Lul Boynton. Washington, DC: Center for Strategic and International Studies.

Brazil, General Accounting Office. 2016. *Tribunal de Contas Da União (TCU).* Brasília: TCU.

Brazil, Ministry of Education. 2012. *Programa Saúde nas Escaolas.* Brasília: Ministry of Education.

Brazil, Ministry of Health. 2005. *Portaria 2313.* Brasília: Ministry of Health.

———. 2006. *Observatory on Chronic Non-communicable Disease: The Case of Brazil.* Brasília: Ministry of Health.

———. 2010. *O que é Transferencia Fundo-a-Fundo?* Brasília: Ministry of Health.

———. 2012a. *Coordenação Geral de Alimentação e Nutrição.* Brasília: Ministry of Health.

———. 2012b. *Programa Saúde na Escola—PSE.* Brasília: Ministry of Health.

———. 2012c. *Secretaria de Educação Continuada, Alfabetação, Diversidade, e Inclusão.* Brasília: Ministry of Health.

———. 2016. *Da Saúde se Cuida Todos os Dias.* http://promocaodasaude.saude.gov.br.

Brazil, Ministry of Planning, Budget, and Spending. 2016. "Portal da Transparência." www.portaldatransparencia.gov.br/PortalSubFuncoes.asp?Exercicio=2016.

Brazil, National AIDS Program. 2007. *Plano Integrado de Enfrentamento da Feminizacão da Epidemia da Aids e outras DST.* Brasília: Ministry of Health.

Bremmer, Ian. 2010. "China vs. America: Fight of the Century." *Prospect*, April.

———. 2012. "Brazil Wants Some Security Council Love. But It Won't Get It (Yet)." *Foreign Policy*, April 3.

Brezhneva, Anna, and Daria Ukhova. 2013. *Russia as a Humanitarian Aid Donor.* Oxford: Oxfam.

Bristow, Michael. 2010. "China Faces Obesity Explosion." *BBC News*, September 25.

Brito, Anna. 2012. Interview with the author, September 19.

Brown, Hannah. 2006. "Russia's Blossoming Civil Society Holds the Key to HIV." *Lancet* 368 (9534): 437–40.

Brown-Polaris, Christopher. 2004. "It's In to Be Thin in India." *TIME Asia*, November 8.

Bruk, Boris. 2013. "TB or Not TB: In Recognition of World TB Day." Institute of Modern Russia, March 25.

Bundy, Colin. 2000. "Survival and Resistance: Township Organizations and Non-violent Direct Action in Twentieth Century South Africa." In *From Comrades to Citizens: The South African Civics Movement and the Transition to Democracy*, ed. Glenn Adler and Jonny Steinberg. New York: St. Martin's Press.

Burges, Sean. 2014. "Brazil's International Development Cooperation: Old and New Motivations." *Development Policy Review* 32 (3): 355–74.

Burki, T. 2016. "Sex Education Chain Leaves Young Vulnerable to Infection." *Lancet* 16 (1): 26.

Burns, Katya. 2007. "Russia's HIV/AIDS Epidemic: HIV/AIDS among Women and Problems of Access to Services." *Problems of Post-Communism* 54 (1): 28–35.

Business Day (Johannesburg). 1997. "Soldiers at Greater Risk of Contracting AIDS Than Others." November 20. Accessed at Access World News, www.newsbank.com.

Butler, Anthony. 2005. "South Africa's HIV/AIDS Policy, 1994–2004: How Can It Be Explained?" *African Affairs* 104 (417): 591–614.

Butler, W. E. 2003. *HIV/AIDS and Drug Misuse in Russia.* London: International Health Family Publishers.

Cai, Thomas. 2006. "Perspectives on Stigma and the Needs of People Living with AIDS in China." In *AIDS and Social Policy in China*, ed. Joan Kaufman, Arthur Kleinman, and Tony Saich, 96–124. Cambridge, MA: Harvard University Asia Center.

Campos, R. 2012. Interview with the author, September 3.

Cannon, Geoffrey. 2004. "Why the Bush Administration and the Global Sugar Industry Are Determined to Demolish the 2004 WHO Global Strategy on Diet, Physical Activity and Health." *Public Health Nutrition* 7 (3): 369–80.

Capuno, Joseph. 2011. "Incumbents and Innovations under Decentralization: An Empirical Exploration of Selected Local Governments in the Philippines." *Asian Journal of Political Science* 19 (1): 48–73.

Cardoso, Fernando H. 2007. Interview with the author, November 1.

Carpenter, Daniel. 2001. *The Forging of Bureaucratic Autonomy: Reputations, Networks, and Policy Innovation in Executive Agencies, 1862–1928.* Princeton, NJ: Princeton University Press.

Carrara, Sérgio. 1997. "A Geopolítica Simbólica da Sífilis: Um Ensaio de Antropologia Histórica." *Historia, Ciencias, Saúde–Minguinhos* 3 (3): 391–408.

———. 1999. "A AIDS e a História das Doencas Venéreas no Brasil." In *A AIDS no Brasil*, ed. Richard Parker, Christiana Bastos, Jane Galvão, and José Stalin Pedrosa. Rio de Janeiro: ABIA.

Carrillo, Susana, Fernanda Lira Goes, Eduarda Passarelli Hamann, Keith Martin, José Flávio Sombra Saraiva, Cromar Lima de Carvalho de Souza, and James Augusto Pires Tibúrcio. 2011. *Bridging the Atlantic: Brazil and Sub-Saharan Africa, South-South Partnering for Growth*. Washington, DC: World Bank Group.

Carter, Gwendolen. 1959. *The Politics of Inequality: South Africa since 1948*. London: Thames and Hudson.

CDC. 2015. "CDC in Brazil." www.cdc.gov/globalhealth/countries/brazil.

Central Eurasia–OSC Report. 2006. "Russia: Epidemiology, Public Health Update for HIV/AIDS for 17–30 October." October 31. Accessed at World News Connection Online.

Centre for Science and Environment. 2017. Center for Science and Environment webpage. www.cseindia.org.

Cerini, Marianna. 2016. "China's Plan to Fight Obesity: Take a College Course." *Financial Times*, May 29.

Cervo, Amando Luiz. 2011. *Inserção Internacional: Formação dos Conceitos Brasileiros*. São Paulo, Brazil: Editora Saraiva.

Chadha, Monica. 2007. "Indian State Bans Sex Education." *BBC News*, April 3.

Chan, Lai-Ha, Luch Chen, and Jin Xu. 2010. "China's Engagement with Global Health Diplomacy: Was SARS a Watershed?" *PLoS Medicine* 7 (4): 1–6.

Chan, Stephen. 1990. *Exporting Apartheid*. New York: St. Martin's Press.

Chandrasekaran, Gina Dallabetta, Virginia Loo, Sujata Rao, Helene Gayle, and Ashok Alexander. 2006. "Containing HIV/AIDS in India: The Unfinished Agenda." *Lancet* 6: 508–21.

Chaturvedi, Sachin. 2015. *Exploring Indian Engagement in Agriculture and Health: A Case of Angola and Mozambique*. Rio de Janeiro: BRICs Policy Centre.

Chen, Huey, Wei Fang, Nanette Turner, and Han-Zhu Oian. 2015. "Promoting HIV Testing through Non-Governmental Organizations in China." *Journal of AIDS and Clinical Research* 6 (3): 1–4.

Chen, Yuyu, and Ginger Zhe Jin. 2011. "Does Health Insurance Coverage Lead to Better Health and Educational Outcomes? Evidence from Rural China." Unpublished manuscript, Guanghua School of Management, Peking University, Beijing.

Cheng, Fuzhi. 2007. "The Nutrition Transition and Obesity in China." In *Food Policy for Developing Countries: Case Studies*, ed. Per Pinstrup-Andersen and Fuzhi Cheng, 11. Ithaca: Cornell University Press.

Cheng, Tsung. 2003. "Fast Food and Obesity in China." *Journal of the American College of Cardiology* 42:773.

———. 2007. "Diabetes and Obesity Epidemics in China: A National Crisis." *International Journal of Cardiology* 123:1–2.

Chequer, Pedro. 2008. Interview with the author, August 5.

Chicago Tribune. 2015. "Russia HIV Infection Rate Rising as World AIDS Day Marked." December 1.

Chilkoti, Avantika. 2014. "Water Shortage Shuts Coca-Cola Plant in India." *Financial Times*, January 19.

China, Ministry of Health. 2012. *China National Plan for NCD Prevention and Treatment (2012–2015)*. Beijing: Ministry of Health.

China, National Health and Family Planning Commission (NHCPC). 2014. *China AIDS Response Progress Report*. Beijing: Ministry of Health.

———. 2015. *China AIDS Response Progress Report*. Beijing: Ministry of Health.

China Daily. 2014. "China to Allocate More Funding for HIV/AIDS." December 1.

Chinese Society for the Study of Sexual Minorities. 1997. "Varying Behaviors, AIDS Risks: Little Known in China."

Chinese University of Hong Kong. 2008. International Conference on Childhood Obesity, Department of Sports Science and Physical Education, Chinese University of Hong Kong, Hong Kong.

Chirambo, Kondwani. 2004. "Introduction." In *Understanding the Institutional Dynamics of South Africa's Response to the HIV/AIDS Epidemic*, ed. Ann Strode and Kitty Barrett-Grant. Pretoria, South Africa: Institute for a Democratic Alternative for South Africa.

Chung Dawson, Kelly. 2010. "Confucius Institutes Enhance China's Int'l Image." *China Daily Online*, April 23.

Churchyard, G. J., I. D. Mametja, L. Mvusi, N. Ndjeka, A. C. Hesseling, A. Reid, S. Babatunde, and Y. Pilay. 2014. "Tuberculosis Control in South Africa." *South African Medical Journal* 104 (3): 244–48.

CIA (Central Intelligence Agency). 2002. *The Next Wave of HIV/AIDS: Nigeria, Ethiopia, Russia, India, and China*. Washington, DC: CIA.

Clark, Fiona. 2016. "Russia Takes One Step Forward, Two Steps Back." *DW*, April 30.

Clements, Benedict, David Coady, and Sanjeev Gupta, eds. 2012. *The Economics of Public Health Care Reform in Advanced and Emerging Economies*. Washington, DC: International Monetary Fund.

Clift, Charles. 2013. *The Role of the World Health Organization in the International System*. London: Chatham House Press.

Clinton, Hillary. 2010. "Leading through Civilian Power." *Foreign Affairs*, November/December.

Cohen, Jon. 2010. "Praised Russian Prevention Program Faces Loss of Funds." *Science* 329:168.

———. 2016. "South Africa's Bid to End AIDS." *Science*, June 29.

Cohen, Stephen. 2002. *India: Emerging Power*. Washington, DC: Brookings Institution Press.

Coitinho, D., Carlos Monteiro, and Barry Popkin. 2002. "What Brazil Is Doing to Promote Healthy Diets and Active Lifestyles." *Public Health Nutrition* 5 (1A): 263–67.

Combes, Katherine. 2012. "Between Revisionism and Status Quo: China in International Regimes." *POLIS Journal* 6 (Winter 2011/2012): 1–37.

Conroy, Mary Schaeffer. 2006. "Civil Society in Late Imperial Russia." In *Russian Civil Society: A Critical Assessment*, ed. Alfred B. Evans Jr., Laura A. Henry, and Lisa McIntosh Sundstrom, 11–27. London: M. E. Sharpe Publications.

Cooke, Jennifer. 2010. "South Africa and Global Health." In *Key Players in Global Health*, ed. Katherine Bliss. Washington, DC: Center for Strategic and International Studies.

Cookson, Clive. 1998. "International: WHO Says 16 Nations Failing to Take World TB Epidemic Seriously." *Financial Times*, March 20.

Correa, Carlos. 2002. *Implications of the DOHA Declaration on the TRIPS Agreement and Public Health*. Geneva: World Health Organization.

Courtwright, Andrew, and Abigail Norris Turner. 2010. "Tuberculosis and Stigmatization: Pathways and Interventions." *Public Health Reports* 125 (4): 34–42.

Coutinho, Janine Giuberti. 2016a. Interview with the author, June 24.

———. 2016b. "Potentials and Challenges for a Common Market Putting Forward the Nutritional Agenda." PhD dissertation, University of Brasília.

Culpeper, Roy. 1997. *Titans or Behemoths?* Boulder, CO: Lynne Rienner Publishers.

Curtis, Glenn, ed. 1996. *Russia: A Country Study* Washington, DC: Library of Congress Press.

Da Costa Marques, Maria Cristina. 2003. *A História de Uma Epidemia Moderna: A Emergencia Política da AIDS/HIV No Brasil.* São Paulo: RiMa/Eduem Press.

Damaceno, Laerte. 2013. President of Sociedade Brasileira de Diabetes. Interview with the author, February 8.

Danishevski, Kirill, Dina Balabanova, Martin McKee, and Sarah Atkinson. 2006. "The Fragmentary Federation: Experiences with the Decentralized Health System in Russia." *Health Policy and Planning* 21 (3): 183–94.

Dasgupta, Rohee. 2005. "The Character and Growth of Indian Diplomacy." Unpublished manuscript, School of Politics, International Relations, and the Environment (SPIRE), Keele University, Keele, UK.

Davenport, Rodney, and Christopher Saunders, eds. 2000. *South Africa: A Modern History.* New York: St. Martin's Press.

D'Avila, Sergio. 2008. Interview with the author, August 14.

Davis, Christopher, and Ben Dickinson. 2005. "Priorities, Government Institutions and Foreign Assistance in the Fight against HIV/AIDS in Russia." *Public Administration and Development* 24:31–40.

Deb, Sutapa. 2014. "HIV/AIDS: Success Becomes the Enemy." NDTV, August 30.

De Bruyn, Tom. 2013. *Adding New Spices to Development Cooperation: Brazil, India, China and South Africa in Health, Agriculture, and Food Security.* Paper no. 9. Leuven, Belgium: HIVA Research Institute for Work and Society.

Dechamp, Jean-Francois, and Odilon Couzin. 2006. "Access to HIV/AIDS Treatment in China." In *AIDS and Social Policy in China*, ed. Joan Kaufman, Arthur Kleinman, and Tony Saich, 126–24. Cambridge, MA: Harvard University Asia Center.

Demikhova, Olga, and Eduard Karamov. 2011. "The Situation of HIV/M. Tuberculosis Co-Infection in Russia." *Open Infectious Diseases Journal* 5:36–50.

De Milliano, Robin. 2007. *India 2020: Rise of the Elephant.* Utrecht, Netherlands: Rabobank.

Dernberger, Brittany. 2014. "A Fluid Two-Way Street: South African HIV/AIDS NGOs and Their Environment." *SPNHA Review* 10 (1).

Devraj, Ranjit. 2005. "Health: HIV/AIDS Campaigns Turning Communal, Say Hindu Leaders." Inter Press Service, May 18.

Dey, Sharmistha. 2010. "Childhood Obesity: A Rising Health Problem in India." *BoloHealth.com*, September 20.

Deyl, Sushmi. 2015. "Global Funding Dips by 90%, May Cripple War on AIDS." *Times of India*, May 23.

———. 2016. "Modi Government Planning Sugar Tax to Fight Obesity and Diabetes." *Times of India*, April 7.

———. 2017. "Rajya Sabha Passes Bill to Ensure Rights of HIV and AIDS Patients." *Times of India*, March 21.

DFID. 2005. *DFID China Briefing Paper: HIV/AIDS.* London: Department for International Development.

Dhalia, C. 2012. Interview with the author, August 31.

Di Ciommo, Mariella, and Alice Amorim. 2015. *Brazil as an International Actor.* Briefing. Rio de Janeiro: Development Initiatives.

Diabetes Foundation (India). 2010. "Recent Events: National Consensus on Dietary Guidelines for Adult Asian Indians for Healthy Living and Prevention of Obesity & Diabetes."

Diário Oficial de União. 2013. Jusbrasil. https://www.jusbrasil.com.br/diarios/DOU /2013/.

Dickinson, Elizabeth. 2010. "China Ups Donations to HIV/AIDS." *Foreign Policy,* October 6.

Dimitrova, B., D. Balabanova, R. Atun, F. Drobniewski, V. Levicheva, and R. Coker. 2006. "Health Service Providers' Perceptions of Barriers to Tuberculosis Care in Russia." *Health Policy and Planning* 21 (4): 265–74.

Downie, Richard, Audry Jackson, and Sahil Angelo. 2016. *Energizing the Fight against HIV/AIDS in South Africa.* Washington, DC: Center for Strategic and International Studies.

Dréze, Jean, and Amartya Sen. 2013. *An Uncertain Glory: India and Its Contradictions.* London: Allen Lane.

Du, Shufa, Bing Lu, Gengying Zhai, and Barry M. Popkin. 2002. "A New Stage of the Nutrition Transition in China." *Public Health Nutrition* 5 (1A): 169–74.

Dugger, Celia. 2010. "South Africa Redoubles Efforts against AIDS." *New York Times,* April 25.

Easterly, William. 2006. *The White Man's Burden.* New York: Penguin Books.

Economic Times. 2010. "The Silent Epidemic." Mumbai, September 9.

———. 2015. "China Makes HIV/AIDS Prevention First Lesson in Beijing Colleges." October 3.

Economist. 2010. "In Lula's Footsteps." July 1.

Edington, Mary. 2000. "TB: Past, Present and Future." *Health Systems Trust Update,* no. 56.

Eley, Brian. 2010. "HIV, TB and Child Health." In *Healthy Children: South African Child Gauge,* ed. Maurice Kibel, Lori Lake, Shirley Pendlebury, and Charmaine Smith, 41–45. Cape Town: Children's Institute, University of Cape Town. www.ci.org.za /depts/ci/pubs/pdf/general/gauge2009-10/sa_child_gauge_09-10_hiv_tb.pdf.

Elliott Armijo, Leslie. 2007. "The BRICs Countries (Brazil, Russia, India, and China) as Analytical Category: Mirage or Insight?" *Asian Perspective* 31 (4): 7–42.

Evans, Alfred B., Jr. 2006a. "Civil Society in the Soviet Union?" In *Russian Civil Society: A Critical Assessment,* ed. Alfred B. Evans Jr., Laura A. Henry, and Lisa McIntosh Sundstrom. London: M. E. Sharpe.

———. 2006b. "Vladimir Putin's Design for Civil Society." In *Russian Civil Society: A Critical Assessment,* ed. Alfred B. Evans Jr., Laura A. Henry, and Lisa McIntosh Sundstrom. London: M. E. Sharpe.

Fan, Maureen. 2007. "They're Big, but Not Yet Stars: With Humanity and Confidence, Chinese Quartet Takes on Bias against the Obese." *Washington Post,* September 6.

FAO. 2013. "Africa to Benefit from Brazil-FAO School Meals Experience." August 13.

Farmer, Paul. 2001. "Russia's Tuberculosis Catastrophe." *Project Syndicate,* January 10.

Feinsilver, Julie. 2008. "Oil-for-Doctors: Cuban Medical Diplomacy Gets a Little Help from a Venezuelan Friend." *Nueva Sociedad* 216 (July/August): 1–15.

Feldbaum, Harley, Kelley Lee, and Joshua Michaud. 2010. "Global Health and Foreign Policy." *Epidemiological Review* 32:82–92.

Feldbaum, Harley, and Joshua Michaud. 2010. "Health Diplomacy and the Enduring Relevance of Foreign Policy Interests." *PLoS Medicine* 7 (4): 1–6.

Fernandes, R. 1931. "Syphilis, Doença Social," *Jornal da Sífilis e Urologia* 20 (10).

Feshbach, Murray. 2008. "The Health Crisis in Russia's Ranks." *Current History*, October.

Fidler, David. 2005. "From International Sanitary Conventions to Global Health Security: The New International Health Regulations." *Chinese Journal of International Law* 4 (2): 325–92.

———. 2009. "Vital Signs: Health and Foreign Policy." *World Today* 65 (2): 27–29.

Figueira, Ariane. 2011. *Introdução á análise de Política Externa*. São Paulo, Brazil: Saraiva Press.

Filho, C. 2012. Interview with the author, September 3.

Filho, Ezio T. 2006. Interview with the author, June 30.

Finch, Christopher. 2007. *China and the World Bank: A Partnership for Innovation*. The World Bank Group. Washington, D.C.

Fitzgerald, Nora, and Oleg Kucheryavenko. 2015. "Spread of HIV in Modern Russia." *Pulitzer Centre on Crisis Reporting*, July 25.

Fleck, Fiona. 2004. "Developing Nations Could Derail Global Anti-Obesity Plan." *BMJ* 328:604.

Flemes, Daniel. 2007. *Conceptualizing Regional Power in International Relations: Lessons from the South African Case*. Working paper no. 53, June. Hamburg: German Institute of Global and Area Studies.

Flynn, Matthew. 2008. "The Evolution of Brazil's Public Production of AIDS Medicines, 1990–2008." *Development and Change* 39 (4): 513–36.

FNDE (Fundo Nacional de Desenvolvimento da Educação). 2016. "Apresentação." www.fnde.gov.br/programs/dinheiro-direto-escola/dinheiro-direto-escola -apresentacao.

Folayan, Morenike. 2004. "HIV/AIDS: The Nigerian Response." In *The Political Economy of AIDS in Africa*, ed. Nana K. Poku and Alan W. Whiteside. Burlington, VT: Ashgate.

Fook, Lye Liang, and Chong Siew Keng, Catherine. 2010. "China's Media Initiatives and Its International Image Building." East Asian Institute background brief no. 555, August 26. Singapore: National University of Singapore Press.

Fourie, Bernard. 2011. "The Burden of Tuberculosis in South Africa." MRC National Tuberculosis Research Programme.

Frederik, Balfour. 2010. "Why China's Weight-Loss Industry Is Gaining." *Bloomberg News*, June 3.

Freitas, D. A., Á. A. Sousa, and K. M. Jones. 2014. "Development, Income Transfer Strategies, and the Nutrition Transition in Brazilian Children from a Rural and Remote Region." *Rural and Remote Health* 14:2632.

French, Paul. 2015. "How Are Policy-Makers Tackling Rising Obesity in China?" *Guardian* (London), February 25.

French, Paul, and Matthew Crabbe. 2010. "Welcome to Fat China . . . A Literally Expanding Market." *Advertising Age*, August 11.

Frontline. 2006. "Russia: Exacerbating a Superpower's Decline." June 19.

Gage, Carrie. 2008. "Toward a Legislative Solution to the Growing HIV/AIDS Epidemic in Russia: A Case for Expanded Health Privacy." *Pacific Rim Law and Policy Journal* 17:157–86.

Gaiha, Raghav, Raghbendra Jha, and Vani Kulkarni. 2010. *Affluence, Obesity, and Non-Communicable Diseases in India*. Working paper no. 8. Canberra: Australia South Asia Research Centre, Australian National University.

Galvão, Jane. 2000. *AIDS no Brasil: A agenda de construção de uma epidemia*. São Paulo, Brazil: ABIA Publishers.

Gandhi, Sonia. 2004. "Sonia Gandhi Says India Can and Will Control AIDS." *Body*, July 16, 1.

Garcia, Eugênio Vargas. 2012. *O Sexto Membro Permanente O Brasil e a Criação da ONU*. Rio de Janeiro: Contraponto Editora Ltda.

Garcia, Jonathan, and Richard Parker. 2011. "Resource Mobilization for Health Advocacy: Afro-Brazilian Religious Organizations and HIV Prevention and Control." *Social Science and Medicine* 72 (12): 1930–38.

Garrett, Laurie. 2005. *HIV and National Security: Where Are the Links?* New York: Council on Foreign Relations.

Gauri, Varun, and Peyvand Khaleghian. 2002. "Immunization in Developing Countries: Its Political and Institutional Determinants." *World Development* 30:2109–32.

Gauri, Varun, and Evan Lieberman. 2006. "Boundary Politics and HIV/AIDS Policy in Brazil and South Africa." *Studies in Comparative International Development* 41 (3): 47–73.

Geldenhuys, J. 1984. *The Diplomacy of Isolation*. Johannesburg: Macmillan.

Gerber, Theodore, and Sarah Mendelson. 2005. "Crisis among Crisis among Crisis: Public and Professional Views of the HIV/AIDS Epidemic in Russia." *Problems in Post-Communism* 52 (4): 28–41.

George, Nirmala. 2006. "Needle Exchange Program on Rise in India." FOX News, November 29.

———. 2016. "India Says Number of Obese Teens Nearly Doubles in Five Years." *Medical Press*, March 9.

Ghosh, Palash. 2012. "Obesity Rates Soaring in Brazil as Prosperity Flourishes." *International Business Times*, April 12.

———. 2013. "Fat of the Land: In India, Obesity Affects the Affluent, Not the Poor." *IB Times*, May 29.

Gill, Bates, Jennifer Chang, and Sarah Palmer. 2002. "China's HIV Crisis." *Foreign Affairs* 81 (2). www.foreignaffairs.com/articles/asia/2002-03-01/chinas-hiv-crisis.

Gill, Bates, J. Stephen Morrison, and Xiaoqing Lu. 2007. *China's Civil Societal Organizations: What Future in the Health Sector*. Report of the Task Force on HIV/AIDS Delegation to China, June 13–20. Washington, DC: Center for Strategic and International Studies.

Gill, Bates, and Susan Okie. 2007. "China and HIV—A Window of Opportunity." *New England Journal of Medicine* 356 (18): 1801–5.

Global Business Council. 2008. *HIV/AIDS Policy Framework and Implementation in China*. Research report. New York: Global Business Council

———. 2009. *HIV/AIDS Policy Framework and Implementation in Russia*. New York: Global Business Council.

Global Fund to Fight AIDS, Tuberculosis, and Malaria. 2009. *India and the Global Fund*. Geneva: GFATM Press.

———. 2011. *Russian Federation: Country Grant Portfolio*. Geneva: GFATM Press.

Goble, Paul. 2011. "Russia No Longer to Provide Free Treatment for Victims of Tuberculosis." *KyivPost*, February 21.

———. 2015a. "HIV/AIDS Epidemic in Russia 'Out of Control,' Health Minister Says." *Euromaidan Press*, October 29.

———. 2015b. "Putin Government Stopped Fighting HIV/AIDS, Russia 'At the Edge of Generalized Epidemic.'" *Euromaidan Press*, July 3.

———. 2015c. "Russian Penal System Incubator of Antibiotic Resistant Tuberculosis." *Window on Eurasia*, October 13.

Goldstein, Avery. 2001. "The Diplomatic Face of China's Grand Strategy: A Rising Power's Emerging Choice." *China Quarterly* 168, 835–64.

Golichenko, Mikhail. 2016. "37 Kamskaya St., Yekaterinburg." Report of the Andrey Rylkov Foundation for Health and Social Justice, Moscow, December 22.

Gómez, Eduardo J. 2006. *The Politics of Government Response to HIV/AIDS in Russia and Brazil: Historical Institutionalism, Culture, and State Capacity*. Working Paper 4, Harvard Initiative for Global Health.

———. 2009. "The Politics of Receptivity and Resistance: How Brazil, India, China, and Russia Strategically Use the International Health Community in Response to HIV/AIDS: A Theory." *Global Health Governance* 3 (1): 1–29.

———. 2011a. "Overcoming Decentralization's Defects: Discovering Alternative Routes to Centralization in a Context of Path Dependent Health Policy Devolution: Lessons from Brazil's Response to HIV/AIDS." *Global Health Governance* 5 (1): 1–35.

———. 2011b. "U.N. Unlikely to Sway Poorer Nations on Obesity, Diabetes." CNN, September 11.

———. 2013a. "Geopolitics, Obesity, and Diabetes: How Brazil, China, and India Responded." *Harvard International Review* 35 (1): 1–8.

———. 2013b. "An Interdependent Analytical Approach to Explaining the Evolution of NGOs, Social Movements, and Biased Government Response to AIDS and Tuberculosis in Brazil." *Journal of Health Politics, Policy and Law* 38 (1): 123–59.

———. 2014. "How Sweet Are the MINTs?" CNN, January 19.

———. 2015a. *Contested Epidemics: How Brazil Outpaced the United States in Its Policy Response*. London: Imperial College Press.

———. 2015b. *Health Spending and Inequalities in Emerging Economies*. Oxford: Oxfam.

———. 2015c. "Responding to Obesity in Brazil: Understanding the Intersect of International and Domestic Politics and Policy through a Nested Analytical Approach." *Journal of Health Politics, Policy, and Law* 40 (1): 73–99.

———. 2015d. "Understanding the United States and Brazil's Response to Obesity: Institutional Conversion, Policy Reform, and the Lessons Learned." *Globalization and Health* 11:24.

Gómez, Eduardo J., and Joseph Harris. 2015. "Political Repression, Civil Society, and the Politics of Responding to AIDS in the BRICS." *Health Policy and Planning* 31 (1): 56–66.

Gómez, Eduardo J., and Fernanda Perez. 2016. "Brazilian Foreign Policy in Health: Transitions and Challenges under the Dilma Rousseff Administration (2011–2014)," *Lua Nova* 98: 171–97.

Gordon, Susie. 2010. "Fat Chance: Solving China's Obesity Problem." *eChinacities.com*, November 15.

Gorry, Conner. 2008. "Cuba's HIV/AIDS Program: Controversy, Care, and Cultural Shift." *MEDICC Review* 10 (4): 10–14.

Gorst, Isabel. 2010. "Prevention and Education Are Grave Blind Spots." *Financial Times*, December 1.

Gouda, Jitendra, and Ranjan Prusty. 2014. "Overweight and Obesity among Women by Economic Stratum in Urban India." *Journal of Health, Population, and Nutrition* 32 (1): 79–88.

Gould, Deborah. 2009. *Moving Politics: Emotion and Act Up's Fight against Aids.* Chicago: University of Chicago Press.

Grangeiro, A. 2012. Interview with the author, September 6.

Grant, Charles. 2008. *India's Role in the New World Order.* Briefing note. London: Centre for European Reform.

Grépin, Karen, Victoria Fan, Gordon Shen, and Lucy Chen. 2014. "China's Role as a Global Health Donor in Africa." *Globalization and Health* 19 (84): 1–11.

Griffing, Sean Michael, Pedro Luiz Tauil, Venkatachalam Udhayakumar, and Luciana Silva-Flannery. 2015. "A Historical Perspective on Malaria Control in Brazil." *Memórias do Instituto Oswaldo Cruz* 110 (6): 701–18.

Grimm, Bill. 2015. "Chinese AIDS Prevention Campaign Faces Battle." *UCANews,* December 16.

Gulati, Seema, and Anoop Misra. 2014. "Sugar Intake, Obesity, and Diabetes in India." *Nutrients* 6:5955-74.

Gupta, R. S. 2015. "The RNTCP: Mission for a TB-Free India." In *Eradicating TB in India,* ed. Harsh Sethi. New Delhi: Global Policy and Observer Research Foundation.

Gupta, Sanjay. 2009. "Why the Brazilian Response to AIDS Is the Envy of the World." CNN, August 27.

Gutterman, Steve. 2008. "Russia Is Losing HIV Fight, Top Official Says." *Virginian-Pilot,* November 23.

Gwalani, Payal. 2014. "NGOs Working for AIDS Control Facing Funds Crunch." TNN, September 8.

Habib, Adam. 2009. "South Africa's Foreign Policy." *South African Journal of International Affairs* 16 (2): 143–59.

———. 2011. "South Africa's Foreign Policy under Zuma." *Broker,* June 3.

Halter, Casey. n.d. "Capitalism-Loving Disease." *Hopes&Fears* (online).

Hancock, W. K. 1962. *Smuts: The Sanguine Years, 1870–1919.* New York: Cambridge University Press.

———. 1968. *Smuts: The Fields of Force, 1919–1950.* New York: Cambridge University Press.

Hardley, J. M. 1999. *A Social History of the Russian Empire, 1650–1825.* New York: Longman Publishing.

Hausler, Harry. 2013. CEO, TB/HIV Care Association, University of the Western Cape, South Africa. Interview with the author, January 22.

Hawkes, C. 2007. "Agro-Food Industry Growth and Obesity in China." *Obesity Reviews* 9 (Suppl. 1): 151–61.

Health & Place. 2004. "Childhood Obesity in China." Letter to the editor, 10 (4): 395–96.

HealthJockey. 2007. "Anti-obesity NGO Launched in Chandigarh, India to Help Overweight People." August 9. www.healthjockey.com.

Heijstek, Esmee. 2015. "Health Diplomacy as a Soft Power Strategy or Ethical Duty? Case Study: Brazil in the 21st Strategy." Master's thesis, Leiden University.

Henderson, Donald. 1988. "Smallpox Eradication—A Cold War History." *World Health Forum* 19:113–19.

Henderson, Emma. 2016. "China Urges Citizens to Eat Less Meat in Bid to Fight Obesity." *Independent* (London), June 1.

Hepler, Kurt. 2012. "Russia's Global Health Engagement." *Johnson's Russia List*, December 26.

Heywood, Marck. 2016. "AIDS 2016." Bhekisisa, Centre for Health Journalism, July 18.

Hindu. 2007. "India Facing Obesity Epidemic." October 12.

———. 2009a. "Red Ribbon Express Aids Spread of Awareness Nation-Wide." December 1.

———. 2009b. "Stress on Role of Government, NGOs in Tackling Obesity." July 12.

Hindustan Times. 2008. "Red Ribbon Express Comes Calling in Tamil Nadu." May 27.

HKASO. 2013. "HKASO Activities Summary 2012–2013." Activities document. www.hkaso.org.

———. 2016. "HKASO Mission Statement." www.hkaso.org.

Ho, Christina. 2010. "Health Reform and De Facto Federalism in China." *China: An International Journal* 8 (1): 33–62.

Hochman, Gilberto. 1988. *A Era do Saneamento: As Bases da Política de Saúde Pública no Brasil*. São Paulo: Editora Hucitec-Anpocs.

———. 2008. "From Autonomy to Partial Alignment: National Malaria Programs in the Time of Global Eradication, Brazil, 1941–1961." *Canadian Bulletin of Medical History* 25 (1): 161–92.

———. 2009. "Priority, Invisibility and Eradication: The History of Smallpox and the Brazilian Public Health Agenda." *Medical History* 53:229–52.

Holacheck, Jeffrey. 2006. *Russia's Shrinking Population and the Russian Military's HIV/AIDS Problem*. Occasional paper. Washington, DC: Atlantic Council.

Hosking, Geoffrey. 2001. *Russia and the Russians: A History*. Cambridge, MA: Harvard University Press.

Huang, Xian. 2013. "The Politics of Social Welfare Reform in Urban China: Social Welfare Preferences and Reform Policies." *Journal of Chinese Political Science* 18:61–85.

Huang, Yanzhong. 2006. "The Politics of HIV/AIDS in China." *Asian Perspective* 30 (1): 95–125.

———. 2010a. "International Actors and China's Health Governance." Paper presented at the Annual Meeting of the American Political Science Association, Washington, DC.

———. 2010b. "Pursuing Health as Foreign Policy: The Case of China." *Indiana Journal of Global Legal Studies* 17 (1): 105–46.

———. 2012. *China and Global Health Governance*. Working paper no. 26. Bloomington: Research Center for Chinese Politics and Business, Indiana University.

———. 2013. *Governing Health in Contemporary China*. New York: Routledge.

Huang, Yanzhong, and Sheng Ding. 2006. "Dragon's Underbelly: An Analysis of China's Soft Power." *East Asia* 23 (4): 22–44.

Human Rights Watch. 2007. "Civil Society Key to Defeating AIDS in China." *News Release Communiqué*, September 27.

Hurrell, Andrew. 2006. "Hegemony, Liberalism, and Global Order: What Space for Would-Be Great Powers?" *International Affairs* 82 (1): 1–19.

Hveem, Helge, and Desmond McNeill. 1994. *Is Swedish Aid Rational? A Critical Study of Swedish Aid Policy in the Period 1968–1993*. Oslo: Centre for Development and the Environment, University of Oslo.

ICDA (International Confederation of Dietetic Associations). 2006. *Country—Brazil*. Toronto: International Confederation of Dietetic Associations Press.

iGoverment. 2008. "India Reworks Obesity Guidelines, BMI Lowered." November 26. www.igovernment.in.

India, Government of. 2004. Letter from Secretary of MHW, Dr. B. P. Sharma, in Response to the Draft Report of the 2004 WHO Global Strategy on Diet, Physical Activity and Health, March 10.

———. 2006. *Recommendations for a National Plan of Action for the Implementation of WHO's Global Strategy on Diet, Physical Activity, and Health in India.* New Delhi: Government of India.

India, Ministry of Health and Family Welfare. 2005. *Financing and Delivery of Health Care Services in India.* National Commission on Macroeconomics and Health (NCMH) background paper. New Delhi: Ministry of Health and Family Welfare.

———. 2010. National AIDS Control Organisation. New Delhi: Ministry of Health and Family Welfare.

———. 2016. *Notes on Demands for Grants, 2017–18.* New Delhi: Ministry of Health and Family Welfare.

India, NACO. 2010. *A Strategy Document: Report of Working Group on ICTC/PPTCT Services for NACP IV.* New Delhi: Ministry of Health and Family Welfare.

Indo-Asian News Service (India). 2011. "Government Mulls Curbs on Junk Food in Schools." July 16. Accessed at Access World News, www.newsbank.com.

Interfax. 2001. "Russia Receives USAID Funding to Combat Tuberculosis." November 26.

———. 2006. "Russian Military Reports 38 HIV Cases in 2006." September 14.

International Federation of the Red Cross. 2015. *Red Cross Raises TB Awareness among Women Held in Russia.* Geneva: International Federation of the Red Cross, March 24.

Irwin, Rachel. 2010. "Chronic Diseases and Marketing to Children in India." Paper presented at the Roundtable on Global Health Diplomacy in Asia, London School of Hygiene & Tropical Medicine, November 17.

ITAR-TASS. 1998. "Russia Approves Federal Tuberculosis-Control Program." February 12.

———. 2000a. "Russian Government Makers Make Proposals for Drug Control Program." November 29.

———. 2000b. "Russian Parliament Approves Bill to Prevent Spread of TB." December 20.

———. 2006a. "Putin Says AIDS Problem to Be Included on G8 Summit's Agenda." April 21.

———. 2006b. "Putin Says HIV/AIDS Control Needs More Efficient Coordination." April 21.

———. 2006c. "Russia to Establish Sub-regional AIDS Center." June 8.

———. 2009a. "HIV/AIDS Rate Growing in Russia." December 6.

———. 2009b. "Russia to Boost HIV, AIDS Funding, Links Infection Growth to Afghan Drugs."

Ito, Toru. n.d. "The Approach to Indian Diplomacy: How to Establish Alternative International Relations Rooted in India." Unpublished manuscript, National Defense Academy of Japan, Tokyo.

Ivanov, Igor. 2009. *The New Russian Diplomacy.* Washington DC: Brookings Institution Press.

Jabeen, Mussarat. 2010. "Indian Aspiration of Permanent Membership in the UN Security Council and American Stance." *South Asian Studies* 25 (2): 237–53.

Jack, Andrew. 2011. "Russia Offers Aid to Help Neighbours Fight HIV." *Financial Times*, October 17.

Jacob, Shiji. 2014. "Prevalence of Obesity and Overweight among School Going Children in Rural Areas of Ernakulam District, Kerala State India." *International Journal of Scientific Study* 2 (1): 16–19.

Jagannivas, Paleru. 2013. Heinz Foundation, Chenai, India. Interview with the author, January 8.

Jaime P., A. Feldenheimer, A. Cavalcante de Lima, and G. Bortolini. 2011. "Ações de Alimentação na Atenção Básica: a experência de organização no Governo Brasileiro." *Revista de Nutrição* 24 (6): 809–24.

Jaime, P., A. Silva, P. Gentil, R. Ciaro, and C. Monteiro. 2013. "Brazil Obesity Prevention and Control Initiatives." *Obesity Reviews* 14:88–95.

James, Philip T. 2003. "The Challenge of Obesity and Its Associated Chronic Diseases." *SCN News* 29:39–43.

James, W. P. T. 2007. "International Association for the Study of Obesity and China." *Obesity Reviews* 9 (Suppl. 1): 2–3.

———. 2008. "WHO Recognition of the Global Obesity Epidemic." *International Journal of Obesity* 32:S120-26.

Jayapal, Pramila. 1996. "AIDS in India. Part 1: A Government in Denial." *ICWA Letters* (Institute of Current World Affairs, Bombay), July, pp. 1-11.

Jayaram, N. 2015. "By Attacking Activists and NGOs, India Is Becoming More like China." *Daily O*, February 12.

Jha, Prabhat. 2013. Interview with the author, January 30.

Ji, Linong. 2010. "Focus on the Frontline—The Chinese Diabetes Society." *Diabetes Voice* 55 (2): 27–29.

———. 2015. Vice President, International Diabetes Federation, Beijing. Interview with the author, June 12.

Jiang, Zhen, Debin Wang, Sen Yang, Mingyue Duan, Pengbin Bu, Andrew Gren, and Xuejun Zhang. 2011. "Integrated Response toward HIV: A Health Promotion Case Study from China." *Health Promotion International* 26 (2): 196–211.

Jiaying, Liu. 2015. "Number of College Students with HIV/AIDS Soars, Official Says." *Caixin Online*, August 12.

Jingxi, Xu. 2015. "Guangzhou Renews Push for HIV/AIDS Prevention." *ChinaDaily .com*, November 12.

Jiwane, Niwrutti, and Sarita Wadhva. 2014. "Prevalence of Overweight and Obesity in Rural School Children of Maharashtra, India." *International Journal of Scientific Research* 3 (5): 405–6.

John, Jacob T. 2008. "NACO and Phony NGOs in India." *Indian Journal of Medical Research*, 128:778–79.

Johnson, Krista. 2005. "The Politics of AIDS Policy Development and Implementation in Postapartheid South Africa." *Africa Today* 51 (2): 107–28.

Jones, Paula. 2016. Interview with the author. June 15.

Jones, Timothy. 2001. "South Africa in Crisis on HIV/AIDS Treatment." *Science* 292 (5526): 2431–32.

Jordan, Pamela. 2010. "A Bridge between the Global North and Africa?" *African Studies Quarterly* 11 (4): 83–115.

Joshi, Charu. 1995. "Fighing Baby Fat." *India Today*, March 15. http://indiatoday.intoday .in/story/parents-schools-tackle-problem-of-overweight-children-with-new -awareness/1/288447.html.

Kadiyala, Suneetha, and Tony Barnett. 2004. "AIDS in India: Disaster in the Making." *Economic and Political Weekly*, May 8, 1888–92.

Kahn, Jeremy. 2009. "India Cleans Up Its Act." *Newsweek*, November 6.

Kalipeni, Ezekiel. 2000. "Health and Society in Southern Africa in Times of Economic Turbulence." In *The Uncertain Promise of Southern Africa*, ed. York Bradshaw and Stephen Ndegwa. Bloomington: Indiana University Press.

Kalra, Aditya. 2015. "India Restores Federal Funding for AIDS Program after Criticism." Reuters, December 1.

———. 2016. "India Sacks Some Foreign-Funded Consultants; Health Programmes May Suffer." Reuters, April 5.

Kalra, Aditya, and Zeba Siddiqui. 2015. "Funding Crisis Puts India's AIDS Program, and Lives, at Risk." Reuters, July 24.

Kapur, Devesh, John Lewis, and Richard Webb, eds. 1997. *The World Bank: Its First Half Century*. Washington, DC: Brookings Institution Press.

Karageorgiadis, Ekaterine. 2016. Interview with the author, June 7.

Karim, Q. A., A. B. Kharsany, J. A. Frohlich, L. Werner, M. Mashego, M. Mlotshwa, B. T. Madlala, F. Ntombela, and S. S. Abdool Karim. 2011. "Stabilizing HIV Prevalence Masks High HIV Incidence Rates amongst Rural and Urban Women in KwaZulu-Natal, South Africa." *International Journal of Epidemiology* 40 (4): 922–30.

Karim, Salim, Gavin Churchyard, Quarraisha Abdool Karim, and Stephen Lawn. 2009. "HIV Infection and Tuberculosis in South Africa: An Urgent Need to Escalate the Public Health Response." *Lancet* 374 (9693): 921–33.

Karim, Salim, Kogieleum Naidoo, Anneke Grobler, Nesri Padayatchi, Cheryle Baxter, Andrew Gray, Tanuja Gengiah, Santhanalakshmi Gengiah, Anushka Naidoo, Niraksha Jithoo, Gonasagrie Nair, Wafaa El-Sadr, Gerald Friedland, and Quarraisha Abdool Karim. 2011. "Integration of Antiretroviral Therapy with Tuberculosis Treatment." *New England Journal of Medicine* 365:1492–1501.

Kassianova, Alla. 2002. *Russian Diplomacy in the 21st Century: Multilateralism Put to Work*. PONARS policy memo no. 262. Washington, DC: PONARS Eurasia.

Katz, Mark. 2005. "Exploiting Rivalries for Prestige and Profit: An Assessment of Putin's Foreign Policy Approach." *Problems of Post-Communism* 52 (3): 25–36.

Kaufman, Joan. 2009. *The Role of NGOs in China's AIDS Crisis*. Cambridge, MA: Hauser Center for Non-Profit Organizations, Harvard University.

———. 2010. "Turning Points in China's AIDS Response." *China: An International Journal* 8 (1): 63–84.

Kaufman, Joan, Arthur Kleinman, and Tony Saich. 2006. "Introduction." In *AIDS and Social Policy in China*, ed. Joan Kaufman, Arthur Kleinman, and Tony Saich, 3–14. Cambridge, MA: Harvard University Asia Center.

Kaufman, Joan, and Kathrine Meyers. 2006. "AIDS Surveillance in China: Data Gaps and Research for AIDS Policy," In *AIDS and Social Policy in China*, ed. Joan Kaufman, Arthur Kleinman, and Tony Saich, 48–71. Cambridge, MA: Harvard University Asia Center.

Kazionny, Boris, Charles Wells, Hans Kluge, Nissa Gusseynova, and Valery Molotilov. 2001. "Implications of the Growing HIV-1 Epidemic for Tuberculosis Control in Russia." *Lancet* 358:1513–14.

Kember, J. L. 1975. "India in the British Commonwealth: The Problem of Diplomatic Representation, 1917–1947." PhD dissertation, University of London.

Keping, Yu. 2009. *Democracy Is a Good Thing: Essays on Politics, Society, and Culture in Contemporary China*. Washington DC: Brookings Institution Press.

Khandelwal, S., and K. S. Reddy. 2013. "Eliciting a Policy Response for the Rising Epidemic of Overweight-Obesity in India." *Obesity Reviews* 14 (2): 114–25.

Khumalo, Thuso. 2014. "TB Is Number One Killer in South Africa." *VOA News*, March 21.

Kironde, S., and J. Nasolo. 2002. "Combating Tuberculosis: Barriers to Widespread Non-Governmental Organisation Involvement in Community-Based Tuberculosis Treatment in South Africa." *International Journal of Tuberculosis and Lung Disease* 6 (8): 679–85.

Kironde, S., and S. Neil. 2004. "Indigenous NGO Involvement in TB Treatment Programmes in High-Burden Settings." *International Journal of Lung Disease* 8 (4): 504–8.

Kiselev, Veronika. 2010. *AIDS Epidemic in the Russian Federation and Policy Reform.* ISP Collection, paper no. 863. Seattle: University of Washington.

Klotz, Audie. 2004. "State Identity in South African Foreign Policy." Paper presented at the Annual Meeting of the American Political Science Association, Chicago, September 2–5.

Knoetze, Daneel. 2015. "Is TB Spinning Out of Control in South Africa?" *GroundUp*, March.

Knutsen, Wenjue Lu. 2009. "Resistance and Radical Shift: An Institutional Account of China's HIV/AIDS Policy Process from 1985–2009." Paper presented at the Annual Meeting of the American Political Science Association, Toronto, September 3–6.

———. 2012. "An Institutional Account of China's HIV/AIDS Policy Process from 1985 to 2010." *Politics and Policy* 40 (1): 161–92.

Kornegay, Francis. 2007. *The Geopolitics of IBSA: The South African Dimension.* London: Center for Policy Studies and Friedrich Ebert Stiftung, August.

———. 2009. "South Africa Excluded as an Emerging Economic Power." *Sunday Independent* (London), June 28.

Kowsalya, T., and R. Parimalavalli. 2014. "Prevalence of Overweight/Obesity among Adolescents in Urban and Rural Areas of Salem, India." *Journal of Obesity and Metabolic Research* 1 (3): 152–55.

Kragelund, Peter. 2010. *The Potential Role of Non-traditional Donors' Aid in Africa.* Geneva: International Centre for Trade and Sustainable Development.

Krishnan, Dharini. 2013. Heinz Foundation, Chenai, India. Interview with the author, January 8.

Krishnan, Vidya. 2014. "AIDS Control Dept to Be Merged with National Health Mission." *LiveMint*, August 15.

Kronstadt, K. Alan. 2004. *India's 2004 National Elections.* Congressional Research Service (CRS) report for the Congress. New Delhi: Indian National Congress, July 12.

Kucheryavenko, Oleg, and Eduardo J. Gómez. 2016. "Agenda-Setting and Political Commitment to HIV/AIDS Policy in Russia." Unpublished manuscript, King's College London.

Kuhn, Anthony. 2009. "In China, AIDS Stigma Proves Difficult to Eliminate." NPR, December 1.

Kyivpost. 1998. "Economic Crisis Saps Ukraine's Resistance to Tuberculosis." December 8.

Labonte, R., and M. Gagnon. 2010. "Framing Health and Foreign Policy: Lesson for Global Health Diplomacy." *Globalization and Health* 6 (14): 1–19.

LaCock, Paul. 2015. *Budget Impact of HIV/AIDS in South Africa.* Paper presented at the ISPOR Africa Network Forum, May 18, Philadelphia.

La Forgia, G. M., and B. Couttolenc. 2008. *Hospital Performance in Brazil: The Search for Excellence*. Washington, DC: World Bank Group.

Lamberti, Taryn, and Pat Sidley. 2000. "Presidential AIDS Panel Appointed." *Business Day* (Johannesburg), May 4. Accessed at Access World News, www.newsbank.com.

Lancet. 2004. "Appropriate Body-Mass Index for Asian Populations and Its Implications for Policy and Intervention Strategies." 363:157–63.

———. 2009. "China's Evolving Response to HIV/AIDS." 373:1.

Leão, Maríla Mendonça, and Renato Maluf. 2012. *Effective Public Policies and Active Citizenship: Brazil's Experience of Building a Food Nutrition Security System*. Oxford: Oxfam.

Lee, Jason. 2009. "Soft Power, Hard Choices." *Sydney Morning Herald*, April 4.

Lee, Kelley. 2009. "Global Health Diplomacy: A Conceptual Review." Globalization, Trade and Health Working Paper Series. Unpublished manuscript, London School of Hygiene and Tropical Medicine.

Lee, Kelley, and Eduardo J. Gómez. 2011. "Brazil's Ascendance: The Soft Power Role of Global Health Diplomacy." *European Business Review*, January-February, 61–64.

Legum, Colin, and Margaret Legum. 1964. *South Africa: Crisis for the West*. New York: Frederick Praeger.

Lei, Sheng, and Cao Wu-Kui. 2008. "HIV/AIDS Epidemiology and Prevention in China." *Chinese Medical Journal* 121 (13): 1230–36.

Leowski, Jerzy, and Anand Krishnan. 2009. "Capacity to Control Non-Communicable Diseases in the Countries of South-East Asia." *Health Policy* 92:43–48.

Lessa de Oliveira, Michele. 2016. Interview with the author, February 26.

Lethbridge, Jane. 2009. "Trade Unions, Civil Society Organizations and Health Reforms." *Capital Class* 33 (2): 101–29.

Levi, C., and M. Vitoria. 2002. "Fighting against AIDS: The Brazilian Experience." *AIDS* 16:2373–83.

Li, M., M. J. Dibley, D. Sibbritt, and H. Yan. 2007. "Factors Associated with Adolescents' Overweight and Obesity at Community, School and Household levels in Xi'an City, China: Results of Hierarchical Analysis." *European Journal of Clinical Nutrition* 62:635–43.

Li, Nana Taona Kuo, Hui Liu, Christine Korhonen, Ellenie Pond, Haoyan Guo, Liz Smith, Hui Xue, and Jiangping Sun. 2010. "From Spectators to Implementers: Civil Society Organizations Involved in AIDS Programmes in China." *International Journal of Epidemiology* 39:65–71.

Lieberman, Evan. 2009. *Boundaries of Contagion: How Ethnic Politics Have Shaped Government Responses to AIDS*. Princeton, NJ: Princeton University Press.

Lijphart, A. 1971. "Comparative Politics and the Comparative Method." *American Political Science Review* 65:682–93.

Likhachev, V. 2010. "Priorities in Modernizing Russia's Diplomacy." *International Affairs* 2:157–64.

LillyPad. 2016. "The Latest on Fighting Tuberculosis in Russia." March 2.

Lim, Meng-Kin, Karen Eggleston, Kun Chen, Yunxian Yu, Sung-Il Cho, Sian Griffiths, Ek Yeoh, Jamal Hisham Hashim, Masamine Jimba, Carl Anderson Johnson, Paula Palmer, Vu-Anh Le, Huu-Bich Tran, Ngoc-Quang La, and Bambang Wispriyono. 2010. *Prevention and Control of Chronic Non-Communicable Diseases in Nine Pacific Rim Countries*. Asia Health Policy Program working paper no. 21, December 10. Stanford, CA: Stanford University.

Little, Matthew, Sally Humphris, Kirit Patel, and Cate Dewey. 2016. "Factors Associated with BMI, Underweight, Overweight, and Obesity among Adults in a Population of Rural South India." *BMC Obesity* 3 (12): 1–13.

Liu, Perilong, Yan Guo, Xu Aian, Shenglan Tang, Zhihui Li, and Lincoln Chen. 2014. "Chinas' Distinctive Engagement in Global Health." *Lancet* 384 (9945): 793–804.

Liu, Yuanli, and Joan Kaufman. 2006. "Controlling HIV/AIDS in China: Health System Challenges." In *AIDS and Social Policy in China*, ed. Joan Kaufman, Arthur Kleinman, and Tony Saich, 75–95. Cambridge, MA: Harvard University Asia Center.

Lo, Ying-Ru, Padmaja Shetty, D. S. C. Reddy, and Salim Habayeb. 2005. "Controlling the HIV/AIDS Epidemic in India." NCMH Background Papers: Burden of Disease in India. Geneva: WHO.

Lodge, Tom. 2015. "The Politics of HIV/AIDS in South Africa." *Third World Quarterly* 36 (8): 1570–91.

Long, Qian, Yan Qu, and Henry Lucas. 2016. "Drug-Resistant Tuberculosis Control in China: Progress and Challenges." *Infectious Diseases of Poverty* 5 (9): 9.

Lou, Z. 2002. "Obesity: A Warning to Chinese Children." *Beijing Review* 45 (26): 14–16.

Loveday, Marian, and Virginia Zweigenthal. 2011. "TB and HIV Integration: Obstacles and Possible Solutions to Implementation in South Africa." *Tropical Medicine and International Health* 16 (4): 431–38.

Low, Marcus. 2016. "SA's New HIV and TB Battle Plan Must Avoid the Mistakes of the Past." *Medical Brief*, August 10.

Loyce, Maturu. 2016. "Despite Russia's Objections, U.N. Member States Plan to End AIDS Pandemic by 2030." *Japan Times*, June 9.

Lu, Xiaoqing, and Bates Gill. 2007. *China's Response to HIV/AIDS and US-China Collaboration*. Washington, DC: Center for Strategic and International Studies.

Lucker, Vicki. 2004. "Civil Society, Social Capital and the Churches: HIV/AIDS in Papua New Guinea." Paper presented at the Governance and Civil Society seminar, Symposium Governance in Pacific States: Reassessing Roles and Remedies, University of the South Pacific, September 30-October 2, 2003.

Luhn, Alec. 2015. "While Russia Grapples with HIV Epidemic, Moscow's Addicts Share Their Filthy Needles." *Guardian* (London), May 24.

Lui, Yuanli, and Joan Kaufman. 2006. "Controlling HIV/AIDS in China." In *AIDS and Social Policy in China*, ed. Joan Kaufman, Arthur Kleinman, and Tony Saich, 75–95. Cambridge, MA: Harvard University Asia Center.

Lum, Thomas, Hannah Fisher, Julissa Gomez-Granger, and Anne LeLand. 2009. *China's Foreign Aid Activities in Africa, Latin America, and Southeast Asia*. Washington, DC: Congressional Research Service.

Luthra, Vandana. 2016. Curls and Curves. "Social Responsibility." September 26.

MacDonald, Victoria. 2013. "The Rising Spectre of Tuberculosis across Russia." 4 News, August 2.

Madurai, Ians. 2016. "Obesity in Children: It's Not Their Fault, Blame It on Poor Parenting." *Hindustan Times*, April 30.

Mahoney, James, and Gary Gertz. 2004. "The Possibility Principle: Choosing Negative Cases in Qualitative Research." *American Political Science Review* 98:1033–53.

Mail Today (Delhi). 2010. "The Hidden Killer and Your Junk Food." April 26. Accessed at Access World News, www.newsbank.com.

———. 2011. "Finding a Way out of the Fat Trap." February 1. Accessed at Access World News, www.newsbank.com.

Makarychev, Andrey, and Licínia Simão. 2014. *Russia's Development Assistance with a Focus on Africa.* Policy brief. Oslo, Norway: Norwegian Peacebuilding Resource Centre.

Maluf, Renato. 2011. "CONSEA's Participation in Building the National Food and Nutrition Security System and Policy." In *The Fome Zero (Zero Hunger) Program: The Brazilian Experience,* ed. José Graziano da Silva, Mauro Eduardo Del Grossi, and Caio Galvão de França. Brasília: Ministry of Health.

Mangu-Ward, Katherine. 2010. "Nestle Barge to Ply the Amazon, Bringing Ice Cream and Rage." *Atlantic,* June 21.

Mannak, Miriam. 2009. "South Africa: Activists Lament Lack of HIV/TB Co-Treatment." Inter Press Service, March 26.

Manor, James. 1999. *The Political Economics of Decentralization.* Washington, DC: World Bank Group.

Marchant, P. W. 2015. "China's Response to HIV/AIDS Epidemic Questioned." *Washington Blade,* October 30.

Marias, Hein. 2000. *To the Edge: AIDS Review 2000.* Pretoria, South Africa: University of Pretoria.

Marshall, Sarah Jane. 2004. "South Africa Unveils National HIV/AIDS Treatment Program." *Bulletin of the World Health Organization* 82 (1): 73–74.

Mascarenhas, Anuradha. 2015. "Fund Crunch Forces NGOs to Quit HIV Prevention Project." *Indian Express,* October 13.

Mathole, T., A. Parsons, J. Cailhol, and D. Sanders. 2010. "GHIs in Africa: Challenges of Implementing Tuberculosis Control Programmes in South Africa." Poster presented at University of Western Cape, Cape Town.

Mattos, R., V. Terto, and R. Parker. 2003. "World Bank Strategies and the Response to AIDS in Brazil." *Divulgação em Saúde para Debate* 27:215–27.

Mawar, Nita, Seema Sahay, Apoorvaa Pandit, and Uma Mahajan. 2005. "The Third Phase of HIV Pandemic: Social Consequences of HIV/AIDS Stigma & Discrimination & Future Needs." *India Journal of Medical Research* 122:471–84.

Maxmen, Amy. 2009. "Salim 'Slim' Abdool Karim: Attracting AIDS in South Africa." *Journal of Experimental Medicine* 26 (11): 2306–7.

Mazower, Mark. 2008. *No Enchanted Palace: The End of Empire and the Ideological Origins of the United Nations.* Princeton, NJ: Princeton University Press.

Mbali, Mandisa. 2005. "TAC in the History of Rights-Based, Patient Driven HIV/AIDS Activism in South Africa." *Passages* (University of Michigan, Ann Arbor), no. 2 (June).

McClellan, Grant. 1962. *South Africa.* New York: H. W. Wilson Company.

McCullough, Marcy. 2005. "How NGOs Respond when the State Does Not: Confronting the Problem of HIV/AIDS in Russia." Paper presented at the conference Public Health and Demography in Russia, Harvard University, March 2005.

McGreal, Chris. 2002. "Mbeki Minister Attacks UN Fund's AIDS Grant." *Guardian* (London), July 22.

McGuire, James. 2010. *Wealth, Health, and Democracy in East Asia and Latin America.* New York: Cambridge University Press.

McNeil, Donald G., Jr. 1996. "Surprising Many, TB Is Found to Be Rampant in South Africa." *New York Times,* June 26.

Mead, Margaret. 1955. *Soviet Attitudes toward Authority.* New York: William Morrow & Company.

Meek, James. 1998. "Killer TB Threat to the World." *Guardian* (London), September 23.

Melorose, J., R. Perroy, and S. Careas. 2015. "We Die of TB." *Statewide Agricultural Land Use Baseline*, December.

Menkiszak, Marek, Rafal Sadowski, and Piotr Zochowski. 2014. "The Russian Military Intervention in Eastern Ukraine." *OSW,* September 3. www.osw.waw.pl/en /publikacje/analyses/2014-09-03/russian-military-intervention-eastern-ukraine.

Menon, Ramesh. 2016. "Bit for Health." *India Legal,* March 15.

Merten, Marianne. 2014. "Leading Causes of Death in SA Revealed." *IOL News,* December 3.

Miller, Mark, Scott Barrett, and D. A. Henderson. 2006. "Control and Eradication." In *Disease Control Priorities in Developing Countries,* ed. Dean Jamison, Joel Breman, Anthony Measham, George Alleyne, Mariam Claeson, David Evans, Anne Mills, and Philip Musgrove. Washington, DC: World Bank.

Milner, Helen, and Dustin Tingley, eds. 2013. *Geopolitics of Foreign Aid.* Northampton, MA: Edward Elgar Press.

Mirovalev, Mansur. 2016. "Is the Kremlin Fuelling Russia's HIV/AIDS Epidemic?" *Al Jazeera News,* July 19.

Misra, Rajiv. 2013. Interview with the author, March 29.

Miti, Andrew. 2013. AIDS Foundation of South Africa. Interview with the author, January 13.

Mitra, Pramit. 2004. "India at the Crossroads: Battling the HIV/AIDS Pandemic." *Washington Quarterly* 27 (4): 95–107.

Mitra, Pramit, Vibhuti Haté, and Teresita Schaffer. 2007. *India: Fitting HIV/AIDS into a Public Health Strategy.* Working paper, pp. 1–13. Washington, DC: Center for Strategic and International Studies.

Monteiro, C. A., and G. Cannon. 2012. "The Impact of Transnational 'Big Food' Companies on the South." *PLoS Medicine* 9 (7): e1001252.

Monteiro, Carlos, Wolney Conde, and Barry Popkin. 2002. "Is Obesity Replacing or Adding to Undernutrition? Evidence from Different Social Classes in Brazil." *Public Health Nutrition* 5:105–12.

———. 2007. "Income-Specific Trends in Obesity in Brazil: 1975–2003." *American Journal of Public Health* 97 (10): 1808–12.

Morrison, J. Stephen, and Jennifer Kates. 2006. *The G-8, Russia's Presidency, and HIV/ AIDS in Eurasia.* Washington, DC: Center for Strategic and International Studies.

Moscow Times. 2008. "Finding a Remedy for Health Care." August 22.

———. 2015. "Russian Incidence of Tuberculosis Falls by 30% over 10 Years." November 4.

Motihar, Renuka, and Vaishali Sharma Mahendra. 2003. "Strengthening India's Response to AIDS." *Sexual Health Exchange.* Journal discontinued.

Motsoeneng, Tilsetso. 2014. "Obesity, South Africa's Emerging Health Crisis." Reuters, December 10.

Mott, Luiz. 2003. *Homossexualidade: Mitos e Verdades.* Salvador, Brazil: Editora Grupo Gay de Bahia.

Mseleku, Thami. 2007. *New TB Plan for South Africa.* Pretoria, South Africa: Department of Health, November 8.

Mudur, G. S. 2008. "Overnight, Many Overweight Indian Figures Revised to Tone up Flab Fight." *Telegraph* (London), November 26.

Musgrave, Richard. 1959. *The Theory of Public Finance.* New York: McGraw-Hill.

Mushtaq, Muhammad Umair. 2009. "Public Health in British India: A Brief Account of the History of Medical Services and Diseases Prevention in Colonial India." *Indian Journal of Community Medicine* 34 (1): 6–14.

NACOSA. 1994. *A National AIDS Plan for South Africa 1994–95.* Pretoria, South Africa: National Secretariat, National AIDS Committee of South Africa.

Naidu, Sanusha. 2009. "Africa's New Development Partners: China and India: Challenging the Status Quo?" Paper presented at the conference Rethinking Development in an Age of Scarcity and Uncertainty, University of York, United Kingdom, September 19–22, 2011.

Nambiar, Devaki. 2012. "HIV-Related Stigma and NGO-isation in India: A Historico-Empirical Analysis." *Sociology of Health and Illness* 34 (5): 714–29.

Nandan Jha, Durgesh. 2014. "NACO No More an Independent Wing." TNN, September 5.

Nascimento, Dilene Raimundo. 2005. *As pestes do século XX: tuberculose e Aids no Brasil, uma história comparada.* Rio de Janeiro: Editora FIOCRUZ.

Nathanson, Constance. 1996. "Disease Prevention as Social Change: Toward a Theory of Public Health." *Population and Development Review* 22 (4): 609–37.

Nature. 2007. "South Africa's AIDS Plan." 447:1.

Nemyria, Hryhoriy. 2002. "Civil Society in Russia." In *Toward an Understanding of Russia: New European Perspective,* ed. Janusz Bugajski. New York: Council on Foreign Relations Press.

New Indian Express. 2010. "The Diva of Beauty and Wellness." May 21.

Newsholme, A., and J. Kingsbury. 1993. *Red Medicine: Socialized Health in Soviet Russia.* New York: Doubleday, Doran & Company.

Ng, Marie, et al. 2014. "Global, Regional, National Prevalence of Overweight and Obesity in Children and Adults 1980–2013: A Systematic Analysis for the Global Burden of Disease Study 2013." *Lancet* 384 (9945): 766–81.

Nicolson, Greg. 2015. "It's Time for Us to Notice: SA's Dying of TB." *Daily Maverick* (Johannesburg), March 25.

Nigam, Shailly. 2015. "India's Foreign AIDS: Social Responsibility or Hegemonic Strategy." *International Journal of Technical Research and Applications* 34:17–25.

Nordling, Linda. 2016. "Rising to the Nutrition Challenge: South Africa's New Obesity Research Centre." *Guardian* (London), February 24.

Norum, Baare. 2005. "World Health Organization's Global Strategy on Diet, Physical Activity and Health." *Scandinavian Journal of Nutrition* 49 (2): 83–88.

Nossel, Suzanne. 2016. "The World's Rising Powers Have Fallen." *Foreign Policy,* July 6.

Nunn, Amy, Samuel Dickman, Nicoli Nattrass, Alexandra Cornwall, and Sofia Grusking. 2012. "The Impacts of AIDS Movements on the Policy Responses to HIV/AIDS in Brazil and South Africa." *Global Public Health* 7 (10): 1031–44.

Nyaka, Owen. 2015. "Global Fund Green-Lights Regional TB Program for Miners in Southern Africa." *Aidspan,* August 18.

Oates, Wallace. 1999. "An Essay on Fiscal Federalism." *Journal of Economic Literature* 37 (3): 1120–49.

Obesity Reviews. 2008. "Special Issue: Obesity in China." 9 (1): 1–161.

O'Brien, Kevin. 2013. "Rightful Resistance Revisited." *Journal of Peasant Studies* 40 (6): 1051–62.

O Estado de São Paulo. 1987. "Aids, um pesadelo para o Brasil." August 9.

———. 1993. "Bird quer reforma urgente de saúde no 3 Mundo." July 7.

O Globo. 1987. "Kits estão acabando e deixarão de ser feitos 40 mil testes contra AIDS." September 27.

O'Hanlon, Oliver. 2012. "HIV Prevention Falls Short of Funding Ends." *Moscow Times,* February 16.

Okuonzi, S., and J. Macrae. 1995. "Whose Policy Is It Anyway? International and National Influences on Health Policy Development in Uganda." *Health Policy and Planning* 10 (2): 122–32.

One World. 2005. "Indian Claims of Decline in HIV Cases Dismays NGOs." *Civil Society Observer,* June 6.

Osadchuk, Svetlana. 2007. "Moscow—The Cabinet Has Tentatively Provided a $2.9 Billion Program Aimed at Raising the Country's Life Expectancy by Tackling AIDS, Diabetes, Tuberculosis and Other Diseases." *St. Petersburg Times,* February 27.

Osih, Regina, and Matshidiso Masire. 2012. "South Africa." In *Shifting Paradigm: How the BRICS Are Reshaping Global Health Development,* 71–75. New York: Global Health Strategies Initiatives.

Ostergard, Robert. 2007. "Leaders and Perceptions in Crisis: An Institutional Framework for Understanding Variations in African Governments Responses to the HIV/AIDS Epidemic." Paper presented at Comparative Politics Workshop, Department of Political Science, University of Pennsylvania.

Osterkatz, Sandra Chapman. 2011. "Capacity and Commitment: How Decentralization in Brazil Impacts Health Policy." Paper presented at the Annual Meeting of the American Political Science Association, Seattle, September 1–4.

Overy, Neil. 2011. *In the Face of Crisis.* International Budget Partnership study no. 7. Washington, DC: International Budget Partnership Press, August.

Oxfam. 2015. *Most Successful Cases of Civil Society Strategies for the Policy Impact in South Africa.* Workshop report. Oxford: Oxfam.

Pahwa, Divya, and Daniel Beland. 2013. "Federalism, Decentralization, and Health Care Policy Reform in India." *Public Administration Research* 2 (1): 1–10.

Paiva, V., L. Pupo, and R. Barboza. 2006. "The Right to Prevention and the Challenges of Reducing Vulnerability to HIV in Brazil." *Revista de Saúde Pública* 40:S1-10.

Palmer, Steven, and Gilberto Hochman. 2010. "A Canadian-Brazil Network in the Global Eradication of Smallpox." *Canadian Journal of Public Health* 101 (2): 113–18.

Pandey, Kundan. 2016. "India's Obesity Doubled in 10 Years." *DowntoEarth,* January 20.

Panina, Maria. 2016. "Russia Activists Struggle to Raise HIV Awareness as Epidemic Grows." Report of the Andrey Rylkov Foundation for Health and Social Justice, Moscow, June 4.

Pape, Maria. 2014. *The Politics of HIV/AIDS in Russia.* New York: Routledge.

Parker, Richard. 2003. "Building the Foundations for the Response to HIV/AIDS in Brazil." *Divulgacão em Saúde para Debate* 27:143–83.

————. 2009. "Civil Society, Political Mobilization, and the Impact of HIV Scale-up on Health Systems in Brazil." *JAIDS Journal of Acquired Immune Deficiency Syndrome* 52:49–51.

Parker, Richard, Jane Galvão, and Marcelo Secron Bessa, eds. 1999. *Saúde, Desenvolvimento, e Política: Respostas frente á AIDS no Brasil.* Rio de Janeiro: ABIA Publications.

Parkhurst, Justin, and Louisiana Lush. 2004. "The Political Environment of HIV: Lessons from a Comparison of Uganda and South Africa." *Social Science and Medicine* 59:1913–24.

Parra, D., C. Hoehner, P. Halal, R. Ris, E. Simoes, and D. Malta. 2013. "Scaling up Physical Activity Interventions in Brazil: How Partnerships and Research Evidence Contributed to Policy Action." *Global Health Promotion* 20 (4): 5–12.

Parry, Hazel. 2010. " 'Pot Bellied' Hong Kongers Warned of Deadly Lifestyles." *China Daily*, February 17.

Parry, Jane. 2008. "China's Pragmatic Approach to AIDS." *Bulletin of the World Health Organization* 84 (4): 1.

Parth, Shubhendu. 2008. "Nutrition Policy for Healthy India on Cards." *iGovernment News*, April 24.

Passarelli, Carlos, and Cristina Pimenta. 2012. "Brazil." In *Shifting Paradigm: How the BRICS Are Reshaping Global Health Development*, 19–29. New York: Global Health Strategies Initiatives.

Patil, Shailaja, Jamie Ports, Malikarjun Yadavanavar, and Solveig Cunningham. 2016. "Physicians' Perceptions about the Emergence of Adolescent Overweight in India." *Journal of Krishna Institute of Medical Sciences University* 5 (1): 37–44.

Patterson, Amy. 2006. *The Politics of AIDS in Africa*. Boulder, CO: Lynne Rienner Publishers.

Peard, Julyan. 1999. *Race, Place, and Medicine: The Idea of the Tropics in Nineteenth Century Brazil*. Durham, NC: Duke University Press.

People's Daily. 2001. "Conference on Obesity Solutions Held in Beijing." June 28.

People's Daily Online. 2009. "The History of AIDS in China." November 22.

Perelman, M. 2000. "Tuberculosis in Russia." *International Journal of Tuberculosis and Lung Disease* 4 (12): 1097–1103.

Perry, Alex. 2005. "When Silence Kills." *TIME*, June 6.

Pfister, Roger. 2000. "South Africa's Post-Apartheid Foreign Policy towards Africa." *Electronic Journal of Africana Bibliography* 6:1–41.

Pierson, Paul. 2003. "When Effect Becomes Cause: Policy Feedback and Political Change." *World Politics* 45 (4): 595–628.

Pilling, David. 2014. "The BRICS Bank Is a Glimpse of the Future." *Financial Times*, July 30.

Pioneer. 2016. "WHO, India Concerned over Rising Obesity." January 28.

Pires, Reibeiro. 2006. "Alguns Apontamentos Sobre o Processo de Descentralização do Programa de Aids." Master's thesis, Universidade do Estado do Rio de Janeiro-Instituto de Medicina Social.

Pontodepauta. 2012. "Ação contra Obesidade Infantil Antingirá 2.593 escolas do Rio Grande do Norte."

Popkin, Barry. 2006. "Technology, Transport, Globalization, and the Nutrition Transition Food Policy." *Food Policy* 31 (6): 554–69.

Portal Brasil. 2016. "Ações do Governo Combatem Obesidade e Sobrepeso." April 10.

Potarazu, Sreedhar. 2015. "Is India Too Fat?" CNN, September 18.

Powell, D. E. 2000. "The Problem of AIDS." In *Russia's Torn Safety Net*, ed. Judith Twigg. New York: St. Martin's Press.

Prasad, Vandana. 2014. "The Fast Food Bomb." *Hindu*, August 1.

Price, Gareth. 2011. *For the Global Good: India's Developing International Role*. London: Chatham House.

Pritchett, Lant, and Michael Woolcock. 2004. "Solutions When the Solution Is the Problem: Arraying the Disarray in Development." *World Development* 32 (2): 191–212.

Provost, Claire. 2011. "The Rebirth of Russian Foreign Aid." *Guardian* (London), May 25.

Prud'homme, Remy. 1995. "The Dangers of Decentralization." *World Bank Observer* 10:201–20.

Przeworksi, A., and H. Teune. 1970. *The Logic of Comparative Social Inquiry.* Medford, MA: Wiley Interscience.

Puhl, Rebecca, and Chelsea Heuer. 2010. "Obesity Stigma: Important Considerations for Public Health." *American Journal of Public Health* 100 (6): 1019–28.

Putzel, James. 2004. "The Politics of Action on AIDS: A Case Study of Uganda." *Public Administration and Development* 24:19–30.

Pye, Lucian. 1996. "The State and the Individual: An Overview Interpretation." In *The Individual and the State in China*, ed. Brian Hook, 16–42. New York: Oxford University Press / Clarendon Paperbacks.

Quinn, Allison. 2014. "Experts Say Russia Ill-Equipped to Fight HIV." *St. Petersburg Times*, August 18.

Radio Free Europe. 2016. "Russia Leads Efforts to Strip Gay De-criminalization from UN Measures." July 26.

Rajshekhar, M. 2015. "AIDS Is about to Explode in Mizaram and the Modi Government Is Partly To Blame." *Scroll.in*, May 1.

Rakhamgulov, M. 2010. "Establishing International Development Assistance Strategy." *International Organizations Research Journal* 5 (31): 50–67.

Rani, Anita. 2013. "India's Supersize Kids." *Huffington Post*, August 13.

Ranjani, Harish, Rajendra Pradeepa, T. S. Mehreen, Ranjit Mohan Anjana, Krishnan Anand, Renu Garg, and Viswanathan Mohan. 2014. "Determinants, Consequences and Prevention of Childhood Overweight and Obesity." *Indian Journal of Endocrinology and Metabolism* 18 (S1): 17–25.

Rao, Krishna, Varduhi Petrosyan, Edson Correia Araujo, and Diane McIntyre. 2014. "Progress towards Universal Health Coverage in BRICS." *Bulletin of the World Health Organization* 92:429–435.

Rao, Sushila. 2004. *The Global Strategy on Diet, Physical Activity, and Health: Relevance and Implications for India.* Policy report. Delhi: WHO India Office.

Ras, G. J., I. W. Simson, R. Anderson, O. W. Prozesky, and T. Hamersma. 1983. "Acquired Immunodeficiency Syndrome: A Report of Two South African Cases." *South African Medical Journal* 64 (4): 140–42.

Rau, Bill. 2006. "The Politics of Civil Society in Confronting HIV/AIDS." *International Affairs* 82 (2): 285–95.

Ravelo, Jenny. 2014a. "For NGOs in South Africa, Reality Gets Tougher." *Inside Development*, May 9.

———. 2014b. "Is Emerging South Africa Ready to Fight TB on Its Own?" *Devex*, March 26.

Recine, Elisabetta. 2016. Interview with the author, June 6.

Reddy, K. Srinath. 2003. *Prevention and Control of Non-communicable Diseases: Status and Strategies.* Working Paper 104. New Delhi: Indian Council for Research on International Economic Relations.

Reddy, K. Srinath, Bela Shah, Cherian Varghese, and Anbumani Ramadoss. 2005. "Responding to the Threat of Chronic Diseases in India." *Lancet* 366:1744–49.

Reis, C. E., I. A. Vasconcelos, and J. Faias de N. Barros. 2011. "Políticas Públicas de Nutrição para o Controle da Obesidade Infantile." *Revista Paulista de Pediatria* 29 (4): 625–33.

Renmin Ribao. 2010a. "China to Establish National Nutrition-Monitoring System." August 13.

———. 2010b. "China, US Separated by Ocean of Fat, but for How Long?" June 14.
Resende-Santos, João. 1997. "Fernando Henrique Cardoso: Social and Institutional Rebuilding in Brazil." In *Technopols: Freeing Politics and Markets in Latin America in the 1990s*, ed. Jorge Dominguez, 145–94. University Park: Pennsylvania State University Press.
Rethinking AIDS. 2000. "India Holds AIDS Reappraisal Conference." 8 (1): 1.
Reuters. 2010. "The Chubby Girl from Ipanema? Brazil Puts on Weight." August 27.
———. 2015a. "Chastity, Filth & Patriotism." October 23.
———. 2015b. "HIV Alarm: Number of Infected in Russia May Double in 4 Years, Experts Warn." May 15.
Reynolds, Kristi, Dongfeng Gu, Paul K. Whelton, Xigui Wu, Xiufang Duan, Jinping Mo, and Jiang He. 2007. "Prevalence and Risk Factors of Overweight and Obesity in China." *Obesity* 15:10–18.
Rich, Jessica. 2010. "Grassroots Bureaucracy: Mobilizing the AIDS Movement in Brazil, 1983–2010." PhD dissertation, Department of Political Science, University of California, Berkeley.
Rich, Jessica, and Eduardo J. Gómez. 2012. "Centralizing Decentralized Governance in Brazil." *Publius: Journal of Federalism* 42 (4): 636–61.
Rigby, Neville. 2006. "Commentary: Counterpoint to Campos et al." *International Journal of Epidemiology* 35 (1): 79–80.
Roberto de Almeida, Paulo. 2012. *Relações Internacionais e Política External do Brasil*. Rio de Janeiro: Livros Técnicos e Científicos Editora.
———. 2013. "Brazil-USA Relations during the Fernando Henrique Cardoso Governments." In *Brazil–United States Relations: XX and XXI Centuries*, ed. Sidnei Munhoz and Francisco Carlos Teixeira da Silva, 217–246. Maringá, Brazil: Eduem.
Rochan, M. 2014. "India: Government Slashes Health Budget by $947m." *International Business Times* (New Delhi), December 23.
Rockefeller Foundation. 2013. *Our Long History in Asia*. New York: Rockefeller Foundation.
Rossiyskaya Gazeta. 1998a. "Russia: Decree on Tuberculosis Program 1998 2004." August 6.
———. 1998b. "Tuberculosis Program for 1998–2004." August 6.
Rozhdestvensky, Ilya. 2015. "Awash in AIDS: How Russia's Economic Crisis Is Skyrocketing HIV Infections Again." *Meduza*, September 15.
RSA (Republic of South Africa). 2007. *Tuberculosis Strategic Plan for South Africa, 2007–11*. Cape Town, South Africa: Department of Health.
———. 2010. "South Africans Praise Latest HIV/AIDS Testing Campaign." Press release, April 27. Accessed at Access World News, www.newsbank.com.
———. 2012a. *Department of Basic Education Integrated Strategic HIV, STI's and TB, 2012–2016*. Pretoria: Department of Basic Education.
———. 2012b. *National Strategic Plan on HIV, STIs, and TB, 2012–2016*. Pretoria: South Africa National AIDS Council.
———. 2013. *Global AIDS Response Progress Report*. Pretoria: Republic of South Africa.
———. 2016. *South African HIV and TB Investment Care*. Pretoria: South Africa National AIDS Council.
RSA, Department of Health. 2011.
Ru, Xiaomei. 2006. "Youth and HIV/AIDS in China." In *AIDS and Social Policy in China*, ed. Joan Kaufman, Arthur Kleinman, and Tony Saich, 96–124. Cambridge, MA: Harvard University Asia Center.

Rubin, Kyna. 2002. "The Butterfly and the Sword: AIDS in China." *Health Affairs* 21 (3): 221–27.

Ruger, Jennifer. 2005a. "The Changing Role of the World Bank in Global Health." *American Journal of Public Health* 95 (1): 60–70.

———. 2005b. "Democracy and Health." *Quarterly Journal of Medicine* 98:229–304.

Ruger, Jennifer, and Nora Ng. 2010. "Emerging and Transitioning Countries' Role in Global Health." *St. Louis University Journal of Health Law and Policy* 3 (2): 253–89.

Ruggie, John. 1998. "What Makes the World Hang Together? Neo-Utilitarianism and the Social Constructivist Challenge." *International Organization* 52 (4): 855–85.

Ruhl, Christof, Vadim Pokrovsky, and Viatcheslav Vinogradov. 2002. *The Economic Consequences of HIV in Russia*. World Bank report. Moscow: World Bank.

Russia, Federal Service for Surveillance on Consumer Rights Protection and Human Wellbeing. 2015. *About a New Sustainable Development Agenda until 2030*. Moscow: Government of Russia, June 6.

Russia, Ministry of Health. 2009. *Tuberculosis in the Russian Federation: An Analytical Review of the TB Statistical Indicators Used in the Russian Federation*. Moscow: Ministry of Health and Social Development.

Russian Federation. n.d. *Official Development Assistance*. National report. Moscow: Russian Federation.

Russian Presidency. 2015. "Russia for Joining BRICS Efforts against Tuberculosis." Official website, October 30. http://brics5.co.za/russia-for-joining-brics-efforts-against-tuberculosis/.

Russo, Giuliano, Lídia Cabral, and Paulo Ferrinho. 2013. "Brazil-Africa Technical Cooperation in Health: What's Its Relevance to the Post-Busan Debate on 'Aid Effectivenss'?" *Globalization and Health* 9 (2): 1–8.

SAARC (South Asian Association for Regional Cooperation). 2009. "SAARC Health Ministerial Meetings."

Sachan, Dinsa. 2014. "India's AIDS Department Merger Angers Activists." *Lancet* 384:842.

Sagar, Gauri. 2001. "VLCC and India Medical Association, Gurgaon Observe Anti-Obesity Day," *BusinessWire*, November 26.

Saich, Tony. 2006. "Social Policy Development in the Era of Economic Reform." In *AIDS and Social Policy in China*, ed. Joan Kaufman, Arthur Kleinman, and Tony Saich, 16–45. Cambridge, MA: Harvard University Asia Center.

Salama, B., and D. Benoliel. 2010. "Pharmaceutical Patents Bargains: The Brazilian Experience." *Cardozo Journal of International and Comparative Law* 18 (3): 633–85.

Salifu, Uyo. 2010. "South Africa's Niche in the United Nations and Africa's Hope for the Future." *Consultancy Africa Intelligence*, December 2.

Saltman, Richard. 2008. "Decentralization, Re-centralization and Future European Health Policy." *European Journal of Public Health* 18 (2): 104–6.

Salve, Prachi. 2014. "How Obesity Is Rising in India & Falling in the West." *IndiaSpend*, January 7.

Sankaran, J. R. 2006. "Current Situation of HIV/AIDS in India and Our Response." *Journal, Indian Academy of Clinical Medicine* 7 (1): 13–15.

Santos Filho, Ezio T., and S. Gomes. 2007. "Strategies for Tuberculosis Control in Brazil: Networking and Civil Societal Participation." *Revista de Saude Publica* 41:111–16.

SAPA (South African Press Association). 1998a. "Democratic Party Wants AIDS to Become a State Priority Concern." Cape Town, October 14. Accessed at Access World News, www.newsbank.com.

———. 1998b. "Deputy President Launches National Anti-AIDS Campaign." Johannesburg, October 9. Accessed at Access World News, www.newsbank.com.

———. 1998c. "RSA: HIV-AIDS Pandemic 'Fuelled by the Apartheid Legacy.'" November 30. Accessed at Access World News, www.newsbank.com.

Scarlatelli, Andrea. 2010. "American Junk Food: Why So Popular?" *eChinacities.com*, October 29.

Schaffer, Teresita, and Pramit Mitra. 2004. *India at the Crossroads: Confronting the HIV/AIDS Challenge.* Report of the CSIS HIV/AIDS delegation to India. Washington, DC: Center for Strategic and International Studies.

Schmidt, Fabiane. 2014. *Ministério da Saúde Lança Guia Alimentar para o População Brasilera.* Brasília: Ministry of Health.

Schneider, Helen. 2002. "On the Fault-Line: The Politics of AIDS Policy in Contemporary South Africa." *African Studies* 61 (1): 145–67.

Schneider, Helen, Hlengiwe Hlophe, and Dingie van Rensburg. 2008. "Community Health Workers and the Response to HIV/AIDS in South Africa: Tensions and Prospects." *Health Policy and Planning* 23:179–87.

Schneider, Helen, and Joanne Stein. 2001. "Implementing AIDS Policy in Post-Apartheid South Africa." *Social Science and Medicine* 52:723–31.

Schwirtz, Michael. 2011. "Inadequate Fight against Drugs Hampers Russia's Ability to Curb H.I.V." *New York Times*, January 16. www.nytimes.com/2011/01/17/world/europe/17russia.html.

Sen, Amartya. 1999. *Development as Freedom.* New York: Knopf.

Sengupta, A. 2013. *Universal Health Care in India.* Occasional paper no. 19, ed. D. A. McDonald and G. Ruiters. Ottawa: Municipal Services Project.

Senthilingam, Meera. 2014. "Beating the Bulge: Brazil's Burgeoning Obesity Problem." CNN, July 9.

Shaffer, M. 2012. Interview with the author, September 13.

Shao, Yiming. 2013. "A Practical Way to Improve Access to Essential Medicines against Major Infectious Disease." In *HIV/AIDS Treatment in Resource Poor Countries: Public Health Challenges*, ed. Yichen Lu, Max Essex, and Chris Chanyasulkit. New York: Springer.

Sharma, Dinesh. 2015. "Budget Cuts Threaten AIDS and Tuberculosis Control in India." *Lancet* 386:942.

Shetty, Prakash. 2002. "Nutrition Transition in India." *Public Health Nutrition* 5 (1A): 175–82.

Shiffman, Jeremy. 2009. "A Social Explanation for the Rise and Fall of Global Health Issues." *Bulletin of the World Health Organization* 87 (8): 608–13.

Shiffman, Jeremy, and Stephanie Smith. 2007. "Generation of Political Priority for Global Health Initiatives: A Framework and Case Study of Maternal Mortality." *Lancet* 370 (9595): 1370–79.

Shilova, Margarita, and Christopher Dye. 2001. "The Resurgence of Tuberculosis in Russia." *Philosophical Transactions of Royal Society of London* 356:1069–75.

Shilts, Randy. 1987. *And the Band Played On: Politics, People, and the AIDS Epidemic.* New York: St. Martin's Press.

Shrivastava, Bhuma. 2008. "350 NGOs Sacked Mega NACO Clean-up." *LiveMint*, January 30.

Shukdev, Mahima. 2008. "Obese India: A Ticking Time Bomb." *India-Forums*, November 25.

Sichieri, Rosely. 2002. "Dietary Patterns and Their Association with Obesity in the Brazilian City of Rio de Janeiro." *Obesity Research* 10 (1): 42–48.

Sidley, Pat. 2000. "Govt Committed to Fighting AIDS." *Business Day* (Johannesburg), March 20. Accessed at Access World News, www.newsbank.com.

Siko, John. 2014. *Inside South Africa's Foreign Policy.* New York: I. B. Tauris & Co.

Silva, Renato, and Carlos Henrique Assunção Paiva. 2015. "The Juscelino Kubitschek Government and the Brazilian Malaria Control and Eradication Working Group: Collaboration and Conflicts in Brazilian and International Health Agenda, 1958–1961." *História, Ciências, Saúde-Manguinhos* 22 (1): 1–20.

Simelela, N. P., and W. D. F. Venter. 2014. "A Brief History of South Africa's Response to AIDS." *South African Medical Journal* 104 (3): 249–51.

Singh, Neelanjana. 2013. Heinz Foundation, Chenai, India. Interview with the author, February 5.

Sjostedt, Roxanna. 2008. "Exploring the Construction of Threats: The Securitization of HIV/AIDS in Russia." *Security Dialogue* 39:7–29.

Skocpol, Theda, and Edwin Amenta. 1986. "States and Social Policies." *Annual Review of Sociology* 12:131–57.

Skolnick, Richard. 2013. Interview with the author, February 8.

Smallman, Shawn. 2007. *The AIDS Pandemic in Latin America.* Chapel Hill: University of North Carolina Press.

Smith, Lydia. 2015. "Why Are Rates of Drug-Resistant TB So High in Russia?" *IB Times*, March 23.

Smoke, Paul, Eduardo Gómez and George Peterson, eds. 2006. *Decentralization in Asia and Latin America.* Northampton, MA: Edward Elgar Publishing.

Soares, Lucila, and Cecília Ritto. 2010. "Pesquisa do IBGE Confirma que Obesidade é Epidemia no Brasil." *Veja.com*, August 27.

Solomon, Suniti, and Aylur Kailasam Ganesh. 2002. "HIV in India." *International AIDS Society* 10 (3): 19–24.

Solomon, Susan Gross. 1990. "Social Hygiene and Soviet Public Health, 1921–1930." In *Health and Society in Revolutionary Russia*, ed. Susan Gross Solomon and John F. Hutchinson, 176–99. Bloomington: Indiana University Press.

Sonke Gender Justice. 2015. "South African Civil Society Groups Call for the Reinstatement of Joint Committee on HIV/AIDS." February 11.

Soto, Alonso, and Peter Murphy. 2011. "Brazil Says BRICS Offer Conditional Help to Europe." Reuters, December 2.

Soul City Research Unit. 2015. *Literature Review of TB in South Africa.* Pretoria, South Africa: Department of Health.

South African History Online. 2011. "South Africa's Foreign Relations during Apartheid (1948–)." March 30.

Souza, S., K. Lima, H. Miranda, and F. Cavalcanti. 2011. "Utilização da informação nutricional de rótulos por consumidores de Natal, Brasil." *Revista Panamericana de Salud Pública* 29:337–41.

Specter, M. 1997. "AIDS Onrush Sends Russia to the Edge of an Epidemic." *New York Times*, May 18.

Spence, Jack. 1975. "South Africa and the Modern World." In *The Oxford History of South Africa*, ed. Monica Wilson and Leonard Thompson. Oxford: Oxford University Press.

Sridhar, Devi, Claire Brolan, Shireen Durrani, Jennifer Edge, Lawrence Gostin, Peter Hill, and Martin McKee. 2013. "Recent Shifts in Global Governance: Implications for the Response to Non-Communicable Disease." *PLoS Medicine* 10 (7): e1001487.

Sridhar, Devi, and Eduardo J. Gómez. 2010. "Health Financing in Brazil, Russia, and India: What Role Does the International Community Play?" *Health Policy and Planning* 25 (6): 1–13.

Sridharan, Eswaran. 2014. "The Emerging Foreign Assistance Policies of India and China: India as a Development Partner." Unpublished manuscript, University of Pennsylvania, Institute for the Advanced Study of India.

Srigyan, Deepankar. 2008. *Social-Hygienic Problems of Public Health and Public Health Systems in Countries around the World: India.* Moscow: Department of Medicine, People's Friendship University of Russia.

Srivastava, Roli, and S. Rukmini. 2016. "Rural India Too Battles Hypertension." *Hindu,* January 22.

Stapleton, D. H. 2005. "Lewis W. Hackett and the Early Years of the International Health Board's Yellow Fever Program in Brazil, 1917–1924." *Parassitologia* 47 (3): 353–60.

Stein, Jeannine. 2009. "China Turns to the US for Help with Overweight Kids." *Los Angeles Times,* April 20.

Stepan, Nancy. 1976. *Beginnings of Brazilian Science: Oswaldo Cruz, Medical Research and Policy, 1890–1920.* New York: Science History Publications.

Stolyarova, Galina. 2010. "Russia Marks World AIDS Day with Protests, Burials." *St. Petersburg Times,* December 3.

Stracansky, Pavol. 2014a. "Outdated Approaches Fuelling TB in Russia, Say NGOs." Inter Press Service, July 14.

———. 2014b. *Outdated Approaches Fueling TB in Society.* Andrey Rylkov Foundation for Health and Social Justice, July 14.

Strachan, Kathryn. 2000. "TB from a Provincial Manager's Perspective." *HST Update* 56:1.

Strand, Per, Khabele Matlosa, Ann Strode, and Kondwani Chirambo. 2007. *HIV/AIDS and Democratic Governance in South Africa: Illustrating the Impact of Electoral Processes.* Pretoria, South Africa: Institute for Democracy in South Africa.

Stuckler, David, Sanjay Basu, and Martin McKee. 2010. "Governance of Mining, HIV and Tuberculosis in Southern Africa." *Global Health Governance* 4 (1): 1–13.

Subramanian, Mangala. 2013. "The Medicalization of HIV/AIDS Policy: The Case of India." In *Global HIV/AIDS Politics, Policy, and Activism: Persistent Challenges and Emerging Issues,* ed. Raymond Smith. Santa Monica, CA: Praeger.

Sun, Helen Lei. 2011. *Understanding China's Agricultural Investments.* Occasional paper no. 102. Johannesburg: South Africa Institute of International Affairs.

Swinburn, B. A., I. Caterson, J. C. Seidell, and W. P. T. James. 2004. "Diet, Nutrition and the Prevention of Excess Weight Gain and Obesity." *Public Health Nutrition* 7 (1A): 123–46.

Tabachnik, Alexander. 2016. "Russia in Ukraine and Syria: Strengths and Weaknesses." *New Eastern Europe,* January 8. http://neweasterneurope.eu/articles-and-commentary /1851-russia-in-ukraine-and-syria-strengths-and-weaknesses.

Takagi, Maya, and José Graziano da Silva. 2011. "New and Old Challenges to Achieve Food Security in the 21st Century." In *The Fome Zero (Zero Hunger) Program: The Brazilian Experience,* ed. José Graziano da Silva, Mauro Eduardo Del Grossi, and Caio Gavão de França. Brasília: Ministry of Agrarian Development.

TakePart. 2015. "India's Obesity Problem Is So Huge, Officials Want to Ban Junk-Food Sales to Students." August 21.

Tatlow, Didi. 2015. "Rise in HIV among China's Youth Draws Attention for World AIDS Day." *New York Times,* November 30.

Teixeira, Paulo. 1997. "Políticas Públicas em Aids." In *Políticas, Instituicões e Aids: Enfrentando a Epidemia no Brasil*, ed. Richard Parker, 43–68. Rio de Janeiro: ABIA Publications.

Tendler, J. 1997. *Getting Good Government in the Tropics.* Baltimore: Johns Hopkins University Press.

Teodorescu, Lindialva Laurindo, and Paulo Roberto Teixeira. 2015. *Histórias da AIDS No Brasil: As Respostas governamentais á Epidemia de AIDS.* Brasília: Ministry of Health.

Thaindian News. 2010. "47 Crore Condoms' Sale Targeted in AIDS Control Programme." August 2.

Thakur, Vineet. 2015. "Foreign Policy and Its People: Transforming the Apartheid Department of Foreign Affairs." *Diplomacy and Statecraft* 26:514–33.

Tharkar, Shabana, and Vijay Viswanathan. 2009. "Impact of Socioeconomic Status on Prevalence of Overweight and Obesity among Children and Adolescents in Urban India." *Open Obesity Journal* 1:9–14.

Thatchenko-Schmidt, E., R. Atun, M. Wall, P. Tobi, J. Schmidt, and A. Renton. 2010. "Why Do Health Systems Matter? Exploring Links between Health Systems and HIV Response: A Case Study from Russia." *Health Policy and Planning* 25 (4): 283–91.

Thekaekara, Mari. 2015. "Indian Schools Told to Junk the Junk Food." *New Internationalist*, May 22.

Thompson, Caitlin. 2014. "Russia's Struggle with Tuberculosis." *Borgen Magazine*, June 27.

Thompson, Drew. 2003. "Pre-empting an HIV/AIDS Disaster in China." *Seton Hall Journal of Diplomacy and International Relations*, Summer/Fall: 29–43.

Thompson, Leonard, and Andrew Prior. 1982. *South African Politics.* New Haven, CT: Yale University Press.

Times Live (South Africa). 2016. "Government, Religious Leaders Join Forces to Fight Scourge of TB." July 17.

Times of India. 2000. "Conference on Obesity in Mumbai." February 2.

———. 2007. "Couch Potatoes on the Rise." April 13.

———. 2012. "Big Food Brands Hid Harmful Effects, Claims Delhi-Based NGO Centre for Science and Environment." March 31.

Tkatchenko-Schmidt, Elena, Rifat Atun, Martin Wall, Patrick Tobi, Jürgen Schmidt, and Adrian Renton. 2010. "Why Do Health Systems Matter? Exploring Links between Health System and Response: A Case Study of Russia." *Health Policy and Planning* 25 (4): 283–91.

Tobergate, David. 2013. "NSP Review Comment." *Journal of Chemical Information* 14.

Toor, Amar. 2015. "Russia Has a Serious HIV Crisis, and the Government Is to Blame." *Verge*, July 2.

Topolev, Andrei, and Elena Topoleva. 2001. "Nongovernmental Organizations: Building Blocks for Russia's Civil Society." In *Russia's Fate through Russian Eyes*, ed. Heyward Isham. Boulder, CO: Westview Press.

Tran, Nhan, Sara Bennett, Rituparna Bishnu, and Suneeta Singh. 2013. "Analyzing the Sources and Nature of Influence: How the Avahan Program Used Evidence to Influence HIV/AIDS Prevention Policy in India." *Implementation Science* 8 (44): 1–11.

Treatment Action Campaign. 2011. "Mobilise against TB." Online report. www.tac.org.za.

Tripathi, Amitava. 2011. "Prospects of India Becoming a Global Power." *Indian Foreign Affairs Journal* 6 (1): 58–69.

Troilo, Pete. 2012. "For Russia Foreign Aid, a Second Act." *Inside Development,* March 19.

Twigg, Judith. 2007. *HIV/AIDS in Russia: Commitment, Resources, Momentum, Challenges.* Report of the Task Force on HIV/AIDS. Washington, DC: Center for Strategic and International Studies.

Twigg, Judith, and Richard Skolnick. 2005. *Evaluation of the World Bank's Assistance in Responding to the AIDS Epidemic: Russian Case Study.* Washington, DC: World Bank Group.

Tyurin, I. 2016. "Fighting Tuberculosis in Russia Remains a Challenge." *Healthcare-in-Europe.com,* March 8.

Uchimura, Hiroko, and Johannes Jütting. 2007. *Fiscal Decentralization, Chinese Style: Good for Health Outcomes?* Working paper no. 264. Paris: OECD Development Center.

UNAIDS. 1999. *UNAIDS and Non-governmental Organizations.* Geneva: UNAIDS.

———. 2002. *HIV/AIDS: China's Titanic Peril.* Geneva: UNAIDS.

———. 2003. *The "Three Ones" Key Principles.* Geneva: UNAIDS.

———. 2004. *2004 Update. South Africa. Epidemiological Fact Sheets.* Geneva: UNAIDS.

———. 2008. *2008 Update. China. Epidemiological Fact Sheet on HIV and AIDS.* Geneva: UNAIDS.

———. 2014. *Antiretroviral therapy coverage.* The World Bank Group Databank. Washington, DC. http://data.worldbank.org/indicator/SH.HIV.ARTC.ZS. Geneva: UNAIDS.

———. 2015. *2015 China AIDS Response Progress Report.* Geneva: UNAIDS.

UNDP. 2015. *The Policy and Legal Environments Related to HIV Services in China.* Geneva: UNDP.

UN General Assembly. 2010. *India: Country Progress Report.* New York: United Nations.

United Kingdom, House of Commons. 2009. *HIV/AIDS: DFID's New Strategy: Government Response to the Committee's Twelfth Report of Session 2007–08.* London: House of Commons.

United Nations. 2006. *Report of the Standing Committee on Nutrition at Its Thirty-Third Session.* Geneva: United Nations.

———. 2007. *Thirty-Fourth Session of the Standing Committee on Nutrition, SCN Working Group on Nutrition, Ethics and Human Rights.* Geneva: United Nations.

Unnikrishnan, Ambika Gopalkrishnan, Sanjay Kalra, and M. K. Garg. 2012. "Preventing Obesity in India." *Indian Journal of Endocrinology and Metabolism* 16 (1): 4–6.

Vandenbosch, Amry. 1970. *South Africa and the World: The Foreign Policy of Apartheid.* Louisville: University of Kentucky Press.

Van der Merwe, Marelise. 2015. "South Africa's Longest Walk to Freedom from HIV/AIDS." *Daily Maverick* (Johannesburg), December 1.

Van der Veen, A. Maurits. 2011. *Ideas, Interests, and Foreign Aid.* New York: Cambridge University Press.

Van der Vliet, Virginia. 2004. "South Africa Divided against AIDS: A Crisis of Leadership." In *AIDS and South Africa: The Social Expression of a Pandemic,* ed. K. D. Kaufman and D. L. Lindauer. Basingstoke, UK: Palgrave Macmillan.

Vangelder, Ben. 2011. "The HIV/AIDS Crisis in Russia." *Yale Journal of Medicine and Law* 7 (2): 1.

Varadharajan, Kiruba, Tinku Thomas, and Anura Kurpad. 2013. "Poverty and the State of Nutrition in India." *Asia Pacific Journal of Clinical Nutrition* 22 (3): 326–39.

Varshney, V. 2006. "Corporate Pressure May Put India's Obesity Prevention Plans on Hold." *DownToEarth News*, October 1. www.downtoearth.org.in/news/corporate -pressure-may-put-indias-obesity-prevention-plans-on-hold-8493.

Vass, Jocelyn. 2005. *A Review of Labour Markets in South Africa: The Impact of HIV/AIDS on the Labour Market in South Africa*. Pretoria, South Africa: Human Sciences Research Council.

Veeken, Hans. 1998. "Russia: Sex, Drugs, and AIDS and MSF." *BMJ* 316:138–39.

Veja. 1985. "AIDS." August 14.

Veloso, I., and V. Santana. 2009. "Impacto nutritional do programa de alimentação do trabalhodor no Brasil." *Revista Panamericana de Salud Publica* 11 (1): 24–31.

Vigitel. 2014. *Vigalência de Fatores de Risco e Proteção para Doenças Crônicas por Inqérito Telefônico*. Brasília: Ministry of Health.

Visão: Revista Semanal de Informação. 1985. "A Verdade onde Estara?" October 16.

Walgate, Robert. 2002. "AIDS Could Dominate Russian Budget by 2020." *Bulletin of the World Health Organization* 80:686–87.

Wallander, Celeste. 2005. *The Politics of Russian AIDS Policy*. PONARS policy memo no. 389. Washington, DC: Center for Strategic and International Studies.

Wang, H., and F. Zhai. 2013. "Programme and Policy Options for Prevention of Obesity in China." *Obesity Reviews* 14 (2): 134–40.

Wang, Hongying. 2003. "National Image Building and Chinese Foreign Policy." *China: An International Journal* 1:46–72.

Wang, Jenny, Minquan Liu, Tao We, and Hang Li. 2013. "Global Health Governance in China." In *Asia's Role in Governing Global Health*, ed. Kelley Lee, Tikki Pang, and Yeling Tan. Oxford: Routledge.

Wang, Longde. 2007. "Overview of the HIV/AIDS Epidemic, Scientific Research and Government Responses in China." *AIDS* 21 (8): S3-7.

Wang, Yan. 2011. *International Health Cooperation in China*. Regional Outlook paper no. 20. Nathan, Queensland, Australia: Griffith Asia Institute, Griffith University.

Wang, Yiwei. 2008. "Public Diplomacy and the Rise of Chinese Soft Power." *Annals AAPS* 616:257–73.

Wang, Youfa, H.-J. Chen, S. Shaikh, and P. Mathur. 2009. "Is Obesity Becoming a Public Health Problem in India? Examine the Shift from Under- to Overnutrition Problems Over Time." *Obesity Reviews* 10:456–74.

Wang, Youfa, Carlos Monteiro, and Barry Popkin. 2002. "Trends of Obesity and Underweight in Older Children and Adolescents in the United States, Brazil, China, and Russia." *American Journal of Clinical Nutrition* 75 (6): 971–77.

Wanjek, Christopher. 2005. *Workplace Solutions for Malnutrition, Obesity and Chronic Disease*. Geneva: International Labour Organization.

Washington Post. 2009. "TB Ravages Putin's Russia." August 26.

Watt, Nicola, Eduardo J. Gómez, and Martin McKee. 2014. "Global Health in Foreign Policy—and Foreign Policy in Health? Evidence from the BRICS." *Health Policy and Planning* 29 (6): 763–73.

Watts, Jonathan. 2005. "China Faces Up to Obesity Epidemic." *Guardian* (London), June 20.

Webster, Paul. 2003. "World Bank Approves Loan to Help Russia Tackle HIV/AIDS and Tuberculosis." *Lancet* 362 (9366): 1355.

Welcome Trust Center. 2009. *Smallpox History*. London: University College London.

Weyland, Kurt. 1996. *Democracy without Equity: Failures of Reform in Brazil*. Pittsburgh: University of Pittsburgh Press.

Whiteside, Alan. 1999. *The Threat of HIV/AIDS to Democracy and Governance.* Briefing paper. Washington, DC: USAID.

Whiteside, Alan, and C. Sunter. 2000. *AIDS: The Challenge of South Africa.* Cape Town, South Africa: Tafelberg and Rousseau.

Whitten, Sarah. 2016. "China Sees Childhood Obesity 'Explosion' in Rural Provinces." CNBC, April 28.

WHO. 1992. *Forty-Fifth World Health Assembly: Global Strategy for the Prevention and Control of AIDS.* Geneva: WHO.

———. 1998. *Obesity: Preventing and Managing the Global Pandemic.* Geneva: WHO.

———. 2000. *Obesity: Preventing and Managing the Global Pandemic.* WHO Technical Report Series no. 894. Geneva: WHO.

———. 2004a. *China's Relationship with the World Health Organization.* Geneva: WHO, April 19.

———. 2004b. *Global Strategy on Diet, Physical Activity, and Health.* Geneva: WHO.

———. 2006. *Conference on Obesity and Related Disease Control in China.* Geneva: WHO, November 20.

———. 2007. "South Africa, Country Profile." In *Global Tuberculosis Control.* Geneva: WHO.

———. 2008. "Consensus during the Cold War: Back to Alma-Ata." *Bulleting of the World Health Organization* 86 (10): 737–816.

———. 2009a. *History of WHO Support to HIV/AIDS in India.* Geneva: WHO.

———. 2009b. *Strengthening Partnerships for Integrated Prevention and Control of Non-Communicable Diseases: The SEANET-NCD Meeting.* New Delhi: WHO Regional Office for Southeast Asia.

———. 2012. *Strengthening National Advocacy Coalitions for Improved Women's and Children's Health.* Geneva: WHO.

———. 2015. *Global Tuberculosis Report.* Geneva: WHO.

———. 2016. *Russian Federation to Promote the Global Action Framework for Tuberculosis Research.* Geneva: WHO Europe.

WHO, Global Infobase. 2012. http://www.who.int/gho/en/.

Williams, Christopher. 1995. *AIDS in Post-Communist Russia and Its Successor States.* Aldershot, UK: Avebury.

Wolfe, Daniel. 2005. *Opportunities Lost: HIV Prevention, Harm Reduction, and the Russian Funding Gap.* New York: Open Society Institute, IHRD, August 31.

World Bank. 1998. *Intensifying Action against HIV/AIDS in Africa: Responding to a Development Crisis.* Washington, DC: World Bank Group.

———. 2009. *China Health Nine Project.* Washington, DC: World Bank Group.

———. 2011. "A Turning Point in the Fight against Tuberculosis in Russia." World Bank, online newsletter.

Wouters, Edwin, H. C. J. van Rensburg, and H. Meulemans. 2010. "The National Strategic Plan of South Africa: What Are the Prospects of Success after the Repeated Failure of Previous AIDS Policy?" *Health Policy and Planning* 25 (3): 171–85.

Wren, Christopher. 1990. "AIDS Rising Fast among Black South Africans." *New York Times,* September 27.

Wu, Zunyou, Keming Rou, and Haixia Cui. 2004. "The HIV/AIDS Epidemic in China: History, Current Strategies, and Future Challenges." *AIDS Education and Prevention* 16:7–17.

Wu, Zunyou, Sheena Sullivan, Yu Wang, Mary Jane Rotheram-Borus, and Roger Detels. 2007. "Evolution of China's Response to HIV/AIDS." *Lancet* 369 (9652): 679–90.

Xiaodong, Wang. 2016. "Obesity Time Bomb Keeps Ticking." *China Daily*, May 16.

Xinhua. 2001. "China May Have 200 Million Obese People in 10 Years." September 30.

———. 2005. "China Plans to Draft Laws on Public Nutrition to Improve Nation's Health." November 24.

———. 2006a. "China Vows to Improve Youngsters' Health." December 24.

———. 2006b. "Health Experts Call for Action to Curb China's Youth Obesity Crisis." August 21.

———. 2007a. "China Takes Measures to Improve Youngsters' Health." May 24.

———. 2007b. "Chinese Government Issues Healthy Eating Advice for Children." October 7.

———. 2008a. "China's School Running Campaign Hits Public Debate Hurdle." October 10.

———. 2008b. "Developing Nations Face Double Burden of Malnutrition, Obesity." April 15.

———. 2010a. "China's Expanding Waistlines to Lead to Lighter Pay Packets." July 28.

———. 2010b. "Interview: China Faces Big Obesity Challenge." July 13.

———. 2015. "Kenyan Officials Benefit from China Funded HIV/AIDS Management Program." November 28.

———. 2016. "Across China: Chinese NGO Explores New Mode of AIDS Prevention Education." July 2.

Xu, Hua, Yi Zeng, and Allen Anderson. 2005. "Chinese NGOs in Action against HIV/AIDS." *Cell Research* 15:914–18.

Yablonski, Peter, Alexandr Vizel, Vladimir Galkin, and Marina Shulgina. 2015. "Tuberculosis in Russia." *American Journal of Respiratory and Critical Care Medicine* 191 (4): 372–76.

Yach, Derek, David Stuckler, and Kelly Brownell. 2006. "Epidemiologic and Economic Consequences of the Global Epidemics of Obesity and Diabetes." *Nature Medicine* 12:62–66.

Yang, Gonghuan, Lingzhi Kong, Wenhua Zhao, Xia Wan, Yi Zhai, Lincoln Chen, and Jeffrey Koplan. 2008. "Health System Reform in China 3: Emergence of Chronic Non-Communicable Diseases." *Lancet* 372:42–49.

Yang Da-hua, David. 2004. "Civil Society as an Analytic Lens for Contemporary China." *China: International Journal* 2 (1): 1–27.

Yapp, Robin. 2010. "Brazil's Obesity Rate Could Match US by 2022." *Telegraph* (London), December 16.

Yardley, Jim. 2003. "China Begins Giving Free AIDS Drugs to the Poor." *New York Times*, November 8.

Yawa, Anele. 2016. "Why Mbeki's HIV Views Have No Place in South Africa." *Newsweek*, March 12.

Yinan, Zhao, and Wang Xiaodong. 2014. "More Funding for HIV/AIDS." *State Council Premier News*, December 1.

Yip, Winnie, William Hsiao, Wen Chen, Shanlian Hu, Jin Ma, and Alan Maynard. 2012. "Early Appraisal of China's Huge and Complex Health-Care Reforms." *Lancet* 379:833–42.

Younas, J. 2008. "Motivation for Bilateral Aid Allocation: Altruism or Trade Benefits." *European Journal of Political Economy* 24:661–74.

Yu, H. 2015. "Universal Health Insurance Coverage for 1.3 Billion People: What Accounts for China's Success?" *Health Policy* 119:1145–52.

Zaardiashvili, Tinatin. 2014. "Russia in Transition from Recipient to Donor of Global Fund Grants." *Aidspan* 236 (5): 3–5.

———. 2016. "Global Fund HIV Grant to Russia Federation Supports TB/HIV Project in the Tomske Oblast." *Aidspan*, July 5.

Zhai, F., H. Wang, Z. Wang, B. M. Popkin, and C. Chen. 2007. "Closing the Energy Gap to Prevent Weight Gain in China." *Obesity Reviews* 9 (Suppl. 1): 107–12.

Zhang, Ernest, and William Benoit. 2009. "Former Minister Zhang's Discourse on SARS: Government's Image Restoration or Destruction." *Public Relations Review* 35:240–46.

Zhang, Fujie, Michael Hsu, Lan Yu, Yi Wen, and Jennifer Pan. 2006. "Initiation of the National Free Antiretroviral Therapy Program in Rural China." In *AIDS and Social Policy in China*, ed. Joan Kaufman, Arthur Kleinman, and Tony Saich, 96–124. Cambridge, MA: Harvard University Asia Center.

Zhang, Heathe Xiaoquan. 2004. "The Gathering Storm: AIDS Policy in China." *Journal of International Development* 16 (8): 1155–68.

Zhang, Juyan, and Geln Cameron. 2002. "China's Agenda Building and Image Polishing in the US: Assessing an International Public Relations Campaign." *Public Relations Review* 29:13–28.

Zhang, Lufa, and Nan Liu. 2013. "Health Reform and Out-of-Pocket Payments: Lessons from China." *Health Policy and Planning* 29 (2): 217–26.

Zhang, Xiaoling. 2008. "China as an Emerging Soft Power: Winning Hearts and Minds through Communicating with Foreign Publics." Discussion paper no. 35, October. Nottingham, UK: University of Nottingham.

Zhang, Xiaoling, Herman Wasserman, and Winston Mano. 2016. *China's Media and Soft Power in Africa: Promotion and Perceptions.* New York: Palgrave MacMillan.

Zhang, Ying-xiu, Zhao-xia, Zhao Jin-Shan, and Chu Zun-hua. 2016. "Trends in Overweight and Obesity among Rural Children and Adolescents from 1985 to 2014 in Shandong, China." *European Journal of Preventive Cardiology* 23 (12): 1314–20.

Zhu, Jane. 2007. "AIDS in South Africa: NGO-State Relations and a Path Towards Reconciliation." *Duke Journal of Public Affairs* 6 (Spring): 1–13.

Ziblatt, Daniel. 2006. "Of Course Generalize, But How? Returning to Middle Range Theory in Comparative Politics." *American Political Science Association, Comparative Politics Newsletter* 17 (2).

Z-News. 2016. "Experts Confirm High Level of Mortality from Tuberculosis in Russia." March 25.

Zou, Guanyang, Barbara McPake, and Xiaolin Wei. 2014. "Chinese Health Foreign Aid and Policy: Beyond Medical Aid." *Lancet* 383:1461.

Zucco, Cesar, and Timothy Power. 2013. "Bolsa Família and the Shift in Lula's Electoral Base in 2002–2006." *Latin American Research Review* 48 (2): 3–24.

Zunyou, Wu, and Sheena Sullivan. 2006. "China." In *Fighting a Rising Tide: The Response to AIDS in East Asia*, ed. Tadashi Yamamoto and Satoko Itoh, 76–95. Tokyo: Japan Center for International Exchange.

Index